FAMILY MEDICINE CLERKSHIP GUIDE

CLERKSHIP GUIDES

Your Essential Guide to Clinical Clerkships

All you need to succeed:

- Practice Cases
- Frequently Asked Questions
- Key Points
- Practice Exam

Other titles in the *Clerkship Guides* Series

Paauw *et al.*
Internal Medicine Clerkship Guide

Woodhead
Pediatric Clerkship Guide

Manley
Psychiatry Clerkship Guide

Adams *et al.*
Surgery Clerkship Guide

Adams
Surgical Subspecialties Clerkship Guide

Forthcoming:

Minassian and Woodland
Obstetrics and Gynecology Clerkship Guide

FAMILY MEDICINE CLERKSHIP GUIDE

Editor-in-Chief

Paul M. Paulman, MD
Professor and Predoctoral Director
Department of Family Medicine
University of Nebraska Medical Center
Omaha, Nebraska

Associate Editors

Jeffrey L. Susman, MD
Professor and Chair
Department of Family Medicine
University of Cincinnati College of Medicine
Cincinnati, Ohio

Jeffrey D. Harrison, MD
Associate Professor and Residency Program Director
Department of Family Medicine
University of Nebraska Medical Center
Omaha, Nebraska

Audrey A. Paulman, MD
Clinical Assistant Professor
Department of Family Medicine
University of Nebraska Medical Center
Omaha, Nebraska

Katherine M. Finkelstein, MLIS
Assistant Director for Education Services
Dahlgren Memorial Library
Georgetown University Medical Center
Washington, District of Columbia

Robert B. Zatechka, MD
House Officer
University of Nebraska Medical Center
Omaha, Nebraska

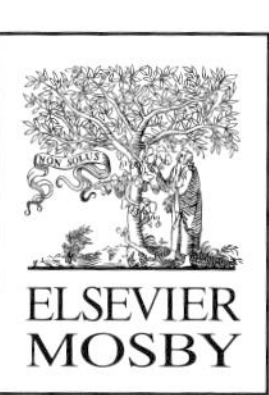
ELSEVIER
MOSBY

ELSEVIER
MOSBY

The Curtis Center
170 S Independence Mall W 300E
Philadelphia, Pennsylvania 19106

FAMILY MEDICINE CLERKSHIP GUIDE ISBN: 0-323-02950-7

Notice

Family Medicine is an ever-changing field. Standard safety precautions must be followed, but as new research and clinical experience broaden our knowledge, changes in treatment and drug therapy may become necessary or appropriate. Readers are advised to check the most current product information provided by the manufacturer of each drug to be administered to verify the recommended dose, the method and duration of administration, and contraindications. It is the responsibility of the treating physician, relying on experience and knowledge of the patient, to determine dosages and the best treatment for each individual patient. Neither the publisher nor the author assumes any liability for any injury and/or damage to persons or property arising from this publication.

Library of Congress Cataloging-in-Publication Data

Family medicine clerkship guide / editor-in-chief, Paul M. Paulman.—1st ed.
p. cm.
Includes index.
ISBN 0-323-02950-7
1. Family medicine—Handbooks, manuals, etc. 2. Clinical clerkship—Handbooks, manuals, etc. I. Paulman, Paul M., 1953–
RC55.F2195 2005
610'.71'1—dc22
2004065604

Acquisitions Editor: Jim Merritt
Developmental Editor: Jacqueline Mahon
Publishing Services Manager: Joan Sinclair
Project Manager: Cecelia Bayruns
Designer: Gene Harris

Printed in China.

Last digit is the print number: 9 8 7 6 5 4 3 2 1

To

Audrey.

Thank you for all the love, laughter,
friendship, and encouragement.

Contributors

Thomas P. Agresta, MD
Associate Professor of Family Medicine
Director of Predoctoral Education
University of Connecticut School of Medicine
Farmington, Connecticut

William A. Alto, MD, MPH
Professor
Department of Community and Family Medicine
Dartmouth Medical College
Hanover, New Hampshire
Faculty
Maine Dartmouth Family Practice Residency
Fairfield, Maine

Kathleen C. Amyot, MD
Associate Program Director, Family Residency Program
Saint Louis University School of Medicine
Belleville, Illinois
Lieutenant Colonel, 375th Medical Group
Scott Air Force Base, Illinois

Steven Bartz, MD, RPh
Assistant Professor of Family Medicine
University of Cincinnati College of Medicine
Cincinnati, Ohio

Linda S. Batck, MD
Department of Family and Community Medicine
University of Illinois College of Medicine at Peoria
Peoria, Illinois

Benjamin Bissell, MD
Clinical Instructor
Department of Orthopaedic Rehabilitation
University of Vermont College of Medicine
Burlington, Vermont

Neil A. Bratney, MD
Department of Pediatrics
University of Minnesota Medical School
Minneapolis, Minnesota

Kathleen Marie Brennan, MD
Department of Obstetrics and Gynecology
University of California Los Angeles, David Geffen School of Medicine
Los Angeles, California

Alan M. Cementina, MD, FAAFP
Medical Director, Practice Center
Associate Professor
Department of Family Practice
University of Connecticut School of Medicine
Asylum Hill Family Medicine Center
Hartford, Connecticut

Chia L. Chang, PharmD
Department of Family Medicine
University of Nebraska Medical Center
Omaha, Nebraska

Jason Chao, MS, MD
Professor of Family Medicine
Case Western Reserve University School of Medicine
University Hospitals of Cleveland
Cleveland, Ohio

Brenda Chrastil, MD
Pennsylvania Hospital
Philadelphia, Pennsylvania

James Crosby, MD
Associate Clinical Professor of Family Medicine
Upstate Medical University
Syracuse, New York
Residency Faculty, Wilson Family Medicine Residency
Johnson City, New York

Anthony A. Day, MD
Clinical Assistant Professor
Department of Family and Community Medicine
University of Illinois College of Medicine
Executive Associate Director
Family Practice Residency Program
Methodist Medical Center of Illinois
Peoria, Illinois

William G. Elder, PhD
Associate Professor of Family Practice
University of Kentucky Family Medicine Center
Lexington, Kentucky

Brian Finley, MD
Assistant Professor
Department of Family Medicine
University of Nebraska Medical Center
Omaha, Nebraska

Nicole Fletcher
University of Nebraska Medical Center
Omaha, Nebraska

Betty B. Gatipon, PhD, MEd
Associate Professor
Department of Family Medicine
Co-Director, Predoctoral Education
Louisiana State University Health Sciences Center School of Medicine
New Orleans, Louisiana

John H. Grebe, MD
Resident Physician
Department of Pediatrics
University of Florida College of Medicine
Gainesville, Florida

John G. Halvorsen, MD, MS
Professor and Thomas and Ellen Foster Chair
Department of Family and Community Medicine
Associate Dean for Community Health
University of Illinois College of Medicine
Peoria, Illinois

Capt. Craig Harms, MD
Assistant Professor
Department of Community and Family Medicine
St. Elizabeth Family Practice Residency Division
Saint Louis University School of Medicine
Belleville, Illinois

David R. Harnisch, Sr., MD
Assistant Professor
Department of Family Medicine
University of Nebraska Medical Center
Omaha, Nebraska

David Henderson, MD
Assistant Professor of Family Medicine
Predoctoral Clerkship Director
University of Connecticut School of Medicine
Farmington, Connecticut

William Y. Huang, MD
Associate Professor
Department of Family and Community Medicine
Baylor College of Medicine
Houston, Texas

Casey Johnston, MD
Department of Orthopaedic Surgery and Rehabilitation
University of Nebraska Medical Center
Omaha, Nebraska

Louis A. Kazal, Jr., MD
Associate Professor and Chief Clinical Officer
Department of Community and Family Medicine
Dartmouth Medical School
Hanover, New Hampshire
Chief, Section of Family Medicine
Dartmouth-Hitchcock Medical Center
Lebanon, New Hampshire

Carol A. LaCroix, MD
Clinical Assistant Professor
Department of Family Medicine
University of Nebraska Medical Center
Omaha, Nebraska

Aaron Lee
University of Nebraska Medical Center
Omaha, Nebraska

Paul Lyons, MD
Associate Professor and Associate Chair for Clinical Education
Department of Family and Community Medicine
Temple University School of Medicine
Philadelphia, Pennsylvania

Homa Magsi, MD
House Officer, Department of Family Practice
University of Nebraska Medical Center
Omaha, Nebraska

Robert Mallin, MD
Associate Professor of Family Medicine
Medical University of South Carolina
Charleston, South Carolina

Katherine L. Margo, MD
Assistant Professor and Director, Student Programs
Department of Family Practice and Community Medicine
University of Pennsylvania Health System
Philadelphia, Pennsylvania

Jim Medder, MD, MPH
Associate Professor
Department of Family Medicine
University of Nebraska Medical Center
Omaha, Nebraska

Glenn D. Miller, MD
Associate Professor of Clinical Family Medicine
University of Illinois College of Medicine
Peoria, Illinois

Katherine Miller, MD
Assistant Clinical Professor
Department of Public Health and Family Medicine
Tufts University School of Medicine
Clinical Instructor in Ambulatory Care and Prevention
Harvard Medical School
Boston, Massachusetts
Cambridge Health Alliance
Cambridge, Massachusetts

Carolyn Murray, MD, MPH
Assistant Professor of Medicine and Community and Family Medicine
Dartmouth Medical School
Hanover, New Hampshire
Chief, Section of Occupational and Physical Medicine
Dartmouth-Hitchcock Medical Center
Lebanon, New Hampshire

Srilakshmi S. Murthy, MBBS, MD
Volunteer Associate Professor
Department of Family Medicine
University of Cincinnati College of Medicine
Medical Staff, Children's Hospital
Cincinnati, Ohio
Active Staff, Fort Hamilton Hospital
Hamilton, Ohio
Active Provisional Staff, Clinton Memorial Hospital
Wilmington, Ohio

Mary Noel, MPH, PhD, RD
Professor, Department of Family Practice
Michigan State University College of Human Medicine
East Lansing, Michigan

Audrey A. Paulman, MD
Clinical Assistant Professor
Department of Family Medicine
University of Nebraska Medical Center
Omaha, Nebraska

Roger Paulman
University of Nebraska Medical Center
Omaha, Nebraska

Layne A. Prest, MA, PhD
Associate Professor
Director of Behavioral Medicine
Department of Family Medicine
University of Nebraska Medical Center
Omaha, Nebraska

Cynthia Rivera-Haft
University of Nebraska Medical Center
Omaha, Nebraska

W. David Robinson, PhD
Family Therapist
Assistant Professor
Department of Family Medicine
University of Nebraska Medical Center
Omaha, Nebraska

Jared C. Rogers, MD
Assistant Professor
Department of Family and Community Medicine
Associate Director
Family Practice Residency
University of Illinois College of Medicine at Peoria
Peoria, Illinois

Joanne Sandberg-Cook, MSN, ARNP, BC
Instructor in Community and Family Medicine
Dartmouth Medical School
Hanover, New Hampshire
Adult/Gerontologic Nurse Practitioner
Dartmouth-Hitchcock Medical Center
Lebanon, New Hampshire

Maj. Peter H. Seidenberg, MD
Program Director, Primary Care Sports Medicine Fellowship
Assistant Professor of Family Medicine
Saint Louis University School of Medicine
Assistant Professor of Family Medicine
Uniformed Services University of the Health Sciences
Belleville, Illinois

Maj. Lowell G. Sensintaffar, MD
Assistant Professor of Family Medicine
Saint Louis University School of Medicine
Assistant Professor of Family Medicine

Uniformed Services University of the Health Sciences
Belleville, Illinois

William B. Shore, MD
Professor of Clinical Family and Community Medicine
Director of Predoctoral Education
University of California, San Francisco, School of Medicine
San Francisco, California

Aamir Siddiqi, MD
Associate Professor of Family Medicine
Associate Director
St. Luke's Family Practice Residency Program
University of Wisconsin Medical School
Vice President of Medical Staff
Aurora Sinai Medical Center
Milwaukee, Wisconsin

John L. Smith, MD
Department of Family Medicine
University of Nebraska Medical Center
Omaha, Nebraska

Gregg D. Stoner, MD
Professor of Clinical Family and Community Medicine
University of Illinois College of Medicine
Peoria, Illinois

Michael P. Temporal, MD
Associate Professor
Department of Community and Family Medicine
Saint Louis University School of Medicine
Belleville, Illinois

Margaret E. Thompson, MD
Family Practice Clerkship Director
Associate Professor
Department of Family Practice
Michigan State University College of Human Medicine
Grand Rapids, Michigan

Richard P. Usatine, MD
Professor and Vice Chair for Education
Department of Family and Community Medicine
University of Texas Health Science Center
San Antonio, Texas

Anthony Valdini, MD, MS
Associate Clinical Professor
Department of Public Health and Family Medicine

Tufts University School of Medicine
Boston, Massachusetts
Director of Research
Director of the Faculty Development Fellowship
Lawrence Family Practice Residency
Lawrence, Massachusetts

Christopher White, MD, JD
Combined Program Resident Physician
Departments of Family Medicine and Psychiatry
University of Cincinnati College of Medicine
Cincinnati, Ohio

Joel Winner
University of Nebraska Medical Center
Omaha, Nebraska

Lawson Wulsin, MD
Associate Professor of Family Medicine and Psychiatry
Training Director, Family Medicine Psychiatry Residency Program
University of Cincinnati College of Medicine
University Hospital
Cincinnati, Ohio

Hakan Yaman, MD
Associate Professor and Chair of Family Medicine
University of Akdeniz Medical School
Antalya, Turkey

Robert B. Zatechka, MD
House Officer
University of Nebraska Medical Center
Omaha, Nebraska

Michael Zionts, MD
Associate Professor
Department of Family Medicine
Associate Residency Director and Faculty Physician
State University of New York at Buffalo
School of Medicine and Biomedical Sciences
Buffalo, New York

Kira Zwygart, MD
Assistant Professor
Department of Family Medicine
University of South Florida College of Medicine
Tampa, Florida

Preface

Welcome to your clerkship years and welcome to the family medicine clerkship!

The *Family Medicine Clerkship Guide* is designed to provide you with information about the specialty of family medicine, the family medicine clerkship, and clinical problems and learning venues you'll likely encounter during this rotation. The chapters are concise and easily read and serve as stand-alone sources of practical information. We've written the Guide primarily for junior and senior students participating in family medicine clerkships. We anticipate that it will be useful for physician assistant and nurse practitioner students, as well.

Because the vast majority of family medicine clerkship training takes place in the offices of practicing community family physicians, away from the medical school, we've included information about adapting to the physician's practice and community. We've also included information about methods to increase your learning during the clerkship.

Medical students value family medicine clerkships for the opportunity to have first contact with a large number of patients, the variety of clinical problems encountered, and the mentoring relationships developed between medical students and family medicine community faculty.

We hope the *Family Medicine Clerkship Guide* facilitates your learning and professional growth during your family medicine clerkship.

Paul M. Paulman, MD
EDITOR-IN-CHIEF

Acknowledgments

This book would not have been possible without the hard work, dedication, and tolerance of the associate editors: Dr. Jeff Susman, Dr. Jeff Harrison, Dr. Audrey Paulman, Ms. Katherine Finkelstein, and Dr. Robert Zatechka. Thank you.

Special thanks to Suellen Dashner for her assistance with this volume and to our chapter authors for producing quality chapters.

Contents

Section 1 Introduction to the Family Medicine Clerkship

Section 2 Patients Presenting with a Symptom, Sign, or Abnormal Lab Value

Section 3 Patients Presenting with a Known Condition

SECTION 1

Introduction to the Family Medicine Clerkship

1

Secrets to Being a Successful Student

Welcome to family medicine! You are likely to be greeted with a similar greeting when you arrive at the clinic site for your first day. Family medicine is relationship oriented. Family physicians interact with their clerical staff, nurses, and of course, their patients every single day. Their people skills tend to be a personal strength, and their staff and nurses tend to exhibit those qualities as well. Don't be surprised if even the receptionist seems to want your life's history before you get into the office. It is their nature, and the nature of family medicine, to be highly interested in people.

Getting off on the right foot is crucial at the start of any clerkship. The key is to be you and to be personable. The clinician and your co-workers will be much more comfortable with you if they get to know you. Treat everyone you meet with respect. Although there is a hierarchy of function, successful family medicine offices don't have a hierarchy of relationships. The physician is likely to be as friendly and respectful to the lowest paid clerical staff as to a colleague. You should emulate that behavior. Everyone in a family medicine office can and will contribute to your understanding of family medicine.

How do I adapt to this new environment?

A family medicine office is unlike any other clerkship setting. The setting combines the speed of an emergency department, the relationship skills of psychiatry, the hand-eye coordination of surgery, and the exam skills of internal medicine. All of this occurs in 10- to 15-minute increments, which encompass the entire breadth of medical knowledge. On top of this, you may also have in-depth experiences in obstetrics, inpatient medicine, and procedures. Your preceptor will have a practice that is unique to his/her individual strengths and interests.

Many techniques will be valuable in adapting to this environment. Ask your preceptor and nurses lots of questions. Because students are seldom quizzed in family medicine, preceptors and nurses may assume that you know things that you don't really know. Ask to be shown how to do something that you aren't sure about. Preceptors expect students to demonstrate a willingness and a desire to learn.

They have a desire to teach, so seek out new experiences and learn new things.

A second technique is to ask for direction when seeing a patient. The preceptor may only give you five minutes to take the basic history and do an abbreviated exam before he/she sees the patient. Ask the preceptor or nurse what information is important for a particular patient's visit. Many patients will have multiple medical problems. A good preceptor will point out a specific area of concern, while the patient may be less focused. It is difficult to discuss four or five medical problems in five minutes, but a focused beginning gives you a better chance to get the information the physician needs.

A third technique is to keep notes about what you see and hear. Many clerkships require a log of your patient encounters. Even if it isn't required, note taking can be very beneficial. You will seldom have time during the day to review medical information. At the end of your day, take a few minutes and read about some of the less familiar things that you experienced. After you've read, pose any remaining questions to your physician teacher. When a student comes in and says "I read about CHF last night and wondered why Mrs. Smith isn't on a beta-blocker," a physician is thrilled to discuss his/her thinking process. Family physicians typically enjoy discussing the art of applying medical knowledge to real patients.

Finally, employ the patients as a source of teaching. Patients that see teaching physicians typically enjoy meeting students. Ask about their lives beyond their medical issues. The number one predictor of patient satisfaction with their physician is the physician's interest in them as a person. When they are comfortable with you, they will tell you the information that they were previously waiting to tell their doctor. You should ask them about your exam findings. If you think you hear a murmur, ask them if they have been told that they have a murmur. If not, reassure them that you'll have their doctor check for sure. Ask them what they think is the cause of the problem, and use open-ended questions. Although it seems like you need to be direct with the time constraints, it is usually faster to allow the patient to tell you all the details.

What about the test?

Family medicine clerkships have very different requirements regarding testing. In many cases, your grade is wholly dependent on your preceptor's evaluation. Others have required reports, tests, or use national shelf exams with board-style questions. The tips above will allow you to do well in your preceptor's eyes. The main challenge with family medicine is the breadth of medical knowledge required. Local tests usually focus on the common illnesses treated by family physicians. Reviewing the conditions of the patients that you've seen should prepare you well for those exams. It also helps with shelf exams, though they will likely include questions regarding conditions you didn't see during your rotation. Anything you've learned on other clerkships may appear on these exams, so reviewing your prior rotations can also help. Finally, students are successful with shelf exam review books. These books contain lots of questions similar to those on the test, as well as explanations of the question and answer choices.

2

Definition and Scope of Family Medicine

What is family medicine?

Also known as family practice and established in 1969 as medicine's twentieth specialty to counter the fragmentation of a subspecialty-oriented system, family medicine is characterized by care that is:

- Primary: first contact and means of entry into the healthcare system
- Continuing: "womb to the tomb"
- Comprehensive: encompassing all ages, both sexes, each organ system, and every disease entity; integrating the biological, clinical, and behavioral sciences
- Coordinated: care by other providers prioritized, facilitated, or redirected and explained
- Compassionate: patient centered
- Family oriented: open to all family members and viewed in the context of the family

A necessary underlying skill is patient management: a family physician confronts large numbers of unselected patients with unknown conditions and carries on a therapeutic role over time. The ideal family physician assumes responsibility, even if peripheral, for all patient problems, current and potential. Assisting the patient through healthcare's complex maze is a needed and welcome role for the family physician. (The American Academy of Family Physicians' website is an excellent resource for obtaining more information about family medicine; it also has a wealth of clinical information.)

Has family medicine been successful in meeting these goals?

Yes and no. Make answering this question, at least as it relates to your practice site, one of the goals of your clerkship, realizing your exposure to family medicine will be limited.

On a quantitative level, as of 2003 approximately 70,000 physicians have completed family medicine residencies. Nearly 50% of all office visits to primary care physicians are to family physicians. However, the primary care workforce in general has shown minimal growth over the past 20 years compared with the much greater growth of other specialties. The number of non–primary care office-based specialists per 1000 people in the United States is nearly twice that of primary care physicians.

On a qualitative level, adequate access to a primary care–based healthcare system has been shown to result in a number of health and economic benefits. However, there is good evidence that the U.S. health system does not have an adequate primary care focus. Compared with our industrialized peer nations, who are much more primary care oriented, we have poorer healthcare outcomes on several key indicators. Furthermore, recent studies of primary care in the United States show that there is substantial room for improvement in realizing the goals of continuity, patient-centeredness, and whole-person care. In an era of increasing subspecialty sophistication and emphasis, a reaffirmation of the initial tenets of family medicine seems warranted.

How does family medicine differ from the other primary care specialties?

Other than the age restrictions, much about family medicine is similar to the other primary care specialties, unless the practice is limited to a specific area. However, in general, family medicine tends to include more procedures (e.g., injections, excisions and biopsies of skin lesions); mental healthcare (e.g., counseling, prescribing psychotropic meds); gynecology (e.g., Pap smears, contraceptives, STDs); orthopedics; obstetrics (approximately 25% of family physicians); and adolescent care.

It sounds like I need to be a specialist in every area and for all ages. How is it possible for one person to do all this with quality?

Knowing your limits is key. It is more important that the family physician be the manager of all problems than the expert. When needed the family physician obtains second opinions, more input (consultations), or transfers primary management of certain problems (referrals). Office references—from paper and computer texts to a number of excellent online resources—become the family physician's second brain. Most family physicians work in groups. These providers cover for each other and may provide consultation and perform procedures. There are a few studies that indicate specialized care programs that focus on a single clinical problem (e.g., diabetes) do better with some indicators of care. However, not all indicators were measured and assuring equal comparison populations is difficult. Nonetheless, referrals to these programs may be best at times. Finally, studies and experience over the past 30 years show that family physicians do give care equal to others for the problems they manage.

What hospital privileges do family physicians have?

Hospital privileges vary, but in general family physicians have privileges comparable to the other primary care specialties. Common are ICU, CCU, and basic OB privileges. Most hospitals have independent family medicine departments.

What procedures do family physicians perform?

Most family physicians do basic skin surgery, tendon and bursa injections, lumbar punctures, endometrial aspirations, simple joint splinting, laceration repair, and wart removal. Some do sigmoidoscopy and colonoscopy, colposcopy, vasectomy, acupuncture, casting, laryngoscopy, and osteopathic manipulation.

Can a family physician develop an expertise in limited areas?

The flexibility available to a family physician is great. There is a formal certification (Certificate of Added Qualifications) available in geriatrics, sports medicine, and adolescent medicine. Some family physicians have limited their practice to geriatrics, school, college, occupational health, or other areas. This deviates from the comprehensive characteristics listed at the beginning of this chapter but illustrates how family physicians can fill important and needed roles in the community.

KEY POINTS

- **Family medicine serves a unique and important role in the healthcare system.**
- **Family medicine aims to care for a patient as a whole, in sickness (as inevitable) or health (as possible), through a broad, multidisciplinary perspective.**
- **The fear that "I can never know enough" is usually unfounded when considering quality care and professional satisfaction in family medicine.**

REFERENCE

Phillips RL, Starfield D: Why does a U.S. primary care physician workforce crisis matter? Am Fam Physician 68:1494–1498, 2003.

USEFUL WEBSITE

http://www.aafp.org

3

Role of the Medical Student in Family Medicine Clerkships

How does your family medicine clerkship differ from inpatient or specialty clerkships?

In contrast to inpatient or specialty clerkships, in which patients present with one or two problems, patients seen in family medicine practices often present as undifferentiated patients with a broad variety of multiple, complex medical and psychosocial problems. There is also the challenge of integrating healthcare maintenance (HCM)—identification of risk factors, disease prevention, and health promotion—in the context of relatively brief office visits. These tasks can seem overwhelming initially to clerkship students, particularly those in early years of their clinical rotations. However, with organization, priority setting, and practice, students learn the skills to approach and manage these challenges in a family medicine setting.

How do I know what history and exam to perform at this visit?

New patient data may be collected over a period of two to three office visits. Begin each visit by asking the patient what he or she would like to address. Address the patient's stated agenda while simultaneously addressing other health needs, e.g., HCM updates and chronic illness issues. After learning the patient's concerns, the student must set priorities (an internal mental task) and address what can be appropriately attended to in that visit. The goal of a first visit with a new patient is to establish rapport, address the patient's presenting issues, and assure that the patient will return for follow-up care.

The focus of your physical examination should be relevant to the patient's presenting complaint, e.g., if a patient is complaining of lower back pain, it is not necessary to do an HEENT exam. If a patient's chronic illness is stable and the acute problem seems to be a greater concern, the chronic problem can receive briefer attention during that visit. If the problem could benefit from more psychosocial or health-related behavior (HRB) information, it is important to obtain it; e.g., in a patient with epigastric pain, ask about alcohol use and stress.

With a new patient, obtain complete history, including family history and genogram, social history, past medical history and HRB, and begin the complete physical exam. By the end of the clinic year, students should be able to complete a new patient history and physical in one 30-minute visit.

How do I present to the attending preceptor?

In your initial meeting with your attendings, ask how they would like you to present patients. Take a few minutes after you see a patient to organize your thoughts before you present the patient. Present in an organized, problem-oriented manner. Include differential diagnoses in your presentations and, when necessary, say "I don't know," if this is based on a background of medical knowledge. Your preceptor may also get to "I don't know." This is an opportunity for you to research information, either online or in textbooks, and bring back information the next time you are at the office. This activity can be a way to give something back to your preceptor—and demonstrates that you are an eager self-learner.

How should I do write-ups?

Write-up interval visits as problem-oriented notes in the **SOAP** (**S**ubjective, **O**bjective, **A**ssessment, **P**lan) format. The plan should include, for each problem, diagnostic plans (tests), therapeutic plans (prescriptions), and patient education (advice). These must be reviewed with your attending before discussing them with the patient because there are issues of costs, patient care, and risks involved, and the preceptors are legally responsible for the patients. Learn to write outpatient prescriptions (cosigned by your attending). All notes and prescriptions must be reviewed and cosigned by your preceptor.

How do I get meaningful feedback?

Schedule a midclerkship feedback meeting and, at the end of each clinic session, ask your preceptor for feedback with specific questions: "How can I improve my presentations/write-ups?" "How can I be more efficient in my use of time?" "How can I do a better knee exam?" As appropriate, give the preceptor some feedback. "I like the way you reviewed the knee exam with me." Make your needs known: "I know you're very busy, but could we find a time to go over the cardiac exam?"

How should I follow-up on patient care?

Follow-up with patients is an important principle of all clinical care and particularly in family medicine. When you order tests, tell the patient when and how you will notify him/her of the results—whether it will be by phone, e-mail, U.S. mail, or at a scheduled follow-up visit. Check on the results of all tests that you order. Early in the clinical year, you may be unsure of what various test results mean and what kind of follow-up they need. Discuss these issues with your attending. All abnormal results should be reviewed with your attending. Scheduling follow-up visits is a good way to learn about the importance and benefits of continuity of care.

When (and what) should I read?

Although this clerkship may be less time demanding than inpatient rotations, it can still be very difficult to read or get information between patients. Arrive at your clinic early and review your assigned patients' charts before the start of a clinic session. From family medicine or primary care resources, online or textbook, review the disease complexes you may be seeing that day and the physical exams you may need to do.

REFERENCE

Rodnick J, Heineken P, Shore W: The Tree of Data Gathering: The Medical History, Physical Examination and Write-up, 5th ed. San Francisco: University of California Press, 1999.

4

Orientation to the Office/Practice/Community

How do I get to know the preceptor?

When you receive the information about your clinic assignment for your family medicine clerkship, follow the instructions about how to contact your preceptor and the office. In contrast to other clerkships in which you work with residents on inpatient teams, on this clerkship you will most often be working individually with practicing family physicians in their offices. Plan to arrive early for your first visit so that you can meet with the preceptor. During this "getting to know you" meeting, review your goals for the clerkship, ask about the office practice, tell the preceptor about your interests and background, and ask the preceptor about his/her interests and life outside of medicine.

During this discussion, ask the preceptor about how he/she would like you to function in the office: for example, how he/she would like you to address him/her (Dr. vs. first name), how students are expected to see patients (do you go in first and introduce yourself or is that done by the preceptor or office staff?), and how he/she would like you to present patients (if the preceptor is also seeing patients, should you interrupt or wait until he/she is finished with a patient?). You should also ask the preceptor whether he/she will go into the exam room with you to review any history and physical findings (students should encourage preceptors to do this). What should you do if you are stumped and need help? How will you get feedback? Asking these questions initially and clarifying the issues can minimize future misunderstandings and false expectations during the clerkship.

How do I get to know the staff?

In a family medicine office, the staff is responsible for the patient flow and the functioning of the office. Each staff person is an important member of the healthcare team in your preceptor's office. The decision to have students in the office is often made solely by the preceptor, and staff may feel that having students slows down the preceptor and the patient flow in busy offices. For this reason, and because you want to become part of the healthcare team at the office, it is important and appropriate to spend time getting to know the staff members and establishing positive professional relationships with them.

On your first day, introduce yourself to all of the staff members and ask about their jobs and professions, how they prefer to be addressed (first name or by professional title), and how you can assist them during your time at the office. Always communicate with all staff members with respect, cultural sensitivity, and professionalism. Staff members who have worked in practices for some time often have a wealth of information about the patients, the community, and the practice. Seek their advice and guidance about how to become part of the clinic team and, as appropriate and in confidence, consult with them about patients.

Remember, you can never say "thank you" too often when people in the office have assisted you. After you have you completed your clerkship rotation, consider sending a thank-you note to the office staff. In addition to showing your appreciation for their assistance, you are paving the way for additional students to be welcomed in the future.

How do I get to know the community?

In contrast to other clerkships, your family medicine assignment likely will be out in the community and not at the medical school. Patients seen in the practice typically come from the surrounding community. If possible, prior to starting your clerkship, try to obtain some information about the demographics of the community, e.g., population, ethnic/cultural composition, any known health problems or environmental hazards, etc. This information often can be obtained online from local health departments. It will be helpful if your clerkship requires a community project.

In your initial discussions with your preceptor and the office staff, ask about the composition of the patients seen in the practice, e.g., gender/age mix, ethnic and cultural backgrounds, languages spoken, socioeconomic status, and variety of problems. It is also helpful to spend some time in the community. You can accomplish this with a drive-through or walk-through analysis of the community. In these activities, be alert to all you are seeing in the community. Notice the housing conditions, whether the neighborhood appears safe, access to public transportation, parking access to the clinic, parks (where people can exercise), presence or absence of full-service grocery stores (where patients can obtain healthy foods that you will be prescribing), schools, and whether you see people out in the neighborhoods. These experiences will help you understand the patients' experiences as they come for their clinic visits. If there is the opportunity and it is safe, talk to people in the community outside of the office setting to get a better understanding of the perceptions about healthcare problems and resources. You can accomplish these "primary informant interviews" by talking to patients and residents in the community, visiting local agencies, and talking to community leaders.

5

Definition of Family

What is a family?

Various authors define "family" from differing viewpoints that reflect their academic discipline, their theoretical framework, and those aspects of the family that they wish to study. When viewed collectively, these multiple viewpoints emphasize several essential attributes that characterize a group of people as a family.

The family is the universal *social unit* in society. It is such an important sociocultural institution that every human society has devised traditional prescriptions and proscriptions to ensure that the family fulfills its biological and enculturating tasks. As the first social environment for every human, the family is also the most potent source for physical, spiritual, emotional, intellectual, and psychological development.

Related to its socialization tasks, the family is also a *functional unit* that is charged to: (1) satisfy the members' needs for affection and intimacy, (2) satisfy the sexual needs of the parents, (3) ensure reproduction, (4) protect and nurture children, and (5) form an economic unit to provide for the material needs of family members.

The family is a *genetic unit* in biological, psychological, and lineage terms. The antecedents for who we become physically and behaviorally stem from our families. Furthermore, the expectations of our lineage family profoundly influence how we think, act, and live out our lives.

The family is the most intense *emotional unit* in society, a unit that paradoxically provides us with our greatest emotional support while it simultaneously produces our greatest emotional distress.

The family is a *dynamic unit.* Change is the norm and is expected as the family progresses through its life cycle, confronting the new challenges of each stage. Since the family exists within a larger culture, however, it must also confront the changes occurring within the culture that influence its own functioning and that threaten its health and well-being.

The family is an *enduring unit* that existed before recorded history and that has continuously and successfully adapted to multiple changes and pressures throughout history.

What is meant by the term "family context"?

The National Academy of Science Institute of Medicine's definition of primary care requires clinicians to practice in "the context of family." How does one define "family context"? The acronym ***CHERESH*** helps to recall these essential components: **C**ulture, **H**ome environment, **E**conomic status, **R**eligion, **E**ducation, **S**ystem dynamics, and **H**ealthcare resources.

Culture focuses on the family's national origin, ethnicity, and the belief systems and behaviors that stem from those influences.

Home environment describes the physical location of the home in the community, the nature of the neighborhood, the type of residence, the physical status of the housing, and the activities that take place within that home. While collecting this information, physicians can inquire about whether people feel safe at home and whether risky behaviors and activities take place within that environment.

Economic status includes data about family income, family savings, employment of family members, and whether they have insurance on their person and/or property to help them withstand a potential disaster.

Religion is often an important part of the family's culture and history. Knowing whether the family actively practices a religion and the extent to which religion influences their lives can help physicians to understand belief systems that may affect family healthcare and to determine whether the family has spiritual resources to help it manage crises.

Education helps define a family. Identifying the highest level of educational attainment by family members, particularly the adults in the family, can help physicians to communicate most effectively with the family. Educational attainment also correlates positively with healthcare outcomes and with access to resources.

System dynamics relate to the rules, roles, and relationships among family members. Where does conflict exist? Where are relationships close? Do family members like each other, support each other, respect each other, and have fun together? Do they communicate effectively? Do they take responsibility for their actions? How flexible is the family in adapting to changes and challenges? (See Chapter 49 for more discussion of family system dynamics.)

Healthcare resources vary among families. Does the family have a medical home—a usual source of primary medical care? Do they have health insurance, and, if so, how adequate is that coverage?

REFERENCES

Campbell TL, McDaniel SH, Seaburn DB: The family system. In Mengel MB, Holleman WL, Fields SA (eds): Fundamentals of Clinical Practice, 2nd ed. New York: Kluwer Academic/Plenum Publishers, 2002.

Rodgers RH: Family Interaction and Transaction: The Developmental Approach. Englewood Cliffs, N.J.: Prentice-Hall, 1973.

6

Patient-Centered Communication

Why is communication important?

Communication is a sine qua non in family practice, where the final diagnosis is apparent 80% of the time from history alone. Good listening promotes adherence and increases patient satisfaction. Malpractice suits correlate with poor communication even when controlled for case complexity. Physician satisfaction is directly related to the quality of communication with patients.

What is the purpose of the family practice interview?

The family practice interview is not just the gathering of information. It involves an effective *exchange* of information. It is also the means by which you will establish a trusting relationship with your patient. The interview has the potential to be a therapeutic intervention, both emotionally and motivationally, for the patient. You should consider the interview a process where you must actively identify what is required for effective communication between you and the patient.

Besides medical knowledge, what do people look for in a doctor?

People like doctors to talk to them in an egalitarian way, listen well, ask lots of questions, answer lots of questions, explain things understandably, and allow patients to make decisions about their care.

What is meant by patient-centered care?

Patient-centered care is a method of communication and clinical decision making. Executed properly, you will follow an interview path that arrives at a point of common ground with the patient. Common ground means that there is a shared view of the patient's and physician's needs and that negotiation occurs between the provider and the patient about the treatment plan, with the patient's willingness and ability to follow the plan incorporated. Physicians typically operate in a context and model that is biomedical and disease based. In contrast, the patient is typically much more focused on health and illness, in terms of suffering and impact on personal and family context. To provide care that is patient centered, you will explore the patient's expectations, beliefs, and concerns about health and illness, including the patient's preferences for alternative treatments. You must adequately explore contextual factors including family, work, culture, gender, age, socioeconomic issues, and spirituality. Patient-centered care involves extreme respect for the patient's autonomy. You will encourage the patient's participation in decisions to the fullest extent the patient desires.

How shall I begin the interview? What is its structure?

The preparation phase begins before you walk in the door. You should review the chart. Try to decide your top priorities, although these may be different from the patient's priorities and should be negotiated. Make sure that you are physically and emotionally ready to interview the patient. Try pausing before you knock on the door to collect yourself. Take a deep breath and begin to focus on the patient. Address the patient formally unless asked to do otherwise. Explain who you are and determine that the patient is comfortable with your training level. Explain that your preceptor will be involved in the medical decisions.

The body of the interview consists of establishing rapport, negotiating priorities, and using appropriate interviewing techniques to conduct the interview. As information is exchanged, you will construct and discuss hypotheses with your preceptor and the patient. Others present, such as family members, must also be involved in this process.

Closure involves summarization and instruction. It is surprising how often providers do the steps of the interview out of order or intersperse them. The patient is much less likely to remember instructions given at times other than the end of the interview. Final steps during closure are assessment of the patient's understanding and arrangements for follow-up care.

How can I be a better listener?

The biggest barrier to good communication is poor listening skills. You can be a better listener if you are certain you are attending to the patient. Again, make sure that you are focused on the patient and not on personal or outside issues. Nonverbal techniques described later in the chapter are incredibly important in creating an environment in which the patient feels heard. Even for medical students there is often a power differential, with the provider perceived as superior to the patient. Interruptions of patients when they are speaking are correlated with these power differentials. Make sure you follow a patient-centered approach and interact with the patient as an equal. Monitor yourself for interruptions of the patient.

How do I gain the cooperation of the patient?

This is a trick question because cooperation [per se] means the patient doing what you want him/her to do. Rather than that, you are seeking a collaborative relationship with most patients—a partnership. Patients will want to collaborate with you if they trust you, perceive you as someone who is warm and caring, and believe you have fully understood their situation. Do not expect your patients to follow instructions unless they believe they are understood by you. Do not expect advice to have any effect unless you clearly understand the patient's situation and context, and have made adjustments accordingly.

How do I know if I am communicating successfully with the patient?

The successful interview consists of information gathered for a correct medical decision and a trusting relationship between the doctor and patient. You will know if things went well if you and the patient are clear about your roles and responsibilities and agree on the plan. It is not always necessary that the doctor and patient feel satisfied or happy, but this should be a goal for your interviewing.

What is the best way to communicate the results of a test?

Communication of test results begins when they are ordered by clearly describing the purpose and potential value of the results. Let patients know when and how they will receive their results. Establish with whom they want the results discussed. You will want to review with your preceptor the rationale for the test and be prepared to discuss in lay terms the accuracy and application of test results. In clinics, normal results are likely to be mailed. On inpatient services, you should report your findings to the patient daily. Always be brief and use language that the patient can understand. You might begin by asking the patient if they remember why the test was ordered. Always check their understanding and the emotional impact of the results.

How do I deliver bad news?

A patient expecting bad news is likely to ask you. If you do not immediately provide an assurance that everything is all right, they will assume that news is bad. You can then help them with the process of acceptance. For patients not expecting bad news, a reasonable approach is to remind them of the purpose for which a test was obtained or ask what they understood was happening when they first presented for care. You should then ask if the patient is ready to hear bad news. They may prefer not to, may wish to wait a while, or may want a family member present. Simple, short, and direct statements are best. Follow a formula such as this: "Here is the difficult part. The (name of test) shows a (result) which could be (condition)."

Everyone needs time to absorb bad news. Pause and wait. Even a few minutes of silence may be appropriate. You can expect some patients to experience strong emotions. You need not do anything other than be present in the face of these emotions and offer your concern. Even negative emotions directed toward you or the health-care team must be accepted with appropriate concern. Patients may have questions or defer them for later. If you do not know the answer, offer to find out. You should let the patient know that not only are you willing to answer questions then, but that it is likely he/she will have questions after he/she has absorbed this news and that you will be available to answer them. Serious bad news should be accompanied by a plan for further discussion later.

How do I handle delayed appointments?

Odds are that you will get behind some days. Your preceptor is likely to have set criteria for the announcement that the "doctor is running late," usually if the patient has been in the room more than 20 minutes. You should keep the initiative for informing patients if you are behind, acknowledge inconvenience, and provide reasons, where applicable. Thank the patients for their patience.

How do I apologize?

Apologies are most effective when done soon, once, and effectively. Always acknowledge the damage. Describe what you will do to rectify the situation.

What are some common interview techniques?

Surely you have covered interviewing techniques in your earlier courses and especially know the importance of *open-ended questions* to invite extended discussion and to bring out the patient's agenda. You also know that *closed-ended questions,* defined as questions that require single word or a short answer, are overused. They allow a very limited range of answers, often address the doctor's agenda, and should be reserved for later in the interview. *Confrontation* is not an aggressive move but rather an honest attempt to understand what is really going on with the patient. This usually works best when you tactfully point out discrepancies in the patient's history. *Silence* can be a type of confrontation. It can help the patient to participate more, give you time to gather your thoughts, and give the patient time to get in touch with his/her feelings. Silence while listening intently demonstrates respect. Silence should be mixed with *facilitations,* which are minimal verbal responses and verbal counterparts to head nodding. They will make you seem warmer. *Clarifications* are an attempt to focus upon or understand the basic nature of a patient's statement. *Reassurance* is a deliberate, somewhat parental statement that can be supportive. It should be accurate, genuine, and reality based. *Summarizing* is a clarifying type of statement by which you synthesize what has been communicated and highlight the major feelings and thoughts.

What should I know about nonverbal communication?

Remember the acronym ***SOFTEN:*** **S**mile, **O**pen posture, **F**orward lean, **T**erritory, **E**ye contact, and **N**od.

Even the brightest and most concise statements will be ineffective and perhaps misconstrued without good nonverbal technique. Personal attitudes and emotions are communicated at the nonverbal level. This begins with your personal appearance, which is seen as a display of your confidence and concern. Patients prefer conventional clothing. They see physicians who wear white coats with conventional clothing as more competent than physicians who wear scrub suits.

Verbal communications may be emphasized or contradicted nonverbally. People have less control over their nonverbal communications; therefore, they are often more genuine. Insincere smiles will ultimately cause difficulties establishing trust, although a patient may not be sure a smile is insincere. A smile can overcome interpersonal distances and help with patient defensiveness or anxiety. Patients are more positively disposed to physicians who smile.

Seek a strong reciprocal affective relationship between you and the patient, where once an affective statement is made by the patient or you, the other responds similarly. Body position is an indicator of affective relationship. High patient satisfaction is associated with body lean and rotation of the torso toward the patient. Relaxed, patient-centered physicians lean forward up to 20 degrees and to the side up to 10 degrees. Changes in body position are more frequent. Tilting the head to one side is not an affectation but is done by animals listening intently; it communicates interest and attention.

Good listeners look at their speakers. Eye contact does not express emotions but does express sincerity and thoughtfulness. Poor eye contact is interpreted as lack of concern. It is appropriate to glance away when formulating your thoughts or selecting phrasing. Prolonged eye contact can be viewed as flirtatious or aggressive.

Touch can promote healing, and infants deprived of touch will suffer physical deterioration. While the majority of patients do not feel better leaving a physician's office if they have not received touch, touching can be viewed as aggressive if it is not accompanied by good verbal and nonverbal communication.

How can I speed up my patient interviews?

Listening effectively—so that the patient becomes comfortable giving his/her history—is almost always quicker than a forced closed-ended interview by the physician. Avoid interruptions and let the patient tell his/her story. Pay attention to structure so that you and the patient do not become confused. At the beginning of the interview, you may need to clarify roles so that the patient understands what information he/she will need to be giving you. You also need to negotiate what complaints and issues will be addressed that day. It is often helpful, and sometimes necessary, for a patient to return another time for less pressing problems. Most practitioners know which patients will take more time. Your preceptor can advise you on this. Some office visits will be routine while others are more dramatic and require more time. Try to experience both.

REFERENCE

Makoul G, Lang F, et al.: Essential elements of communication in medical encounters: The Kalamazoo Consensus Statement. Acad Med, 76:390–393, 2001.

USEFUL WEBSITES

Bayer Institute for Healthcare Communication
http://www.bayerinstitute.com
American Academy on Physician and Patient
http://www.physicianpatient.org

7

Learning Contracts

What are learning contracts?

A learning contract is an educational plan "negotiated" between you and your faculty adviser that allows you to identify particular areas of knowledge, skills, and attitudes on which to concentrate during your clerkship. It is a process that can be used to assist you in tailoring your clerkship to meet your own recognized needs. You might develop a plan to focus specifically on an area of knowledge, e.g., management of low back pain, or on a skill, e.g., interpretation of EKGs. More challenging to develop are objectives related to attitudes and values. One example might be developing cultural sensitivity in patient encounters by allowing patients to express what a problem means to them. For each identified area, you would then outline a plan to achieve your goal, including a mechanism for determining that you have done so.

What should be included in a learning contract?

The first step is to identify your academic needs within the framework of the course goals and objectives—areas in which you feel weak or in which you have a special interest. The plan itself usually includes the following elements:

- What you plan to accomplish—your objectives. These should be specific enough so that you can measure their achievement.
- How you plan to accomplish your objectives—the resources you will use and the activities in which you will engage.
- Evidence that you will gather to show that you have accomplished your goals.
- Criteria against which to measure your achievement.

The learning contract should list your name, the course, and the time frame in which the objectives are to be accomplished. This could be a simple form that includes all elements named in the preceding list presented in a horizontal table. Here is an example:

Student: Faculty Adviser:
Course: Date:

Learning Objectives	Resources/ Activities	Documentation	Assessment Criteria

Such a tabular arrangement would allow you and your faculty adviser to review and edit your plan, as well as monitor your progress and complete the final assessment. You might consider developing a template using database software, which would offer several advantages. You and your faculty adviser could communicate electronically for ongoing management and final evaluation. Additionally, you could begin to build a "Learning Portfolio," which would assist you in organizing your overall learning and in managing your progress toward clinical competence.

How will completing a learning contract assist me in learning what I need to know?

First and foremost, a learning contract respects you as an adult learner and allows you to assume responsibility for your own learning. It encourages you to become a reflective learner, focusing on what you most need to learn in each educational experience. It also gives you a structure to use in continuing your education beyond medical school.

Most immediately in your clerkship, a learning contract can be used to help you focus on your specific needs in the busy ambulatory clinic. It also gives you a mechanism for planning with your preceptor how to make the clerkship most beneficial to you.

A learning contract can be used anywhere in the educational process. In planning clerkships in special settings and with special populations, it can make that experience most meaningful and contribute most to your overall education.

REFERENCES

Anderson G, Boud D, Sampson J: Learning Contracts. London: Kogan Page, 1996.

Cohen EB: Electronic learning contracts. Acad Med 17(5):529, 1996.

Knowles MS, Horton EF, Swanson RA: The Adult Learner. Houston: Gulf Publishing, 1998.

McDermott M, McGrae C, Raymond H, Stille F, et al.: Use of learning contracts in an office-based primary care clerkship. Med Educ 33:374–381, 1999.

Stanton F, Grant J: Approaches to experiential learning, course delivery, and validation in medicine. Med Educ 33:282–297, 1999.

8

Biopsychosocial Model

What is the biopsychosocial model?

Until the 1970s, the biomedical model was the prevailing conceptual framework for what was being taught in medical school. Its foundation was the notion that disease can be explained on the basis of measurable biological variables. Correspondingly, treatment interventions targeted biological and physiological factors. But there often was a disconcerting disconnect between this reductionistic model and the realities of both physicians' practice and patients' illness experiences. Practitioners had long recognized that more than biology was at work in their patients' lives. Psychological (cognitive and emotional), social (family, community, economic), cultural, and spiritual factors were identified as important in the etiology of, and patient responses to, disease.

In the last 25 years, the biopsychosocial (BPS) model has become the predominant conceptual framework in family medicine and, to a lesser degree, all of primary care. It is a holistic framework for understanding the etiology, onset, course, and outcome of illness. This model is rooted in general systems theory, which considers life as being comprised of overlapping system levels ranging from the subatomic to the biosphere (Box 8–1). Each of these system levels is characterized by parts that have roles, are governed by rules of operation, and tend toward homeostasis. The system levels are connected by positive and negative feedback loops providing communication and corrective action in order to maintain this homeostasis. The system level may go through periods when change is required (morphogenesis), but homeostasis eventually will be reestablished.

The generation of symptoms occurs when the system is out of balance. There are often reciprocal connections among the system levels so that it is difficult or impossible to point to one or more causal factors that, isolated from other influences, cause disease.

How does the BPS model influence assessment, diagnosis, and treatment?

Because clinical problems are thought of as resulting from the interaction of multiple variables, the assessment (history, physical, lab, and diagnostic procedures) ought to reflect an investigation of the biopsychosocial territory.

BOX 8–1

Systems Hierarchy

- Biosphere
- Society/nation
- Culture/subculture
- Community
- Family
- Two person
- Person
- Nervous system
- Organs/organ systems
- Tissues
- Cells
- Organelles
- Molecules
- Atoms
- Subatomic particles

How do I adapt the BPS model to the typical office visit and patient interview?

The typical office visit ranges between 10 and 30 minutes. This is a relatively brief amount of time, especially if the presenting complaint has its roots in a complex interplay of BPS factors. How much time is spent exploring these factors will depend on whether or not the problem is acute or chronic and how urgent or debilitating it is. Your most pressing objective is to help the attending physician discover information that will help relieve suffering or prevent a condition from worsening acutely. But the BPS factors in complex or chronic conditions may take some effort, over time, to sort out. You will have to negotiate and prioritize items on the agenda for each visit with the patient and/or family members (see Chapter 6). For example, a patient with bronchitis and asthma may also be a smoker or live with smokers. Helping her with managing an immediate flare-up so that she can breathe more easily is the first order of business. But changing her exposure to tobacco smoke should be addressed as soon as possible.

What kinds of questions should I ask patients?

Follow the advice provided in Chapter 6 and ask open-ended questions, followed by closed-ended questions where necessary, to help clarify the various factors that contribute to the development, exacerbation, and amelioration of the condition. Asking questions that elicit the patient and family members' perspectives will be very helpful in fleshing out the biopsychosocial explanation for the condition. Examples of good questions to ask include:

What do you think is causing this problem?
Are there things going on in your life that worsen (or improve) your symptoms?
How is this problem affecting (being affected by) your life (family, living situation, coping, etc)?
Sometimes our bodies react to things going on in our lives—kind of signaling us that something is wrong. Could that be happening in your situation?
Having this kind of problem can be very difficult, especially if there are a lot of other things going on in our lives. Are there things going on that make it difficult to care for yourself (or do the things you need to in order to manage this disease)?

How does the BPS model affect treatment?

As with some biological, anatomical, and/or physiological states, some psychosocial factors are difficult or impossible to change. But, for those areas that have the potential for change and are implicated in the disease process related to the presenting condition, change needs to be negotiated with the patient and/or family members. This begins with helping the patient gain an appreciation of what is going on from a holistic perspective.

KEY POINTS

- **The biopsychosocial model is based on general systems theory, including the idea that clinical problems are the result of the interaction of variables at multiple system levels.**
- **This holistic model provides an integrated perspective for understanding and treating problems commonly presented by patients of family physicians.**
- **Accurate assessment and effective treatment depend on the physician, over time, discussing a variety of issues and negotiating the treatment plan with the patient (and family, where appropriate).**

9

Prevention of Disease in Family Medicine

Family medicine is about relationships, especially when it comes to caring for patients. Most family physicians treat patients the way they would treat their spouse or their mother. Because of that, preventive medicine is a major component of family medicine.

While we are trained to treat our patients when they have a heart attack, we would much prefer to help them prevent that heart attack. Many illnesses are completely preventable. Many that are not preventable can be controlled to prevent complications from developing. In some conditions we are very successful, but in others it is very difficult. The relationship between the physician and patient is paramount to creating a successful environment.

Preventive medicine is typically broken into three broad categories: health promotion or counseling, disease surveillance or screening, and disease prevention including immunizations.

HEALTH PROMOTION OR COUNSELING

Health promotion encompasses much of the educational role of a family physician. It is dependent on the age and medical condition of the patient. We counsel patients to stop smoking, maintain an ideal body weight, eat a nutritious diet, exercise regularly, and address many other lifestyle issues. These are based on the medical evidence that specific lifestyle changes decrease the risk of acquiring illness or increase the quality of overall health. The U.S. Preventive Task Force is a review committee that sets evidence-based guidelines for the nation. Many other independent organizations also set guidelines for prevention. Some of these have an evidence base, while others are simply opinions of the physicians and policymakers of those organizations. The U.S. Preventive Task Force recommendations can be found on the Internet at http://www.ahrq.gov/clinic/prevenix.htm.

DISEASE SURVEILLANCE OR SCREENING

Disease surveillance or screening should also be based on the best medical evidence available. Much controversy occurs in this area of preventive medicine. While the U.S. Preventive Task Force guidelines are evidence-based, many organizations disagree on many screening tests. The purpose of a screening test is to identify all of the patients at risk for a disease while minimizing the number of patients falsely labeled as at risk. Commonly recommended screening tests include colonoscopy for colon cancer, clinical evaluation for depression, pap smears for cervical cancer, mammograms for breast cancer, and laboratory tests for *Chlamydia* infections. Some of these (and others) are recommended for certain populations at higher risk—such as *Chlamydia* screening for women under 26 years old that are sexually active. Others are recommended for larger groups—such as screening for depression in all adults. Some screening tests require a great deal of discussion and application to the individual patient. It may be very appropriate for an individual to decline some screening tests. Great family physicians teach their patients and help them decide what is best for them.

DISEASE PREVENTION

Disease prevention takes many forms. Immunizations are perhaps the most obvious form of prevention. The Advisory Committee on Immunization Practices (ACIP), of the U.S. Centers for Disease Control (CDC), sets the national guidelines for immunizations. The most recent guidelines can be found at http://www.cdc.gov/nip/publications/acip-list.htm. Infants in America receive as many as four or five injections at some of their routine well-child visits, with more in stages of development and testing. Our success rate at immunizing children is very high, since immunizations are required for children to be able to attend school. Adults tend to not be up-to-date with their recommended immunizations. People often forget that immunizations against tetanus, influenza, and pneumococcal infections are recommended for many adults as well.

Disease prevention also includes treatment of many conditions that increase a patient's risk for a more serious illness. We treat hypertension primarily to decrease the risk of a stroke or heart attack later in life. Many other diseases are managed this way, including hyperlipidemia, diabetes, and strep throat. Commonly, this approach is called secondary prevention. Secondary prevention involves treating an existing illness with the purpose of preventing a complicating illness. Removing colon polyps before they become malignant or treating cervical dysplasia before it becomes invasive cancer are two other examples of secondary prevention.

Disease prevention has been divided into primary, secondary, and tertiary prevention. Primary prevention really refers to both health promotion and immunizations. For example, physicians help patients quit smoking before they have enough lung damage to be diagnosed with emphysema. Of course, physicians also help patients quit smoking after they begin to have symptoms of emphysema. This is really tertiary prevention, because its purpose is to prevent the severity of the disease from progressing. Tertiary prevention is focused on improving quality of life in the midst of disease. Other examples include the treatment of CHF, chronic pain, and arthritis.

Our model of medical care is still very much defined by the treatment of diseases and symptoms. But family physicians strive to take that extra minute or two at every visit to educate, screen, encourage, counsel, and support patients in their efforts to live longer, healthier lives. Americans are living longer lives, but we are challenged to make as many of those years as healthy as possible. The Put Prevention into Practice (PPIP) initiative, started in 1994, attempted to put preventive tools in the hands of family physicians. Their website, http://www.ahrq.gov/clinic/ppipix.htm, lists many of these tools. Age-based clinical guides are particularly helpful as a quick reference to recommended prevention interventions. Other tools include office posters, chart flow sheets, educational materials, and the *Clinician's Handbook of Preventive Services*.

Most electronic medical records now include reminders to offer preventive services to patients. Prescriptions for exercise or other wellness activities are more common in family physicians' offices. Local organizations offer many wellness services, exercise programs, and confidential testing and treatment. National ad campaigns have been used to increase screening with mammograms, Pap smears, and prostate cancer. Our culture has definitely become more interested in prevention, though many individuals struggle to be successful. Family physicians must play a leading role in helping patients live healthier lives.

10

Remote Information Access

What is patient-centered information mastery at the points of care?

The fluid environment in which modern medical care is delivered demands that physicians provide care that is up-to-date and evidence-based. Providers must rapidly and efficiently sort through an expanding medical knowledge base and apply that information in a patient-centered manner. Information mastery incorporates the practice of evidence-based medicine (EBM), defined as the capacity to obtain information that has high validity and relevance to a specific patient encounter with minimal effort. Access to information at the "point of care" is the ability to get the correct information while in the room with the patient, from a web-connected computer, a handheld computer, or other resource.

Patient-centered care is the ability to focus on the whole patient within his/her individual concept of illness and to partner with him/her to develop a plan of care. Technology can be a potential barrier to patient-centered care if not explicitly integrated in a thoughtful manner, or it can dramatically enhance and focus response to the specific needs of an individual.

Why is it important to have these skills?

A healthcare provider's information-access skills can help improve the overall quality of care, decrease the cost of care, and increase satisfaction of both the patient and physician. In 1986 approximately 100 articles based on research from randomized controlled trials were published. By 1995 that number had increased to over 10,000 publications annually, and has grown significantly since. This represents an explosion of information that is relevant to daily patient care. At the same time physicians are being challenged to reduce medical errors, provide evidence-based care, and focus on the unique needs of individual patients. The only way to meet these challenges is to use electronic resources judiciously. Physicians today struggle to stay current in many aspects of patient care. A 1999 study showed that practicing family physicians average 3.2

questions for every 10 patients. Reasonable answers were available 80% of the time but were sought only 36% of the time.

How does information mastery improve care?

Good EBM resources should provide current, useful information, accessible at the point of care. This information should include data helpful in making a diagnosis, such as the relative utility of certain diagnostic studies, and best treatment options. This information can be provided in a number of formats including clinical rules and calculators, peer-reviewed summaries of meta-analyses, practice guidelines, and recommendations. In addition, an information master should be conversant with resources that provide valid, relevant information to patients in a format that is easily understood and patient-friendly. Such resources may include, but should not be limited to, disease-specific information (patient handouts), health maintenance recommendations, and information on local resources such as support and advocacy groups. For example, students should be able to rapidly provide a victim of domestic violence with information on local shelters, or find the current Centers for Disease Control travel recommendations for a patient planning a trip to West Africa.

What skills and strategies are crucial to patient-centered information mastery?

The practice of EBM is integral to information mastery. Students must have a working knowledge of basic EBM principles, the potential applications of EBM, and its limitations at the current state of development. Taking an EBM course is one way to acquire such skills. Many schools provide training in this area (Box 10–1).

To facilitate information mastery in the clinical setting, students should assess the site to identify computer and internet access and software resources. Resources compatible with point-of-care access include rapidly searchable brief summaries that facilitate medical decision making. Handheld computers and the Internet are both tools suitable for patient-centered information retrieval. Comprehensive resources are important but most useful outside specific patient encounters.

How does one evaluate the quality of web-based medical information?

Assessing the quality of information can be difficult. One strategy is to limit searches to peer-reviewed sources of information, if possible. Some sources rate the material according to the level of evidence, which aids assessment of quality. In the absence of appraised resources, one may evaluate medical literature using the ***POSSE*** acronym:

- Is the evidence **P**atient oriented?
- Is the **O**utcome an important one?
- What is the **S**ize of the study? Is it underpowered?
- Are the **S**tatistics and the analysis of data sound?
- Is the **E**vidence relevant to my clinical setting/practice?

Many of the major medical specialties, subspecialties, and societies have websites that provide peer-reviewed articles. However, it is often useful to consider the sponsor of the research, and also the qualifications and associations of the author(s), in an effort to detect the possibility of underlying bias. Resources should be updated quarterly at a minimum.

What about handheld computers? Should I own one and what should be on it?

Students should consider owning a mid- to high-range handheld computer with an expandable memory option. High-yield software resources that can be updated on an ongoing basis can be easily

BOX 10–1

Web-Based Evidence-Based Medicine (EBM) Resources

Web-based EBM/Information Mastery Learning Resources

Michigan State University FP Dept.	http://www.poems.msu.edu/InfoMastery
USC Norris Medical Library	http://www.usc.edu/hsc/nml/lis/tutorials/ebm.html
Florida State University	http://www.med.fsu.edu/library/GuidelinesEBM.asp
New York Academy of Medicine	http://www.ebmny.org/teach.html

Open High-Yield EBM Databases and Search Engines

Oxford Center for EBM	http://www.cebm.net/toolbox.asp
Trip Database	http://www.ceres.uwcm.ac.uk/section.cfm?section=trip
Cochrane Database	http://www.cochrane.org/index2.htm
Bandolier	http://www.jr2.ox.ac.uk/bandolier
National Guideline Clearinghouse	http://www.guideline.gov
DARE	http://nhscrd.york.ac.uk/darehp.htm
SUMSearch	http://sumsearch.uthscsa.edu

loaded at about the same cost as many bound medical textbooks. At a minimum a drug reference program and a medical calculator should be loaded. An EBM resource is strongly recommended as well. Many medical schools now require students to own handheld computers, or provide them for use. Schools will often provide some software to students for free and negotiate reduced costs for others. Nearly 50% of practicing physicians and more than 80% of residents use handhelds in their care of patients, underscoring their value to the quality of care.

The choice of operating system (Palm or Pocket PC) should be weighed with the local medical environment in mind, taking into consideration that most devices will last two to four years and that residencies might require a change. While the Palm operating system has the largest market share, the environment is changing as hospitals, private practices, and health centers adopt electronic medical records and try to provide access to handheld devices (Box 10–2).

BOX 10–2

Handheld Computer Information Resources

University of Arizona	http://educ.ahsl.arizona.edu/pda/index.htm
University of Iowa	http://www.lib.uiowa.edu/hardin/pda/resources.html#guidelines
University of Connecticut	http://library.uchc.edu/pda

KEY POINTS

- **Patient-centered information mastery is an important skill for students to learn.**
- **Evidence-based medicine resources should provide current, useful information at the point of care.**
- **It is important to assess the clinical site soon after arrival to identify potential resources.**
- **Review the quality of the resource, using the POSSE model if no other appraisal methods are available.**

REFERENCES

Ely JW, Osherhoff JA, Ebell MH, et al.: Analysis of questions asked by family doctors regarding patient care. BMJ 319:358–361, 1999.

Leung GM, Johnston JM, Tin KY, et al.: Randomized controlled trial of clinical decision support tools to improve learning of evidence-based medicine in medical students. BMJ 327:1090, 2003.

Peterson MW, Rowat J, Kreiter C, Mandel J: Medical students' use of information resources: Is the digital age dawning? Aca Med 79:89–95, 2004.

White B: Making evidence-based medicine doable in everyday practice. Family Practice Management 11:51–58, 2004.

11

Practical Skills for the Medical Student

What procedures are done in a family medicine office?

The scope of clinical procedures varies a great deal from one family medicine office to another. Some of the most common office procedures are injections, phlebotomy, IV infusions, EKGs, splinting, and simple suturing. These procedures will be described in this chapter. Other offices may offer colposcopy, antenatal testing, radiology, flexible sigmoidoscopy, spirometry, and exercise treadmill testing, among other procedures.

Should I tell the patients that I am just learning?

It is important to always introduce yourself as a medical student, and explain to the patient that you and your supervisor (be it a nurse, medical assistant, or physician) will perform the procedure together.

What are universal precautions?

Universal precautions are the procedures used by healthcare professionals to prevent transmission of disease. They come into play any time there is reasonable likelihood of exposure to blood or other body fluids. Barrier protection (which may include gloves, safety glasses, face shields, and lab coats) may be used to prevent skin and mucous membrane contamination with blood or body fluids. When contact is only likely to be with the patient's intact skin (such as during a routine chest or abdominal exam), then these measures are not necessary. In the event of skin contamination, wash the area with copious amounts of clean water and soap. Eyes or mucous membranes should be irrigated with clean water. Hands should always be washed immediately after removal of gloves. In addition, all sharp instruments, including needles, syringes, scalpel blades, and glass slides, should be disposed of in approved, puncture-resistant sharps containers. While it may be ungainly at first to perform such procedures as phlebotomy and injections while wearing gloves, it is important to learn to manipulate the instruments as well as to palpate veins through the gloves, in order to maintain safety.

What should I do if a patient feels woozy or passes out during a procedure such as a blood draw or an injection?

Vasovagal responses (hypotens ive bradycardic responses) are fairly common during routine procedures such as injections or blood draws. If the patient complains of dizziness or light-headedness, stop the procedure (if possible), offer reassurance, and get help to move the patient to a supine position as soon as possible. If the patient loses consciousness, call for help, assess ABCs (airway, breathing, and circulation), and move the patient into a supine position with the legs elevated as soon as possible. Generally these symptoms will pass spontaneously within a few minutes, and the procedure can be retried or resumed (if needed) with the patient supine.

What should I do if I receive a needle stick or other injury with a contaminated sharp?

Stop the procedure and wash the affected area with copious amounts of soap and water. Speak immediately to your supervisor, who can help you to assess the potential risks for communicable disease (especially HIV and viral hepatitis) and plan the next steps. Antiretroviral medications may be indicated in the case of a high-risk HIV exposure, and these must be started within a couple of hours of the stick in order to be most effective.

VENIPUNCTURE

What is the best site for drawing blood?

The easy answer is "where the veins are"—but seriously, the antecubital fossa is often the first place to look for a "good vein" (more on this later). Other common sites are the radial forearms, dorsal hands, feet, and occasionally larger central veins (brachial, femoral). If your patient has few accessible veins (often true of chemotherapy patients or IV drug users), be sure to ask the patient where the best veins are. For this chapter we will address only peripheral veins.

How do I select the best vein?

Generally speaking, a "good" vein is one that is full, easily palpable, and fairly straight. Don't be fooled by ropy prominent veins—

they often roll away from your needle. These veins are most stable at the point where they divide (the point of the "V"). Similarly, given a visible vein that is tortuous or fine and a nonvisible but palpable large, straight vein, choose the latter.

▶ WHAT YOU WILL NEED

- Gloves (not sterile)
- Tourniquet
- Sterile 2×2 gauze
- Alcohol pads (or povodine iodine wipes if a blood culture is to be drawn)
- Vacutainer tubes for the requested tests (two sets)
- Adapter to connect the needle to the vacutainer tube
- Three sterile venipuncture needles; 20-gauge or 22-gauge is usually fine (the larger the number, the more fine the needle)
- Band-Aids®

▶ TO PREPARE

Check the patient's name against the lab request form, and be sure that you have the correct number and types of tubes for the requested analyses. Label the tubes before starting.

▶ THE PROCEDURE

1. Place the tourniquet about halfway up the upper arm. It's best to loop the tubing under itself so that you can release quickly.
2. Ask the patient to open and close the hand to distend the veins, then locate your vein of choice on the arm. If it is not easily visible, mark the skin with your fingernail or the top of a pen to keep track of where the vein travels. Then cleanse the area with an alcohol swab.
3. Put on your gloves, and prepare your needle and vacuum collection tubes. This procedure will vary a little depending on whether you are using a butterfly or a straight needle—in either case, do not push the tube into the collecting hub until you have accessed a vein.
4. Warn the patient, then insert the needle, bevel up, at about a 15-degree angle to the skin along the route of the vein (point proximal). When you see a flash of blood in the hub of your needle, hold steady and push the vacuum tube onto the hub/tubing using your other hand. Do not tent the skin up or move the needle around as you fill as many tubes as are required.

5. IF you do not get a blood flash and there is no visible subcutaneous bleeding around the vessel, withdraw the needle until just the tip is beneath the skin, redirect slightly and try again.
6. IF you get an initial flash, and then the flow of blood stops:
   a. Try to slightly redirect the needle
   b. Withdraw the needle very slightly (sometimes it can be against a valve)
   c. If still no flow, remove the vacuum tube, release the tourniquet, and remove the needle. You will have to try again at a different site.
7. Once the last tube is nearly full, release the tourniquet, disconnect the tube when it is full, hold sterile gauze over the puncture site, and remove the needle, immediately placing pressure on the site.
8. Place a Band-Aid® on the puncture site (once bleeding has stopped), and be sure that all sharps are properly disposed of.

INJECTIONS

▶ WHAT YOU WILL NEED

- Gloves
- Alcohol swabs
- Appropriate-sized syringe
- Injectate
- 2×2 gauze
- Needles (22-gauge or 24-gauge half-inch for subcutaneous, 22-gauge five-eighths-inch or 1-inch for IM for most patients)
- Consents/patient information pages, if applicable

▶ TO PREPARE

Get appropriate informed consent from the patient if required. Prepare syringes with injectate. If using multidose vials, draw up only the required dose plus about 0.2 mL, after first passing an alcohol swab over the top of the vial. For single-use vials, reconstitute the injectate if necessary, then draw up the full volume into the syringe. Record lot number, expiration date, and the site of the injection in the medical record. In general, for infants and children less than six years of age the thighs are easiest, upper arms for older children and adults. In the case of a large-volume (more than 1 mL) IM injection, the thigh or gluteal muscles are preferred.

▶ THE PROCEDURE

Intramuscular

1. Put on gloves, and prepare injection site with alcohol swab. For an arm injection, use the deltoid muscle, about three fingerbreadths below the lateral border of the clavicle. Be careful to stay low enough to avoid the shoulder joint and the subacromial bursa. For thigh injection, use the midthigh slightly lateral to midline. For gluteal, using a four-quadrant model use the upper outer quadrant of the buttock.
2. Ensure that there is no air trapped in the syringe, and push the plunger to the required volume to be injected.
3. Holding the syringe like a dart, warn the patient and briskly insert the needle perpendicular to the skin into the muscle—usually up to the hub of the needle. In a very thin patient, you may need to go less deep. In contrast, for an obese patient a 1.5-inch needle may be necessary.
4. Draw back the plunger briefly, and if there is no blood return then quickly and smoothly inject the syringe contents and pull out the needle. If there IS blood return, withdraw the needle about a quarter inch and try again—repeat until there is no blood return, then inject as above.
5. Place the used needle in a sharps container.
6. Use pressure with 2×2 sterile gauze to stop any bleeding (rare) and cover with a Band-Aid®.

Subcutaneous

The instructions are the same as for intramuscular injection, except use a half-inch needle, and the site is usually the posterior upper arm for children over six years of age and adults and the thigh for infants. Follow the instructions for an intramuscular injection, but for the actual injection pinch up the skin over the area to be injected and insert the needle at about a 45-degree angle, shallow to the muscle. Draw back the plunger, and if no blood return, inject and remove the needle as you would for an intramuscular injection.

INTRAVENOUS ACCESS

Where do I place an IV catheter?

The location depends on the situation at hand. If the patient is to have an IV for many hours or days, it is best to place it where it will least interfere with other activities. Radial forearm or dorsal hand are often good options. If the goal is to infuse fluids quickly and for a short duration, then the larger antecubital vessels are often easier to access, although are considerably less convenient for the patient. In the case of infants, foot, hand, and scalp veins are often used. For this discussion we will present IV access for adults. Be sure that you familiarize yourself with the specific tubing and infusion pumps at your site, as well as the kit for starting heparin locks (an IV access site that is capped off, for intermittent or later use).

▶ WHAT YOU WILL NEED

- Gloves
- Tourniquet
- Alcohol swabs
- IV catheters (Angiocath is one brand)—two or three; 18-gauge or 20-gauge usually fine—for large volume infusions (like urgent blood transfusions or fluid resuscitation) consider a 16-gauge.
- Tape
- 2×2 sterile gauze
- Op-site or other sterile covering for the IV site
- Band-Aids®
- Consider using 1% lidocaine *without* epinephrine for local anesthesia—0.5 mL in a tuberculin or insulin syringe with the smallest gauge needle you have.

If you are placing a heparin lock:

- Saline flush
- Heparin flush
- Appropriate cap

If you are starting an infusion:

- Extension tubing
- IV tubing
- Solution to be infused
- Infusion pump for fixed rate infusions

▶ TO PREPARE

Be sure that you have all materials at hand. If you are running an infusion, connect the infusion fluid to the tubing, run the air out of the tubing, and reclose the valve.

▶ THE PROCEDURE

1. Apply tourniquet and choose your site based on the recommendations at the beginning of this section. It is best to try

for the nondominant hand whenever possible. The ideal vein is large, straight, and without a lot of branches.

2. Put on gloves.
3. Swab the site with alcohol and inject a *small amount* of local anesthetic (0.1 mL or so) shallow to the vein where you plan to place the IV.
4. Holding the entire catheter (with the needle protruding from the flexible catheter), follow the same basic technique as for a venipuncture. Warn the patient, then advance the needle along the course of the vein at about a 15-degree angle to the skin (pointing proximal) until you see a flash of blood in the hub of the catheter.
5. Advance the needle about 2 mm further, then holding the needle steady, use the index finger to advance the soft catheter over the tip of the needle and into the vein as far as possible. Once you do this, *never* push the needle back into the catheter because you could shear off the tip.
6. Release the tourniquet.
7. Hold firm pressure just proximal to the IV site, and fully withdraw the needle.
8. Attach tubing/syringe and be sure that either saline will flush through or that your infusion fluids are running in freely once the valve is released.
9. If all is well, place an op-site over the IV, note the date and time on the op-site, and secure tubing to the patient with tape.
10. If it is a heparin lock, flush one syringe (usually 10 mL) of saline through the catheter, followed by about 10 mL of the prepared heparin solution, then cap the tubing.
11. If it is an infusion, run the fluids at the indicated rate. If the patient feels pain at the IV site, check to be sure that the fluids are still running into the vein and are not infiltrating the subcutaneous tissues. If you detect infiltration (pain and swelling around the catheter site), then immediately stop the infusion, remove the IV catheter, and start again at a new site.

BASIC SKIN SUTURING

What are the methods of closing a skin wound?

While suturing is the most traditional method of skin-wound closure, surgical adhesive (such as Dermabond) and skin staples are becoming increasingly common. Skin staples are particularly useful for operative closure of abdominal incisions, and for repair of simple scalp lacerations. They are quick, and for small scalp lacerations (requiring only one to three staples) are often placed without anesthesia. Surgical skin adhesive is particularly useful in areas of low skin tension, such as the face. It should not be used on areas of stress, such as across joints or near the eye. The description in this section applies to simple skin lacerations.

How should I select suture material?

The two basic types of suture material are absorbable (such as gut, chromic, braided polygalactan [Vicryl], and others) and nonabsorbable (such as nylon and Ethilon). The absorbable sutures will dissolve in four to eight weeks in most cases and are used internally. For the skin surface, nonabsorbable suture is used. Sutures are removed from 5 to 14 days after placement, depending on the location. Facial sutures are left for less time, sutures in the thick skin of the back or extremities may be left for 7 to 10 days. The coarseness of suture is measured from O (coarse suture used for very high-tension closures or tying off of vessels) to 7-O (extremely fine suture used for vascular or plastic surgery) and smaller. For most skin closures 3-O to 6-O will be sufficient: 3-O for high-tension areas (such as across a joint), 6-O for the face or other delicate skin.

How shall I select the needle?

Each suture material may come with several possibilities for a needle, usually various sizes of curved needle, and possibly a straight needle. The smaller the needle, the easier it will bend and break, and the smaller the stitches will need to be. A cutting needle is best for skin and other tough structures, while a smooth or tubular needle is best for fragile tissues. In addition, each manufacturer has a different nomenclature for describing needle sizes. Look at the suture packages, and in general choose a cutting needle that is curved and about 1.5 cm in length. PS2 and FS2 are two of the commonly used needle sizes for skin closures.

What is best to use for local anesthesia?

In general, 1% or 2% lidocaine with epinephrine will provide excellent anesthesia, and the vasoconstriction from the epinephrine will diminish bleeding. Do *not* use epinephrine on digits, earlobes, the nose, or the penis because the associated vasoconstriction can cause distal ischemia.

▶ WHAT YOU WILL NEED

- Local anesthetic of choice, in appropriate-sized syringe with a 22-gauge or smaller needle
- Sterile gloves
- Suture material of your choosing
- Sterile fields—one fenestrated, one nonfenestrated
- Mayo stand

- Sterile saline
- Sterile 4×4 gauze (several)
- Needle driver
- Pick-ups without teeth
- Suture scissors

► TO PREPARE

1. Be sure that there is adequate light, and that both you and the patient are fairly comfortable.
2. Put on gloves. If the wound is traumatic rather than surgical, irrigate copiously with sterile saline. A 50-mL syringe with a splashguard can be useful for deep injuries. If scrubbing is necessary, inject local anesthesia first. Cleanse the wound and surrounding skin with an antiseptic such as dilute povodine-iodine, then rinse with sterile saline.
3. Prepare syringe with local anesthetic and inject along the edges of the wound. It is usually best to inject into the wound edge itself, rather than through intact skin. Don't be afraid to distend the tissues a bit with the anesthetic.
4. Using sterile technique, open the nonfenestrated field onto the mayo stand and empty your sterile instruments, second drape, and gauze onto the field.

► THE PROCEDURE

1. Don sterile gloves, and place the fenestrated field on the patient to expose only the wound.
2. Open the corner of the suture material (look at the package) and grasp the base of the needle with the needle drivers.
3. For interrupted sutures, each stitch follows an arc beneath the skin, in order to evert the wound edges (Figure 11–1). You can either bring the needle back out through the wound, regrasp, and send through to the other side, or, to make the entire stitch in one arc, use rotation at the wrist to follow the curve of the needle. When regrasping or otherwise manipulating the needle, use forceps and the needle driver, rather than your fingers. Sutures should be evenly spaced, close enough to prevent gaping of the wound edges.
4. In order to tie each stitch, tie sequential square knots—2.5 or 3 knots is sufficient per stitch. There are many ways to accomplish this, such as an instrument tie (Figure 11–1).
5. Cut the suture for each stitch to about 0.5 cm in length.
6. When finished, cover with a dry dressing. Do not use any ointments or creams.

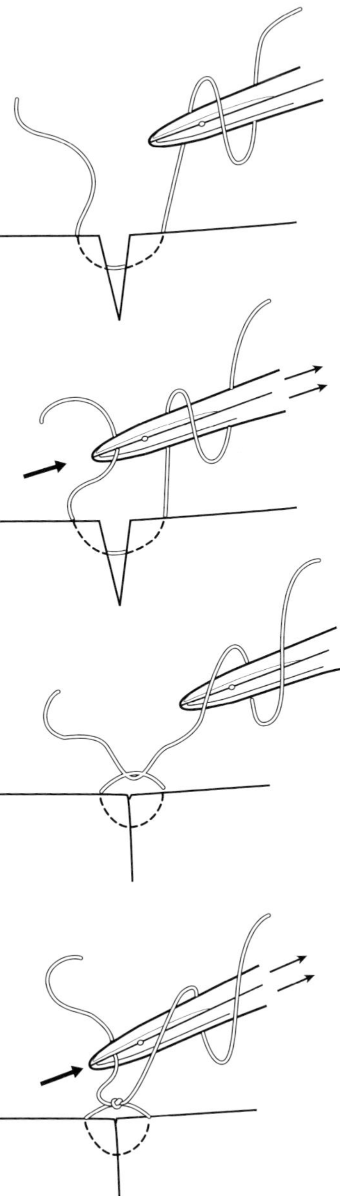

Figure 11–1. Four steps to tie a square knot using instrument ties. Path of needle through tissue follows an arc to promote eversion of skin edges. After each knot throw, maintain slight tension on suture to prevent knot from loosening. Most knots will be four or five throws, and suture ends are usually trimmed to about 0.5 cm.

ELECTROCARDIOGRAMS

Under what circumstances will I need to do an EKG?

EKGs are most commonly done to evaluate patients with chest pain, hypertension, palpitations, or other suspected cardiac problems. They are especially useful for detecting cardiac arrhythmias, anomalous conduction, acute and old ischemia, and heart chamber enlargement.

▶ WHAT YOU WILL NEED

- EKG machine with 10 leads
- 10 new electrodes
- EKG recording paper
- A razor (if the patient has a lot of body hair)

▶ TO PREPARE

Be sure that you record the patient's identifying information on the EKG tracing. Have the patient undress from the waist up and put on a gown open in front. Also be sure that you can access the skin of the lower legs (removal of tights, panty hose, or compression stockings will be necessary).

▶ THE PROCEDURE

1. With the patient in the supine position (okay to raise the head of the bed 20–30 degrees for patient comfort), place the two arm electrodes on the anterior forearms and the two leg electrodes on the medial lower legs. For the chest:
   - V1—fourth intercostal (IC) space, right sternal border;
   - V2—fourth IC space, left sternal border;
   - V3—midway between V2 and V4;
   - V4—fifth IC space, left midclavicular line;
   - V5—fifth IC space, left anterior axillary line;
   - V6—fifth IC space, left midaxillary line

   Some body hair may need to be shaved if there is inadequate adherence of the electrodes.
2. Attach the leads to the electrodes (double-check each one).
3. Instruct the patient to lie quietly, and activate the 12-lead option on the EKG machine. Most modern machines will produce a single page with all 12 leads on it; however, some machines will produce a long strip that has a short segment of each lead, one after the next. These strips can later be

mounted in sections. In the case of an arrhythmia, you can also request a rhythm strip—a longer recording of a single lead (usually lead II).

What if the tracing is very uneven across the page?

This is most commonly due to motion artifact. Ask the patient to remain still and quiet, and repeat the tracing.

What if some of the tracings are completely flat or with excessive noise?

This is usually due to poor electrode contact with the skin or with the lead. Recheck all electrode placements and lead connections. Occasionally, excessive noise can also come from electrical interference in the clinical area, and moving the patient to another room (if possible) can be helpful.

How is the EKG interpreted?

Many family physicians read their own EKGs. Basic EKG interpretation skills are beyond the scope of this chapter, but one good resource is Dale Dubin's book *Rapid Interpretation of EKGs*.

BASIC SPLINTING PRINCIPLES

What are the usual reasons for placing a splint?

The most common reason is to prevent further injury and pain after a bone or joint injury, such as a fracture or a severe sprain. In addition, splinting can be used to prevent further injury to crushed digits, to prevent wound dehiscence where sutures have been placed across an area of flexion, to prevent excessive motion around soft tissue infection, and to speed recovery in the case of tendonitis, acute arthritis, or other inflammatory condition.

How do I choose the most appropriate splint type?

In general, in the case of a fracture the goal is to immobilize the joints proximal to and distal to the injury. For instance, in the case of a forearm fracture, the ideal splint will immobilize both the wrist and the elbow in order to keep the fracture stable until the swelling subsides and a cast can be placed. For soft tissue injuries or inflammatory conditions, the goal is to immobilize the area in question while maintaining maximum function.

What are the most common splint materials?

Currently the most commonly used splints are made of vacuum-sealed fiberglass, often with attached padding on one side; these harden on exposure to air and water. They come in various widths from 2-inch to 6-inch, and in varying lengths. These are secured in place with elastic wraps. If there is no included padding, then a stockinette, along with cotton padding, must be placed beneath the splint to prevent skin injury. Some offices still use plaster splints, but this is increasingly rare. In addition, premade finger splints, volar wrist splints, thumb spica splints, and ankle splints are available in a variety of sizes. For fingers most offices stock aluminum splints with foam on one side, which can be cut to varying lengths.

How do I know the best splint to use?

Table 11–1 lists some common injuries and the preferred splint type for each.

What is the best way to shape a splint?

In general, splints are meant to protect an injury while maintaining maximum functionality. For a thumb spica splint, this comprises maintaining the thumb in a position that allows it to oppose with the rest of the fingers. For a volar wrist splint, it is important to maintain independent movement of the thumb, and movement of the fingers distal to the distal palmar crease. See Figure 11–2 for more details on these two splints. Most splinting materials harden in a few minutes, so once the material is exposed to air/water, efficiency is very important. In general, it is best to wear gloves while casting and splinting. When working with fiberglass, using hand lotion on the splint can reduce sticking to your gloves. Mold the splint around bony prominences (like the malleoli or the contours of the wrist) using palms or the pads of several fingers together. Do not mold

TABLE 11–1

Injury	Splint
Suspected or actual wrist fracture, carpal tunnel syndrome	Volar wrist splint—neutral position (see Figure 11–2)
Thumb injury, de Quervain's tenosynovitis, suspected navicular fracture	Thumb spica splint (see Figure 11–2)
Fourth or fifth metacarpal fracture (boxer's fracture)	Ulnar gutter splint
Forearm fracture	Sugartong splint with sling
Malleolar fracture or severe ankle sprain	Posterior lower leg splint
Nondisplaced foot phalanx fracture	Buddy-tape to adjacent toes, hard-sole shoe

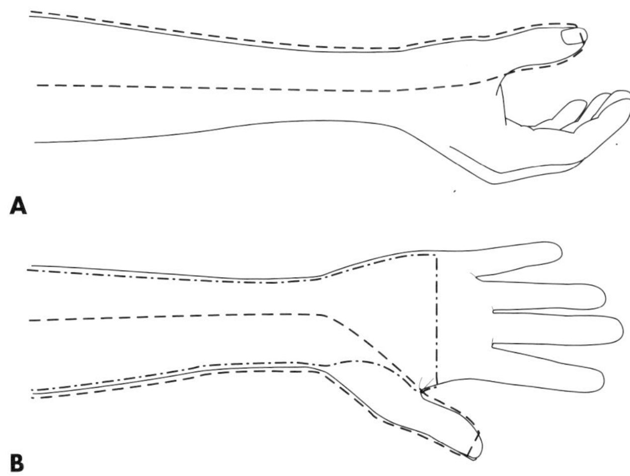

Figure 11–2. **A,** Radial view, wrist position in slight extension for both volar and thumb-spica splints. For thumb spica, thumb is in flexion and abduction to allow opposition with other fingers. **B,** Volar view, volar splint, extends along anterior forearm from distal palmar crease to about 4 cm distal to the antecubital crease, with cutout to allow full thumb motion (*dashed line*). Thumb spica splint extends from tip of thumb along radial forearm to 4–5 cm distal to antecubital crease. Tip of thumb is exposed to assess neurovascular status (*dash-dot line*).

with single fingers or other small areas of pressure, because the resulting indentation can cause a pressure sore beneath. Similarly, do not allow the patient to rest the splint on any hard surface until it is completely hardened.

REFERENCE

Pfenninger J, Fowler G (eds): Procedures for Primary Care Physicians. St. Louis: Mosby, 2003.

SECTION

2

Patients Presenting with a Symptom, Sign, or Abnormal Lab Value

12

Abdominal Pain

▶ ETIOLOGY

What are the types of abdominal pain?

Visceral pain results when visceral pain receptors are stimulated by stretch, distension, traction, compression, or torsion. This type of pain is dull and difficult to localize. Other symptoms such as sweating, nausea, and vomiting may occur with it. Parietal pain occurs when pain receptors in the parietal peritoneum are stimulated. This type of pain is more localized and severe and increases with movement or coughing. The patient with appendicitis may initially notice visceral pain in the periumbilical area but later feel a more distinct parietal pain in the right lower quadrant. Referred pain is perceived in a location different from the diseased organ because visceral afferent neurons join with parietal afferent neurons from different anatomic regions in the spinal cord at the same level. For example, cholecystitis may result in pain felt in the scapula. Conversely, abdominal pain may originate from an extra-abdominal site: a patient may feel upper abdominal discomfort with myocardial ischemia or infarction.

What are common causes of abdominal pain in the family physician's office?

Many cases of abdominal pain in the primary care setting remain undiagnosed and either resolve spontaneously or persist despite exhaustive evaluation. Other common causes of abdominal pain are gastrointestinal (acute gastroenteritis, irritable bowel syndrome, gastroesophageal reflux, gastritis, peptic ulcer disease, or cholelithiasis), urinary (urinary tract infection), or gynecologic (pelvic inflammatory disease, ovarian cyst). Remember that uncommon causes of abdominal pain may still occur in the family physician's office and always consider a complete differential diagnosis.

What serious causes of abdominal pain should I not miss?

Many inflammatory or infectious causes of abdominal pain, such as appendicitis, pelvic inflammatory disease, and diverticulitis, will continue to worsen if undiagnosed and may lead to peritonitis, abscess formation, sepsis, and other complications. A delay in diagnosing cancer of abdominal organs (e.g., the stomach or colon) may result in diagnosis at a more advanced stage with metastasis to other organs. Mesenteric ischemia, a condition more common in elderly patients, may present with a normal physical examination, but may lead to bowel infarction, sepsis, and other organ failure if undiagnosed. Taking a careful history and physical examination and maintaining a high index of suspicion will help avoid missing these important causes of abdominal pain.

▶ EVALUATION

What is an appropriate history?

In eliciting the chief complaint and history of present illness, you should ask standard questions such as location, duration, radiation, quality/character, severity, associated symptoms, alleviating and exacerbating factors, progression of pain, and time of onset. In particular, knowing the exact location of the pain will help narrow your differential diagnosis. It is also important to understand the chronologic development of the patient's presentation including the sequence of different symptoms and the time frame in which these symptoms occurred.

You should ask about pertinent aspects of the patient's past medical history including previous episodes of abdominal pain and gastrointestinal symptoms (e.g., nausea, vomiting, jaundice, and bowel movement abnormalities), previously diagnosed gastrointestinal or other abdominal diseases, previous surgery, and current medications and allergies.

In taking a review of systems, you should remember that disorders in a variety of systems may cause abdominal pain. Questions about other gastrointestinal symptoms such as bowel movement changes, melena or hematochezia, urinary symptoms such as dysuria or hematuria, and gynecologic symptoms such as amenorrhea or other menstrual irregularities are important. Finally, consider systems whose conditions may result in referred pain to the abdomen and ask about cardiac and respiratory symptoms including chest pain and shortness of breath.

What elements of the physical examination should I perform?

The appearance of the patient and the vital signs provide you with valuable information on the acuity of the patient's illness as well as possible causes for the pain. A patient in obvious distress or with abnormal vital signs such as fever, tachycardia, and hypotension indicates a serious condition that warrants your immediate attention. A patient who wishes to be quiet and avoids movement may have peritonitis while a patient constantly writhing or moving about may have biliary or renal colic.

Examination of areas other than the abdomen may give clues to the severity of the illness or show signs of other disorders that may cause abdominal pain. A dry mouth with decreased skin turgor may indicate dehydration due to vomiting or poor oral intake. Weight loss may suggest a chronic condition such as cancer. Rales on the lung examination may suggest pneumonia.

A careful abdominal examination is necessary. Inspection may reveal distension or the presence of a hernia. Auscultation may reveal high-pitched bowel sounds suggesting an early bowel obstruction or absent bowel sounds suggesting an adynamic ileus. Before proceeding to palpate the abdomen, you should ask the patient to identify the area of discomfort. Generally, it is useful to begin palpation away from the area of discomfort and gradually but gently palpate in both a light and deep manner all areas of the abdomen, leaving your examination of the area of discomfort until last. Your goal is to identify areas of tenderness and any masses. The maneuver to check for "rebound" tenderness by using deep palpation and then suddenly letting go is extremely uncomfortable for the patient. Gentle percussion over a suspected area of peritonitis will enable you to more accurately and humanely localize an area of peritoneal inflammation. Percussion may also enable you to identify an enlarged liver or other abdominal mass.

In addition, you should examine the flank and costovertebral angles with gentle palpation or light fist percussion. Check hernial orifices and if a hernia is present, establish whether it is tender or difficult to reduce. In most cases, a rectal and pelvic examination is indicated. The rectal exam may show tenderness and also is an opportunity to obtain stool for occult blood testing. A pelvic examination helps clarify if a gynecologic etiology of the pain is present (such as pelvic inflammatory disease or an ectopic pregnancy).

What laboratory and diagnostic studies should I order?

After you complete your history and physical examination, you should have a differential diagnosis in mind. Laboratory and diagnostic tests should *selectively* be ordered to confirm or rule out possibilities in your differential diagnosis. A standard battery of tests for all patients with abdominal pain is neither efficient nor cost-effective. In ordering laboratory and diagnostic tests, it is important to remember that most family physicians' offices are only able to do a few simple tests and most other diagnostic tests are either sent to an outside laboratory or performed in a hospital or testing center. For the patient needing urgent diagnosis, it may be best to admit the patient to the hospital rather than waiting for test results that may not be immediately available.

Specific indications for commonly used diagnostic tests are explained in this section. You may wish to order a *CBC with differential* to check for anemia resulting from a bleeding lesion in the gastrointestinal tract or to demonstrate an elevated white blood cell count with a left shift to confirm suspicion of an infectious or inflammatory process (e.g., appendicitis). An abnormal *urinalysis* may diagnose a urinary tract infection (a positive nitrate test or bacteria and white blood cells in the sediment) or suggest the passing of a ureteral stone (red blood cells in the sediment). A *serum or urine pregnancy* test may help confirm or rule out pregnancy (but remember no test is infallible). *Liver function tests* are useful in evaluating suspected cases of hepatic or biliary disease. An elevated *amylase or lipase* may confirm inflammation of the pancreas.

An *EKG* may be indicated if the patient has cardiac risk factors or known coronary artery disease and has upper abdominal pain. A *chest x-ray* may show a lower lobe pneumonia or free air under the diaphragm suggesting a perforated abdominal viscus. A *flat and upright abdominal x-ray* series may show air-fluid levels or other signs of a small bowel obstruction. A *barium enema* may be used in stable patients to investigate the cause of a large bowel obstruction. It may also be useful in reducing an intussusception or sigmoid volvulus in some patients. An *intravenous pyelogram* may demonstrate a ureteral stone. An *ultrasound of the abdomen/pelvis* is most helpful in evaluating patients with suspected cholelithiasis or cholecystitis and females with lower abdominal/pelvic pain. It may clarify patients with appendicitis whose presentation is not clear, but it is not recommended as a routine test for this condition. A *CT scan of the abdomen/pelvis* can demonstrate an intra-abdominal neoplasm, appendicitis, diverticulitis, mesenteric ischemia, or pancreatitis.

Upper endoscopy may reveal esophagitis or peptic ulcer disease or cancer of the esophagus or stomach. *Flexible sigmoidoscopy or colonoscopy* may show the cause of a colonic obstruction (e.g., cancer) or changes of inflammatory bowel disease. *Laparoscopy* may be useful in clarifying whether the patient has appendicitis or a gynecologic condition (ovarian cyst, tubal pregnancy, salpingitis).

How should I manage the patient's condition?

The management plan is dependent on the differential diagnosis of the condition you have formulated based on the patient's symptoms, signs, and laboratory test results. Generally, consideration should be given to diet, activity, and use of medications. Surgery may be a consideration in patients with an acute abdomen.

Diet

For the ambulatory patient with nonacute abdominal pain, any diet that the patient tolerates is generally acceptable. Specific diets that are useful include a low-fat diet for the patient with suspected cholelithiasis or biliary colic and a high-fiber diet for the patient with irritable bowel syndrome. For the patient with acute abdominal pain that is severe or unclear in its etiology, admission to the hospital for giving intravenous fluids and withholding oral intake is often warranted.

Activity

Generally, most patients with nonacute abdominal pain may continue their usual activity as tolerated. Patients with acute abdominal pain may be advised to rest.

Medications

The type of medication used in treating a patient with abdominal pain depends on the cause. For example, H_2 blockers or proton pump inhibitors may alleviate symptoms in acid-related disorders including gastroesophageal reflux, peptic ulcer disease, and gastritis. These medications along with antibiotics also comprise the regimen of medications used to treat patients with confirmed *Helicobacter pylori* infection. Fiber supplements or antispasmodic medication may benefit the patient with irritable bowel syndrome.

Surgery

For some conditions such as appendicitis, immediate surgery is the only means of treating the condition. For others such as uncomplicated cholecystitis, you may treat with antibiotics until the infection subsides and then the gallbladder can be removed electively at a later date.

KEY POINTS

- Evaluation of a patient with abdominal pain begins with a careful history and physical examination. You should be able to formulate a differential diagnosis after completing your history and physical examination.
- In a family physician's office, you must be open-minded and consider conditions from a variety of systems as potential causes for the patient's abdominal pain.
- Use gentle palpation in examining the patient's abdomen and be mindful of the patient's comfort. Use gentle percussion rather than the "rebound" maneuver to check for peritonitis.
- Selective use of diagnostic tests helps confirm or rule out conditions listed in your differential diagnosis. A standard battery of tests for all patients is not indicated.
- Not all patients with abdominal pain in the family physician's office have a clear diagnosis. Some may have an acute, self-limited illness. Others may have a functional disorder such as irritable bowel syndrome or a more serious condition that has not yet been diagnosed. Paying attention to the symptoms and signs over the course of different visits will suggest if you need to pursue further diagnostic evaluation.

CASE 12–1. **A 32-year-old female presents with a history of abdominal pain that initially was vague and diffuse, but now is increasing and moving to the right lower quadrant. She reports no fever but after the pain started she also noted the onset of nausea and vomiting.**

A. What additional history and physical exam would be most helpful?
B. What is your differential diagnosis?
C. Assuming the patient is stable and your family physician's office can do basic laboratory tests, what tests will you order now?

CASE 12–2. **A 45-year-old female complains of a long history of abdominal pain, described as a crampy and bloating sensation, which is relieved by defecation. She at times suffers from diarrhea and on other occasions has constipation.**

A. What additional history and physical exam would be most helpful?
B. What is your differential diagnosis?
C. What laboratory tests will you order?

REFERENCES

Adelman A: Abdominal pain in the primary care setting. J Fam Pract 25:27–32, 1987.

Fishman MB, Aronson MD: Approach to the patient with abdominal pain. In UpToDate Online, version 11.3 (online textbook). Available at http://www.uptodateonline.com. Accessed on December 19, 2003.

Glasgow RE, Mulvihill SJ: Abdominal pain, including the acute abdomen. In Feldman M, Sleisenger MH, Scharschmidt BF (eds.): Sleisenger and Fordtran's Gastrointestinal and Liver Disease: Pathophysiology, Diagnosis, Management, 6th ed., vol. 1, Philadelphia: WB Saunders Company, 1998, pp 80–89.

Klinkman MS: Episodes of care for abdominal pain in a primary care practice. Arch Fam Med 5:279–285, 1996.

Silen W: Cope's Early Diagnosis of the Acute Abdomen, 20th ed. New York: Oxford University Press, 2000.

USEFUL WEBSITES

The National Library of Medicine/National Institutes of Health Medline Plus Health Information webpage on abdominal pain at *http://www.nlm.nih.gov/medlineplus/ency/article/003120.htm*

American Colleges of Emergency Physicians Clinical Policy: Critical Issues for the Initial Evaluation and Management of Patients With a Chief Complaint of Nontraumatic Acute Abdominal Pain. Available at *http://www.acep.org/library/pdf/cp402130.pdf.*

Takeyesu JM: Abdominal pain. In Emedicine (online textbook). Available at *http://www.emedicine.com/wild/topic69.htm.*

Abdominal pain. In The Merck Manual of Diagnosis and Therapy, 17th ed. (online textbook). Available at *http://www.merck.com/mrkshared/mmanual/section3/chapter25/25a.jsp.*

13

Anemia

▶ ETIOLOGY

What is anemia?

Anemia is a reduction in the volume of red blood cells (RBCs) in circulation. RBC volume is approximated by hemoglobin (Hb) concentration and hematocrit (Hct) level. In men, anemia is defined as Hb less than 13 g/dl or Hct less than 39%; in women, the cutoffs are Hb less than 12 g/dl or Hct less than 36%.

Which populations may have lower baseline Hb/Hct values?

While African-Americans, endurance athletes, elders, and patients with chronic disease may have lower hemoglobin levels, it is important to rule out other important problems.

Which populations may have higher baseline Hb/Hct values?

Smokers and residents of high altitudes may have higher baseline Hb/Hct values.

How is anemia classified?

Anemia is often classified by the mean corpuscular volume (MCV), which is the average volume of individual RBCs. The three classifications are microcytic (MCV < 80), normocytic (MCV 80–100), and macrocytic (MCV > 100).

What are the most common causes of microcytic (MCV < 80) anemia?

The most common causes of microcytic (MCV < 80) anemia are iron deficiency (most common type of anemia), thalassemia, sideroblastic anemia (e.g., congenital, lead, alcohol, drugs), anemia of chronic disease (late in the course), hemoglobin E, and copper deficiency/zinc poisoning (rare).

What are the causes of iron deficiency anemia?

Common causes of iron deficiency anemia include gastrointestinal bleeding, menstrual bleeding, increased physiologic needs (e.g., infants, adolescents, pregnancy, lactation), malabsorption (e.g., celiac sprue, subtotal gastrectomy), and inadequate nutrition.

What are the most common causes of normocytic (MCV 80–100) anemia?

Common causes of normocytic (MCV 80–100) anemia include acute blood loss, anemia of chronic disease (e.g., malignancy, infection, inflammation), iron deficiency (early in course), bone marrow suppression (e.g., aplastic anemia), endocrine dysfunction (e.g., hypothyroidsim, hypopituitarism), and chronic renal insufficiency.

What are the most common causes of macrocytic (MCV > 100) anemia?

Common causes of macrocytic (MCV > 100) include alcohol abuse, vitamin B_{12}/folate deficiency, liver disease, myelodysplastic syndromes, acute myeloid leukemias, reticulocytosis (e.g., hemolytic anemia), and drug-induced (e.g., hydroxyurea, zidovudine, methotrexate, chemotherapeutic agents).

▶ EVALUATION

List the components of the patient's history that are particularly important.

Evaluate the following relevant components: current illness (history of bleeding or infection, duration of illness), past medical history (chronic diseases), past surgical history (transfusions), current medications (hydroxyurea, zidovudine, methotrexate, chemotherapeutic agents), family history (ethnicity, history of anemia, hemoglobinopathy), social history (age, smoker, alcohol abuse, nutrition), and review of systems (fatigue, malaise, weakness, headache, weight loss, dizziness, light-headedness, shortness of breath, dyspnea on exertion, chest pain, palpitations).

What is important on physical examination?

Important points include pallor (skin, conjunctivae, mucous membranes, nail beds, palms), jaundice (scleral icterus), tachycardia, flow murmur, fever, postural hypotension, lymphadenopathy, hepatosplenomegaly, bone tenderness, petechiae, and fecal occult blood.

Which lab tests should be ordered?

Anemia must always be evaluated thoroughly. Initially, a CBC will identify whether anemia is present (based on the Hb/Hct) and the type of anemia present (based on MCV). An elevated reticulocyte count indicates appropriate response of the bone marrow to try and compensate for anemia by increasing RBC production. A positive stool guaiac indicates gastrointestinal blood loss. A peripheral smear identifies abnormal RBC morphology.

What additional work-up is necessary?

If microcytic anemia is identified, check serum ferritin, total iron binding capacity (TIBC), and iron levels. Normal iron studies should prompt evaluation for hemoglobinopathies. A low ferritin (indicating low stored iron), high TIBC (protein that transports iron is not saturated with iron), and low total iron indicates iron deficiency. If normocytic anemia is present, also check a TSH. If macrocytic anemia is present, check serum B_{12} and folate levels. If the CBC shows pancytopenia or if the peripheral smear has blasts, a bone marrow biopsy may be indicated.

▶ TREATMENT

How is anemia treated?

It is important to identify and treat the underlying cause of anemia. Iron deficiency anemia can generally be treated with oral iron replacement. It may up to take six months to replenish iron stores. Parenteral iron is only indicated if side effects of oral therapy are not tolerated, inflammatory bowel or peptic ulcer disease is present, or if there is documented iron malabsorption. Vitamin B_{12} deficiency is usually treated with B_{12} shots.

KEY POINTS

- ▶ **Anemia is never considered normal and must always be evaluated.**
- ▶ **A thorough history is essential in the evaluation and treatment of anemia.**
- ▶ **Initial testing for anemia includes a CBC (Hb, Hct, MCV), reticulocyte count, and peripheral smear. Further evaluation is based on the history, physical examination, and laboratory testing.**

CASE 13–1. **A 26-year-old gravida 2 para 2 woman comes into your office complaining of increased fatigue over the past few weeks. She has not been ill and denies recent dietary or weight change or any other stressors. Her periods are regular and last about five days with heavy flow. She is not currently taking any birth control. Physical exam is within normal limits.**

A. What type of anemia is most likely in this patient?
B. What laboratory testing should be done?

CASE 13–2. **A 74-year-old male smoker with a history of chronic obstructive pulmonary disease presents to the office complaining of increased weakness.**

A. If he were anemic, what would you expect his lab values to show?
B. How would you treat his anemia?

14

Arthralgia/Joint Pain

▶ ETIOLOGY

What are common causes of joint pain?

Joint pain has a broad differential diagnosis. When a patient has a chief complaint of joint pain, more questions are needed to narrow the diagnosis and to guide the history collection, physical examination, and diagnostic approach. A good beginning is to confirm that it is actually the joint that is painful and determine whether the joint pain is monoarticular or polyarticular.

What are common causes of acute monoarticular joint pain?

Acute joint pain is typically thought of as having been present for less than two weeks. The most common causes are trauma, infection, and crystal deposition. It is important to determine if the pain is acute, because infection should be immediately ruled out. A septic joint is rapidly destructive. Risk factors for a septic joint include trauma to the skin or skin infection, intravenous drug use, an artificial joint, previous joint surgery, rheumatoid arthritis, diabetes mellitus, and older age. The knee is the most common joint involved, and the most common pathogen is *Staphylococcus aureus*. In atraumatic, young sexually active patients, one must think of gonococcal arthritis. Women are three times more likely than men to be affected with gonococcal arthritis.

Common adult orthopedic injuries include shoulder dislocation (usually anterior), hip dislocation, Colles' fracture (most common wrist fracture: patient falls on an outstretched hand and fractures the distal radius, ulna styloid process in 50% of cases, and the scaphoid less often), scaphoid fracture (most commonly fractured carpal bone), boxer's fracture (fracture of the fifth metacarpal neck from a closed-fist injury), humerus fracture (rule out radial nerve damage), Monteggia's fracture (fracture of the ulna and dislocation of the radial head), Galeazzi's fracture (fracture of the radius and dislocation of distal radioulnar joint), hip fracture, femur fracture, tibial fracture, and ankle fracture.

Helpful Hint: Use the acronym ***GRUM*** to distinguish Monteggia's and Galeazzi's fracture: **G**aleazzi and **r**adial fracture; **u**lnar fracture and **M**onteggia.

Crystal-induced disease includes gout and pseudogout. Gout results from the deposition of intra-articular monosodium urate crystals. This disorder is much more common in men. Calcium pyrophosphate dihydrate (CPPD) crystals are the etiology of pseudogout, which is more common in middle age to elderly women. Calcium oxalate crystals, which may be found in patients undergoing renal dialysis, can also cause joint pain.

■ **Red Flag:** Be sure that the joint is the actual origin of the pain, not the surrounding soft tissues. The surrounding area may be inflamed and therefore painful, and may fool both the patient and the physician. Examples are olecranon bursitis of the elbow and prepatellar bursitis of the knee.

What are some other causes of monoarticular joint pain?

Some other common etiologies include avascular necrosis of bone, hemarthrosis, Lyme disease, viral synovitis, osteoarthritis, osteomyelitis, metastasis, and overuse.

What are common causes of polyarticular joint pain?

There are many causes of polyarticular joint pain (Box 14–1).

BOX 14–1

Differential Diagnosis of Polyarticular Joint Pain

Infectious

Viral (e.g., parvovirus B19, enterovirus, adenovirus)
Bacterial (e.g., gonococcal, meningococcal, Lyme disease, bacterial endocarditis)
Fungal
Tuberculosis
Reactive (e.g., Whipple's disease [*Tropheryma whippelii*], Reiter's syndrome [*Chlamydia* species, *Campylobacter* species], rheumatic fever [group A *Streptococcus*])

continued

BOX 14–1. Differential Diagnosis of Polyarticular Joint Pain *continued*

Crystal-Induced

Gout
Pseudogout
Hydroxyapatite

Osteoarthritis

Inflammatory
Hemachromatosis
Acromegaly

Seronegative Spondyloarthropathies

Ankylosing spondylitis
Psoriatic arthritis
Inflammatory bowel disease

Systemic Rheumatoid Disease

Rheumatoid arthritis
Systemic lupus erythematosus
Systemic sclerosis
Behcet's disease
Polymyositis/dermatomyositis
Polymyalgia rheumatica
Sjögren's syndrome

Systemic Vasculitis Disease

Schönlein-Henoch purpura
Polyarteritis nodosa
Wegener's granulomatosis
Giant cell arteritis

Endocrine Disorders

Hyperparathyroidism
Hyper/hypothyroidism

Other

Sarcoidosis
Malignancy (e.g., multiple myeloma, leukemia, metastasis)
Hyperlipoproteinemias
Amyloidosis
Hemophilia

▶ EVALUATION

What can I do to narrow the differential diagnosis when evaluating a patient with joint pain?

A thorough history and physical exam is essential. A helpful approach is to always ask about distribution, disease chronology, extra-articular manifestations, disease course, and patient demographics (Box 14–2). Distribution of the joint pain is helpful for several reasons; for example, certain etiologies are more likely to be monoarticular versus polyarticular. The pattern of joints involved may be specific for a disease process. For instance, rheumatoid arthritis most often involves the metacarpophalangeal (MCP) and proximal interphalangeal (PIP) joints, while osteoarthritis and psoriatic arthritis typically affect the distal interphalangeal (DIP) joints. Certain disorders are more likely to involve small joints (rheumatoid arthritis) versus large joints (spondyloarthropathies, such as Reiter's syndrome). Migratory arthritis may suggest an infectious etiology, such as Lyme disease or rheumatic fever.

The physician should think of joint pain as acute versus chronic. The criteria for acute monoarticular joint pain is pain of less than two weeks duration, while polyarticular joint pain is usually not considered chronic until six weeks. Therefore, the systemic rheumatologic diseases such as rheumatoid arthritis cannot be diagnosed in a patient unless the arthralgias have been present for six weeks.

Helpful Hint: Keep in mind that infectious etiologies generally tend to be acute and monoarticular.

Extra-articular manifestations are not diagnostic by themselves but often provide helpful clues. A thorough review of systems is

BOX 14–2

Helpful Patient Demographic Information

Women: More likely to develop SLE, rheumatoid arthritis, fibromyalgia, gonococcal arthritis, and viral-related arthritis
Men: More likely to develop ankylosing spondylitis, reactive arthritis, HIV-related arthritis, hemochromatosis, polyarteritis nodosum, and gout
Young: Rheumatic fever, SLE, rheumatoid arthritis, reactive arthritis, spondyloarthropathies, and Lyme disease
Elders: Osteoarthritis, pseudo-gout, polymyalgia rheumatica, and giant-cell arteritis
Blacks: Increased prevalence SLE and sarcoidosis and decreased prevalence ankylosing spondylitis and polymyalgia rheumatica

necessary when assessing for rheumatologic diseases, reactive arthritis, endocrine disorders, systemic vasculitidies, and other important conditions.

What are the most important tests to order?

The most important factor in deciding tests is the epidemiology of disease based on the patient's circumstances. In the acute setting, trauma is likely to be evident from the history (although not necessarily true in patients with fractures secondary to osteoporosis). In such an individual the exam will reveal worsening pain with movement. Plain-film radiographs will be the most helpful initial diagnostic test. Without a history of trauma, acute monoarticular arthritis requires arthrocentesis. Blood cultures should also be ordered if septic arthritis is suspected. Table 14–1 presents the interpretation of synovial fluid. Crystals within leukocytes upon microscopic exam are a good clue to crystal-induced arthropathy.

■ **Red Flag:** Superimposed cellulitis is a contraindication to arthrocentesis (but warfarin therapy is not).

Work-up for chronic joint pain also relies on a careful history and physical exam. Suspected systemic disease requires basic blood work, including complete blood count, urinanalysis, metabolic panel, and erythrocyte sedimentation rate. If applicable, more specific tests such as Lyme and HIV titers can be drawn. Rheumatologic tests such as ANA and rheumatologic factor should only be ordered in the context of suspected disease because of high false-positive rates. Radiographic studies may reveal sacroiliitis and other

TABLE 14–1

Synovial Fluid Values

WBC* per mm^3	Category	Associated Pathologic Processes
Zero to 200	Normal	
201 to 2,000	Noninflammatory	Osteoarthritis, trauma, avascular necrosis, hemochromatosis
2,001 to 100,000	Inflammatory	Crystal-induced, systemic rheumatoid diseases, spondyloarthropathies, Lyme disease, possibly septic arthritis*
More than 100,000	Septic	Septic arthritis, typically more than 90% neutrophils†

* WBC, white blood cells

† Fluid with a high WBC count or high percentage of neutrophils should be cultured to exclude septic arthritis.

diagnostic clues. However, x-ray findings typically are late disease manifestations.

▶ TREATMENT

Treatment is highly variable, depending on the underlying disease process. Ideally, a quick literature search will reveal any new therapeutic modalities that might benefit the patient. This is especially important with the rheumatologic diseases, because new disease-modifying agents are being developed. Because of the limited space of this chapter, this section will be limited to therapeutic injection of the knee joint.

When should I therapeutically inject a joint with steroids?

Here are the indications for steroid injection:

- When there is inflammation of only a limited number of joints
- As adjunct to systemic therapy in polyarthritis disease (such as rheumatoid arthritis)
- To assist in rehabilitation and prevent deformity
- In the presence of osteoarthritis exhibiting local inflammation
- For soft-tissue disorders such as bursitis

■ **Red Flag:** Infection must be excluded before injecting a joint with steroids.

What is the technique for knee injection?

The most common technique is the lateral approach (Figure 14–1). The patient should be in the supine position with the affected knee slightly flexed, and a pillow or towel placed underneath the knee for support. The skin may be sprayed with ethyl chloride solution, or the skin and subcutaneous tissues may be infiltrated with lidocaine for adequate pain control. For a lateral approach, a line is drawn between the lateral and proximal borders of the patella. The needle is aimed at a 45-degree angle toward the joint and inserted near the intersection of the lines, and between the patella and the femur. Aspiration will insure proper placement into the joint capsule. Release of medication should be firm but not forceful. After the medication is delivered, the joint can be gently moved and massaged to enhance delivery.

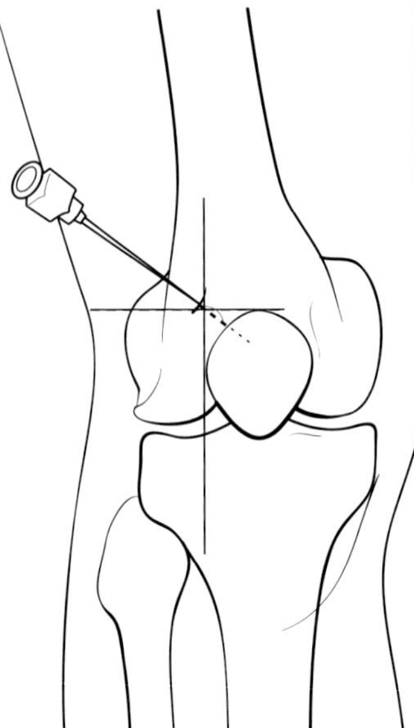

Figure 14–1. Knee aspiration using a lateral approach. The needle should enter at a 45-degree angle toward the joint.

KEY POINTS

- A thorough history and physical exam are necessary for evaluation of joint pain.
- Assess distribution, disease chronology, extra-articular manifestations, disease course, and patient demographics to help guide physical exam and diagnostic tests.
- In the absence of trauma, immediate arthrocentesis of acute monoarticular joint pain is necessary.
- Rheumatologic tests are necessary only if there is high clinical suspicion. Remember, these tests have high false-positive rates.
- Remember your anatomic landmarks when injecting a joint.
- Injection of the knee takes practice, but is straightforward and provides pain relief and improved function.

CASE 14–1. An 80-year-old woman presents to clinic with pain in her right knee that began two days ago. She has a right knee prosthesis from two years ago. She does not recall falling or other trauma to her knee. Other health problems include osteoporosis, hypertension, and non–insulin-dependent diabetes mellitus.

A. What is the differential diagnosis for this patient?
B. What history would you elicit from this patient?
C. What would you look for on physical exam?
D. Which tests, if any would you order?

CASE 14–2. A 52-year-old Hispanic man with a 20-year history of rheumatoid arthritis treated with methotrexate and NSAIDs presents with acute swelling of his right knee. The knee has been "acting up" for several days and is interfering with his job in a factory. He does not recall any trauma and states that this has happened occasionally over the past ten years. On physical exam, the joint has extremely limited and painful range of motion.

A. Describe what you would do for this patient.
B. Describe and be able to demonstrate the procedure you would use on this patient.

REFERENCES

Cardone DA, Tallia AF: Diagnostic and therapeutic injection of the hip and knee. Am Fam Physician 67(10):2147–2152, 2003.

Ike RW: Therapeutic injection of joints and soft tissues. In Klippel JH, Crofford LJ, Stone JH, Weyand CM: Primer on the Rheumatologic Diseases, 12th ed. Atlanta: Arthritis Foundation, 2001: pp 579–582.

Pinals RS: Polyarticular joint disease. In Klippel JH , Crofford LJ, Stone JH, Weyand CM: Primer on the Rheumatologic Diseases, 12th ed. Atlanta: Arthritis Foundation, 2001: pp 160–165.

Richie AM, Francis ML: Diagnostic approach to polyarticular joint pain. Am Fam Physician 68:1151–1160, 2003.

Siva C, Velazquez C, Mody A, Brasington R: Diagnosing acute monoarthritis in adults: A practical approach for the family physician. Am Fam Physician 68:83–90, 2003.

USEFUL WEBSITE

http://www.arthritis.org

15

Low Back Pain

▶ ETIOLOGY

What are the most common causes of low back pain?

Nonspecific mechanical causes account for more than 70% of low back pain episodes, with the pain thought to arise from injury to the muscles and ligaments of the lumbosacral spine. The terms *lumbar strain* and *lumbar sprain* are most often applied, but an exact anatomic cause is often not readily identifiable. Other common terms are defined in Box 15–1. Identified risk factors include heavy lifting and twisting, obesity, whole body vibration, and lack of physical conditioning, but low back pain is common even in people without these risk factors. Age-related degenerative changes to the spine and disk herniations are the next most common causes of low back pain but account for only 10% to 15% of patients.

Describe the natural history of low back pain.

Two-thirds of all adults experience back pain symptoms at some point in their life. Fortunately, recovery from nonspecific low back pain is generally rapid, with 30% of patients better in one week and 75% to 90% improved at one month. Recurrences are common but not usually disabling. Herniated disks also have a favorable natural history but at a slower pace than low back pain alone. Nevertheless, only 10% of patients are affected sufficiently at six weeks to warrant consideration of surgery.

What serious underlying diseases can present as low back pain?

Infection, cancer, especially metastatic disease, and diseases of other organ systems, such as kidney disease, pelvic masses, abdominal aneurysm, or gastrointestinal disorders, can present with back pain but account for less than 5% of cases. The history and physical examination can accurately rule out such problems.

BOX 15–1

Common Diagnostic Labels Used to Describe Low Back Pain

- Nonspecific low back pain: symptoms occurring primarily in the back without significant leg symptoms
- Sciatica: back-related lower limb symptoms suggesting nerve root compromise
- Acute low back pain: symptoms present for less than four to six weeks
- Chronic low back pain: symptoms present for greater than three months
- Lumbar disk herniation: disruption of the fibrous rim of the disk with extrusion of small amounts of disk material outside of the disk
- Cauda equina syndrome: rare condition caused by severe compression of the distal spinal cord usually from a tumor or massive disk herniation. Patients with cauda equina syndrome present with variable features including acute urinary symptoms, numbness in the perineum and medial thighs, and bilateral leg pain and weakness. This condition is a surgical emergency.

▶ EVALUATION

What are the key points in the history?

How long have symptoms been present? Focus on the intensity and distribution of the pain, and rule out risk factors for serious underlying medical conditions. Presence or absence of leg pain, or other leg symptoms such as weakness or numbness will help guide your physical exam. Red flags for infection include fever, current steroid use or other immune suppression, and/or intravenous drug use. Ask about any previous history of cancer or recent trauma such as a fall. Bowel or bladder symptoms, especially an inability to empty the bladder or incontinence, may suggest acute neurological issues.

Which exam findings are most helpful?

Symptoms lasting four weeks or less, confined to the low back, with limitations in range of motion and absence of leg symptoms or red flags, suggest mechanical low back pain. For patients with leg symptoms, a neurological exam of the lower extremities can identify signs of nerve root compression, generally from a lumbar disk herniation. Look for asymmetry by checking the reflexes at the knees and ankles, muscle strength, and sensation. The straight leg raising test (Figure 15–1), if positive, suggests compression of the S1 nerve root.

What tests should I order?

No tests would be indicated if symptoms have been present for less than a month and there are no red flags for underlying illness and no history of trauma. If the patient has a history of cancer, then obtain a CBC, ESR, and plain x-ray films of the spine. If risk factors for infection are present, start with the CBC and ESR and consider further testing. In elders, the physician should have a lower threshold for further testing given the risk of such problems as cancer, compression fractures, and systemic disease.

When should imaging studies be ordered? What kind should they be?

If there is no history of acute trauma, or if clinical findings do not suggest a serious underlying disease, plain x-rays are not indicated unless back pain symptoms have persisted for more than four to six weeks. MRI and CT scans of the spine should be ordered only if there is a strong suspicion of underlying cancer, infection, or systemic disease, or if abnormalities persist on a neurological exam for longer than four weeks.

▶ TREATMENT

How should I treat acute low back pain?

Acetaminophen, aspirin, and NSAIDs are effective for relief of low back pain symptoms. Muscle relaxants may be helpful in some patients but sedation is a common side effect. Encouraging patients to stay as active as possible is the best recommendation. Bed rest of more than two days impedes recovery and should be discouraged. Reassurance about the natural history of back pain and encouraging activity, even in the face of discomfort, will help allay patient concern and speed recovery. Physical therapy or spinal manipulation may provide symptomatic relief, but since over half of patients improve spontaneously in the first two to three weeks, it is reasonable to wait and reassess the need for referral after two weeks.

What if I suspect a disk herniation?

If the neurological findings are stable and there are no red flags, early treatment for disk herniation is the same as for patients with nonspecific low back pain. Opioid analgesics may be used selectively and for short periods of time. Bed rest does not speed

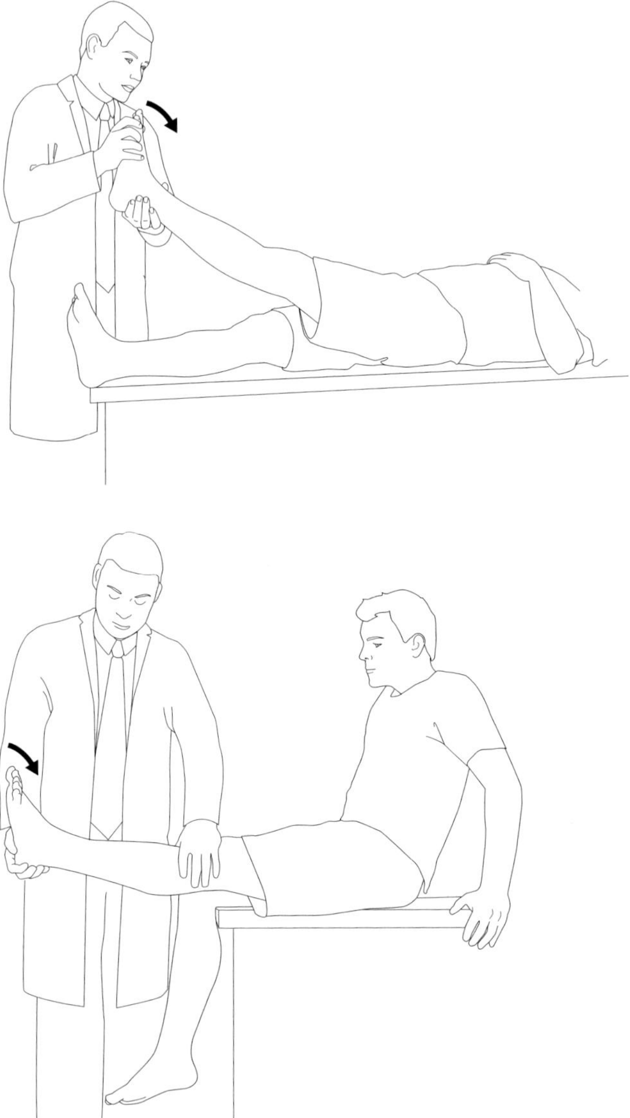

Figure 15–1. Straight leg raising test.

recovery. Physical therapy may be of benefit in restoring function and assisting with symptom control.

When should I refer?

If a disk herniation is suspected and severe pain and neurological changes persist for more than four to six weeks, imaging and a surgical referral are appropriate to offer. The cauda equina syndrome, though rare, is a surgical emergency.

CASE 15–1. A 48-year-old woman presents with one week of low back pain (LBP) symptoms she attributes to working in the garden. She has had previous episodes of LBP that improved with one to two days of rest. Pain is worse with forward bending and prolonged sitting. She denies leg pain, bowel or bladder symptoms, and leg weakness. She is in otherwise good health, has no history of cancer, and is up to date on her preventive health care. On examination, she is in moderate discomfort when sitting, has decreased range of motion of her lumbar spine, tenderness to the low back muscles, and a normal neurological exam of her lower extremities.

A. What are possible etiologies for her low back pain?
B. What would be the most appropriate treatment at this time?

CASE 15–2. A 70-year-old woman presents with worsening low back pain over the past month. She denies any specific trauma. Her past medical history is significant for hypertension. She has had a 10-lb weight loss over the past six months she attributes to decreased appetite. Pain is worse at night and she is most comfortable sleeping in a recliner.

A. What would prompt you to evaluate this patient further?
B. What tests would you do?

CASE 15–3. **A 33-year-old old bricklayer reports the onset of intense right-sided low back pain after lifting a large piece of concrete two days ago. The pain radiates down the posterior thigh to the lateral calf and foot. He is in good health otherwise. He has had a few episodes of back strain in the past but never as intense as this episode. Bladder and bowel function are normal. He denies alcohol or drug abuse and is on no routine medications.**

A. What physical findings would help clarify his diagnosis?
B. Which tests are indicated at this time?
C. How will you treat him?

REFERENCES

Atlas SJ, Deyo R: Evaluating and managing acute low back pain in the primary care setting. J Gen Intern Med 16:120–131, 2001.

Bigos S, Bowyer O, et al: Acute low back problems in adults. Clinical Practice Guideline No. 14, AHCPR Publication No. 95-0642, 1994.

Deyo RA, Weinstein JN: Primary care: Low back pain. N Engl J Med 344(5):363–370, 2001.

USEFUL WEBSITES

Mayo Clinic: A helpful patient-oriented overview of low back problems.*http://www.mayoclinic.com/invoke.cfm?id=DS00171*

American Academy of Orthopedic Surgeons: An easy-to-understand, illustrated site targeting the consumer.*http://orthoinfo.aaos.org/brochure/thr_report.cfm?Thread_ID=10&topcategory=Spine*

16

Children's Behavioral Problems

► ETIOLOGY

What is the nature of children's behavioral problems? Why should I be concerned about them?

Many children develop transitory problems about which their parents become concerned. Among all American school-age children, 13% of preschoolers and 12% to 25% of older students have significant behavioral or emotional disorders. One study showed that 90% of mothers had at least some concern about their children's behavior. After teachers, primary care physicians are the professionals to whom parents turn with concerns about their children's behavior. However, only about 50% of these children are correctly identified, treated, or referred for appropriate intervention. The informed family physician can screen, identify, diagnose, treat, and/or refer, as well as provide advocacy with other systems (e.g., school, legal authorities, community agencies).

The most common complaints made to physicians by parents regarding their children's behavior fall into four main categories: discipline and parenting problems, inadequate school performance, sleep disturbance, and toileting problems. The behaviors can be situational or global (confined to one or two settings versus across settings) and primary or secondary (a problem in and of itself or as a result of another condition). Global and primary problems are often more difficult to treat.

Why do children develop behavioral problems?

In general, behavioral problems are a normal part of growing up, a process that involves children responding to their environment, attempting to get needs met or desires satisfied, and negotiating developmental tasks. And most children are doing the best they can with the skills they have, in the environment in which they find themselves. However, the difficulty that a child has can be quite serious and indicative of one or more underlying problems in the child, in his or her environment, or in the fit between the two. Children misbehave because of a combination of comorbid physical and emotional health conditions, biological sensitivity/ reactivity to the environment, temperament, prior learning (or lack thereof), situational distress, family structural problems, inadequate resources for coping and support, poor parenting techniques, and patterns of interaction established with family members, peers, and others.

Misbehavior is manifested through passive, passive-aggressive, active resistance, or aggressive defiance of authority, rules, and the rights of others. The intentionality varies from situation to situation; some children are more cognizant and in control of their behavior than others. Among the most important child characteristics to consider is temperament—the hard-wired set of emotional and behavioral tendencies related to adaptability, mood, responsivity, distractibility, receptivity, locus of control, etc. Temperament seems to be genetically influenced. And extremes in these traits can cause great difficulty, especially if adults and other individuals important in the child's life do not understand why the child behaves as he or she does.

Situational and developmental stressors (e.g., a move, addition to the family, death, significant interpersonal conflict, separation, or divorce) often explain behavioral changes in children. If this is the case, the child may need support and guidance during the adjustment period. The rates of emotional and behavioral disorders are higher among children in families with high or chronic levels of stress and structural problems (e.g., single-parent or stepfamilies). The most significant chronic stressors include illnesses; psychiatric or substance abuse impairment in one or more parent figures; emotional and physical neglect; emotional, physical, or sexual abuse; high levels of crime, or threats of violence/bullying in the peer group or neighborhood; and unemployment or other financial problems.

► EVALUATION

How do I know if the behavioral problems are normal ("just a phase") or clinically significant?

While an exhaustive review of children's behavioral issues is outside the scope of this chapter, any problem that is causing significant distress to the child or family member(s) or is chronically impeding the child's social or academic progress warrants evaluation. This is especially the case if one or more adults, in more than one setting, are concerned. The most common problems are typically manifested through developmentally inappropriate academic achievement, social interaction, responses to authority, aggression, or sexual exploration. Common diagnoses include oppositional defiant disorder, conduct disorder, attention deficit hyperactivity disorder, mood and anxiety disorders, learning disabilities, and developmental disorders. It is important for the student physician to inquire about changes in mood, sleep, appetite, friendships, activities, school performance, and other behaviors.

What parts of the history are particularly important for me to pay attention to?

Find out what you can about the views of parent(s), other caregivers, teacher(s), and other adults involved; their views are as effective as, or more effective, than existing instruments in helping with screening and diagnosis. You should ask about their perception of the problem, what makes it worse or better, and their expectations of treatment. Asking about recent changes or stressors in the child's life is helpful. In the family and social history, it is important to ask about a history of similar problems in the family tree and the presence of the family and social problems mentioned above (e.g., abuse, substance abuse). You also should ask about prenatal exposure to drugs and alcohol, whether or not the child has developed normally from an early age, and the presence of chronic medical problems such as asthma.

Which screening tests are helpful in determining the nature of problems that may underlie behavioral issues?

In addition to familiar medical procedures (i.e., lab, physical, and neurological exams), there are a number of screening tests that can be helpful. These include the Battelle Developmental Inventory Screening Test (receptive and expressive language, fine and gross motor, adaptive, personal/social, and cognitive/academic), Family Psychosocial Screening (asks about physical abuse, substance abuse, maternal depression), Connors Parent and Teacher Rating Scales (oppositional behavior, problems with inattention and hyperactivity), and the Eyberg Child Behavior Inventory (presence of disruptive, externalizing behavior problem, e.g., disorders of attention, conduct, oppositional defiance).

▶ TREATMENT

What can I do to help parents and children with behavioral problems?

Once you have recognized a potential behavior problem in a child, parents will need to be educated about the nature of the problem and treatment options. Treatment of behavioral issues usually involves a combination of education; behavioral management including a system of clearly defined and age-appropriate expectations, consequences, and rewards; coordination of efforts among the adults in the settings the child spends time (e.g., home and school or daycare); and possibly medication.

Unless the parent has brought the behavior problem to your attention, you may encounter resistance to your assessment and recommendations. Watch the parents' verbal and nonverbal responses in order to assess their "readiness to change" their previous view of the child and his/her behavior. Use these principles in addressing the problem. For example, if the parent is still in precontemplation, provide a summary of your assessment and recommendations for treatment; allow the opportunity for the parent(s) to ask questions and express their reaction to what you have had to say; discuss further if time allows; and suggest the parent(s) think about things or seek a second opinion. On the other hand, if the parent(s) had suspected or even knew all along that this was the problem, then it will be time to discuss and negotiate the next steps in the treatment plan.

There is often a temptation for providers to get pulled into offering advice to parents about managing their child's behavior. Do this only after assessing the problem (including the parents' and child's perspectives), stages of readiness for change, and any solutions the parent(s) may have previously attempted, *and* whether you have expertise in this area. The problem with offering advice before assessing the parents' stage of readiness and their previously attempted solutions is that you may waste a lot of time with frustrating interchanges such as "Try X," countered by "But I already tried that and it didn't work."

To whom should I refer children and their parents?

A referral is an appropriate step to take if the parent requests one or if you have negotiated an agreement that one may be helpful. Referrals should be made to mental health professionals who specialize in treating problems of childhood. Qualified professionals include family therapists, child psychologists, child psychotherapists (professional counselors, clinical social workers), and child psychiatrists (especially regarding medical management).

How can I manage behavior problems in the clinic?

Children with behavioral problems are often less than perfectly well behaved in the clinic setting. The following strategies may help to forestall unmanageable problems:

- Establish yourself as a benign authority figure and the territory (e.g., the clinic room) as yours.
- Support the parent(s) in their position as the child's primary authority figure by deferring to the parent if the child asks you for something (e.g., "If you need to leave the room, you need to ask your mom first") or when guidance or discipline is called for (e.g., Mrs. Jones, I need to examine Josh but I can't when he is upset and kicking, so I am going to leave while you

calm him down and get his cooperation. I will be back in a few minutes).

- Provide available age-appropriate toys or other materials that can be used to constructively occupy the child's interest and energy.
- Give directions in a gentle but firm manner, clearly stating expectations (e.g., "The otoscope is not a toy and you may not play with it").

Are medications helpful for behavioral problems?

The type of child behavioral problem most frequently treated with medication is inattention and hyperactivity. Stimulant medications are the most often prescribed. There is much controversy concerning the use of other medications (e.g., for mood and anxiety disorders) as part of a comprehensive treatment plan for behaviorally disturbed children.

KEY POINTS

- **Behavioral problems in children are common.**
- **Those problems about which adults in the child's life are concerned and which seem to be causing significant delay in development, socialization, or performance ought to be explored further.**
- **Treatment plans usually consist of some combination of education, reassurance, and medical or behavioral treatment. The underlying or comorbid condition(s) can be treated with medication, behavior modification, parent training, and/or family therapy.**

CASE 16–1. A 10-year-old boy is brought in by his single-parent mother who complains that he is frequently in trouble in school, and to a lesser degree at home. He seems to have difficulty paying attention, completing assigned work, and complying with the teacher's directives. He has difficulty falling asleep at night and often does not want to go to school the next day, saying "I hate school." He is irritable with his siblings, sometimes breaks things when he doesn't get his way, and doesn't appear to have any close friends.

A. What additional information would you like from the mother?
B. What is your differential diagnosis at this point?

CASE 16–2. **A 4-year-old girl is brought to the clinic by her parents. They are concerned that she seems overly shy and withdrawn in settings outside the home. They worry that she may not make a smooth transition to preschool and kindergarten. She has a younger sister (2 years old) with whom she plays well. She is reportedly very responsive to the parents' affection and correction at home and you observe that they all interact supportively while in the clinic.**

A. How do you decide if the child has a clinically significant problem?
B. What other information would be helpful to know?

REFERENCES

Campbell SB: Behavior problems in preschool children: A review of recent research. J Child Psychol Psychiatry Allied Disciplines 36(1):1113–1149, 1995.

Gardner W, Kelleher KJ, Pajer KA, Campo JV: Primary care clinicians' use of standardized tools to assess child psychosocial problems. Ambul Pediatr 3(4):191–195, 2003.

The Working with Families Institute. Working with families: Case-based modules on common problems in family medicine. Watson W, McCaffery M (eds). Toronto, Canada, Department of Family & Community Medicine, University of Toronto, 2003.

USEFUL WEBSITES

The American Psychological Association website covers topics ranging from anger to divorce and includes many excellent links to specific disorders. *http://www.apa.org/topics*

The National Resource Center on ADHD website has links to news items, professional resources and patient education materials. *http://www.help4adhd.org*

The American Academy of Pediatrics website has a host of professional- and patient-oriented materials covering the differential diagnosis of children's behavioral issues. *http://www.aap.org*

17

Chest Pain

▶ ETIOLOGY

What are the most common causes of chest pain in the outpatient setting?

Musculoskeletal, gastrointestinal, cardiac, psychiatric, and pulmonary are among the most common causes of chest pain in the outpatient setting. However, cardiac disease may be the cause in as many as 50% of elderly patients presenting with chest pain.

List the most common causes of life-threatening chest pain.

Myocardial infarction, pulmonary embolus, aortic dissection, tension pneumothorax, and esophageal rupture may result in sudden death.

What causes pleuritic chest pain?

Viral pleurisy, pneumonia, acute pulmonary embolus, pneumothorax, pericarditis, systemic lupus erythematosis (SLE), rheumatoid arthritis (RA), drug-induced lupus, inflammatory bowel disease, radiation pneumonitis, and pulmonary histoplasmosis cause pleuritic chest pain (pain that increases with deep breathing).

List the causes of chest wall pain.

Musculoskeletal pain, rheumatic diseases (e.g., SLE, RA), systemic disorders (e.g., multiple myeloma, bone cancer), skin/sensory nerve disorders (shingles, post-radiation neuralgia) are common causes of chest wall pain.

What are cardiac causes of chest pain?

Cardiac causes of chest pain include coronary heart disease, aortic dissection, valvular heart disease, pericarditis, and myocarditis.

What are gastrointestinal (GI) causes of chest pain?

Gastrointestinal causes of chest pain include gasteroesophageal reflux disease (GERD), esophageal hyperalgesia, abnormal motility/achalasia, esophageal rupture, and drug-induced esophagitis; these also may cause referred pain.

What are pulmonary causes of chest pain?

Common pulmonary causes of chest pain include pulmonary embolism, cor pulmonale, pneumonia, cancer, sarcoidosis, pneumothorax, pleuritis, and pleural effusion.

What are psychological causes of chest pain?

Psychological causes of chest pain include panic attacks, depression, and hypochondriasis.

► EVALUATION

What is important in the patient's history?

When evaluating chest pain, the first step is to rule out imminent, life-threatening diseases. Initially, a problem-focused history should be obtained. It is important to determine duration, location, radiation, character, intensity, and rate of onset of the chest pain. What was the patient doing at the onset of pain? Are there any exacerbating or relieving factors? Have there been similar episodes of chest pain in the past? Is there associated nausea, vomiting, diaphoresis, palpitations, dyspnea, orthopnea, edema, cough, dysphagia, syncope, parasthesia, or an impending sense of doom? Any recent fever or chills? Cardiac risk factors? Risk factors for hypercoagulability (e.g., prolonged immobility, trauma, malignancy, hormone replacement therapy, birth control pills)? Past medical history of coronary artery disease, diabetes, stroke, GERD, anxiety/depression, or panic attacks? Social history of smoking, alcohol, cocaine, or other illicit drugs? Family history of cardiac disease?

List cardiac risk factors.

Cardiac risk factors include age, hypertension, hyperlipidemia, diabetes, smoking, family history of coronary artery disease (CAD) in a first-degree relative (male < 45 years old, female < 55 years old).

What is important on physical examination?

Patients having a myocardial infarction are classically diaphoretic and pale and have tachycardia. Vital signs are extremely important—monitor blood pressure closely and check it in both arms; fever may indicate an infectious disease process. Look for distended neck veins and labored breathing. Listen for new murmurs, equal breath sounds, and pulmonary crackles or rales. Palpate the chest wall to determine if the pain is reproducible. Palpate the epigastric area to determine if the pain is reproduced. Palpate peripheral pulses and determine capillary refill time. Palpate lower extremities for pain and document any asymmetry or unilateral edema.

What lab tests should be ordered?

All patients with chest pain should have an initial EKG. If abnormal, the patient should immediately be sent to the emergency room for further evaluation. Emergency room evaluation should include chest x-ray, cardiac enzymes, CBC with differential, and a comprehensive metabolic panel. If the EKG is normal in the outpatient setting, further testing is guided by history and physical exam.

What additional work-up is needed?

Patients with cardiac risk factors will need serial cardiac enzymes and EKGs. They will likely undergo stress testing with or without an echocardiogram, or they may need cardiac catheterization for further evaluation. Patients with sudden onset of pleuritic chest pain may need a D-dimer, V/Q scan, or spiral CT to rule out pulmonary embolism. Those with chest wall pain generally do not need an extensive work-up. Patients with GERD are generally prescribed a trial of medications to relieve their pain; they may eventually need upper endoscopy on an outpatient basis if medical management fails. Patients with pleural effusions may need diagnostic or therapeutic thoracenteses. Patients with acute stressors may need screening for depression or anxiety.

▶ TREATMENT

Describe the treatment for myocardial infarction.

Administer oxygen, aspirin, nitrate (initially sublingual until IV access is obtained, then switch to a nitroglycerin drip if needed), morphine (if pain not controlled with nitrates), β-blockers (if blood pressure is elevated), thrombolytic (if within three hours of onset of chest pain), and anticoagulant (fractionated or low molecular weight heparin) for selected patients. The patient should be admitted to the intensive care unit and monitored closely in a telemetry bed.

What is the treatment for pulmonary embolus?

Administer oxygen and anticoagulation drugs. Surgical placement of an inferior vena cava filter may be necessary, if indicated, to prevent recurrence.

What is the treatment of aortic dissection?

An aortic dissection requires emergency surgery.

What is the treatment of tension pneumothorax?

A tension pneumothorax requires emergency chest tube placement.

What is the treatment of esophageal rupture?

An esophageal rupture requires emergency surgery.

Describe the treatment of musculoskeletal pain.

Treatment of musculoskeletal pain involves administration of an NSAID or COX-2 inhibitor if there is a history of GI bleeding. If there is evidence of bone cancer, administer appropriate opioid medication.

What is the treatment of gastroesophageal reflux disease (GERD)?

Treatment of GERD involves the use of an H_2-blocker or proton pump inhibitor. The patient should avoid caffeine, soda, and spicy foods.

What is the treatment of pneumonia?

Administer antibiotics and oxygen (if needed).

What is the treatment of panic attacks?

Administer anxiolytic such as benzodiazepines.

■ RED FLAGS

Elderly and diabetic patients may have atypical presentations of myocardial infarction, such as back pain or isolated nausea/vomiting.

History of heart disease should increase suspicion for myocardial infarction.

KEY POINTS

- **The most common cause of chest pain in a primary care clinic is musculoskeletal, but a high degree of suspicion should be maintained in patients with cardiac risk factors.**
- **Life-threatening causes of chest pain include myocardial infarction, pulmonary embolus, aortic dissection, tension pneumothorax, and esophageal rupture. These causes must be ruled out prior to discharge from the hospital.**
- **Not all patients with chest pain need to be hospitalized. Several chest pain evaluation and treatment protocols exist to evaluate patients presenting with chest pain.**

CASE 17–1. A 29-year-old woman presents to her primary care physician's office with a three-week history of substernal chest pain that does not radiate to her neck or left arm. It is a dull ache that often keeps her up at night. The pain is worse at night and typically begins 30 minutes after dinner. She smokes and drinks alcohol occasionally, both of which appear to aggravate the pain. She tried some Tums™ once, which seemed to help the discomfort.

A. What is the most likely cause of this patient's chest pain?
B. Describe the work-up and treatment you would recommend at this time.

CASE 17–2. A 65-year-old man is rushed to the emergency department at 3 AM with crushing substernal chest pain radiating to his left jaw and shoulder. The pain started suddenly, awakening him from sleep, and it is increasing in intensity. Nothing seems to help, and activity makes the pain worsen. The patient denies any similar episodes in the past. He does have a history of hypertension and hyperlipidemia, for which he takes daily medications. He has a 30-year history of smoking but quit two weeks ago. He denies alcohol or illicit drug use. His father died of a heart attack at age 68.

A. What are this patient's cardiac risk factors?
B. What work-up and treatment are recommended at this time?

USEFUL WEBSITES

UpToDate, Wellsley, MA. A subscription-based clinical information resource, written by physicians for physicians. Provides a comprehensive review of the management of chest pain. *http://www.uptodate.com*

Another broad resource concerning chest pain and myocardial infarction is *http://www.emedicine.com*

18

Cough and Congestion

Upper respiratory tract infections (URIs) are the most expensive and widespread illnesses in the United States. They represent 9% of the practice of the average family physician or pediatrician. Antibiotics are often prescribed for URIs, although viruses cause the vast majority of URIs and antibiotics do not enhance the resolution of symptoms. This practice has been implicated in the growing antimicrobial resistance.

▶ ETIOLOGY

What are the signs and symptoms of upper respiratory tract infections?

URI is associated with rhinorrhea, sneezing, nasal congestion, sore throat, cough, fever, headache, and myalgia. The duration of the illness is generally less than a week. The diagnostic challenge is to distinguish viral URI infection, allergic inflammation, and bacterial infection, because the symptoms are similar. URI signs are generally mild and include nasal discharge, injected conjunctiva, and mild pharyngitis.

How do I differentiate URI from allergic rhinitis?

Allergy symptoms are similar to URI symptoms but generally do not result in a fever or myalgia. It is often helpful to visualize the nasal mucosa, which usually reveals a boggy, pale appearance with allergic inflammation. Allergic rhinitis is associated with an increased number of eosinophils on nasal smear.

What are the most common viruses implicated in URI?

Rhinovirus and coronavirus are the most common viruses associated with the cold. Other causative agents include parainfluenza virus, respiratory syncytial virus, influenza virus, adenovirus, and enterovirus. The route of transmission can be airborne by aerosolization, by skin-to-skin contact, or by direct contact with fomites.

With the rhinovirus, a very small amount of virus is necessary for infection. Viral deposition occurs through aerosol inoculation or direct deposition on the nasoepithelium, the eye, and the lacrimal duct. This deposition causes infection. An inflammatory response is triggered, which results in vasodilation, vascular transudation, mucous gland secretion, pain, cough, and sneezing. There is minimal damage to the nasal epithelium. Symptoms begin approximately 16 hours after inoculation, and viral shedding continues for up to three weeks.

What are the common causes of cough?

Cough is a physiological mechanism that protects the pulmonary system. The pathological source of a cough can be at any point along the respiratory tract from the tip of the nose to the lungs. Common causes of cough and congestion (Box 18–1) are often categorized as acute (less than three weeks), subacute (three to eight weeks), or chronic (longer than eight weeks). Subacute coughs, which are not associated with an acute infection, can usually be evaluated as a chronic cough. Those subacute coughs that began with a URI are most often a postinfectious cough, a symptom of asthma, or secondary to sinusitis.

▶ EVALUATION

Which conditions often are not apparent and therefore are initially missed?

Underlying sinusitis must be considered with prolonged URI symptoms. Gastroesophageal reflux disease (GERD), asthma, mild congestive heart failure (CHF), occupational illnesses, HIV infection, tuberculosis, and side effects of ACE inhibitors should be considered when a patient presents with acute onset of a cough.

How do I identify more serious causes of cough and congestion?

Color or quantity of sputum or nasal discharge does not predict etiology. Symptoms of hemoptysis, shortness of breath, chest pain or tightness, weight loss, and a previous history of smoking suggest a more serious etiology. Signs of hypoxia (cyanosis, tachypnea, tachycardia), abnormal auscultatory findings (rales, rhonchi, wheezing), lymphadenopathy, and peripheral edema require further investigation. Smoking increases the probability of pneumonia, bacterial bronchitis, and neoplasm.

What additional tests should be performed if a more serious cause is suspected?

If persistent symptoms of sinusitis occur, plain sinus x-rays or CT scans should be obtained to exclude another underlying cause for

BOX 18–1

Common Etiologies of Cough and Congestion

Acute

- Allergic rhinitis
- Aspiration
- Asthma
- Bronchitis
- Congestive heart failure (CHF)
- Croup
- Foreign body aspiration
- Influenza
- Inhalation of irritants
- Laryngitis
- Pharyngitis
- Pneumonia
- Pulmonary edema
- Pulmonary embolism
- Respiratory distress syndrome
- Sinusitis
- Upper respiratory tract infection (URI)

Chronic

- Aspiration
- Benign endobronchial neoplasm
- Bronchiectasis
- Bronchogenic carcinoma
- Chronic obstructive pulmonary disease (COPD)
- Fungal disease
- Gastroesophageal reflux disease (GERD)
- Lung abscess
- Medication side effect
- Sarcoidosis
- Tobacco use
- Tuberculosis

the sinus symptoms. Peak flow determination is helpful to assess the severity of bronchospasm. Oximetry should be preformed if there are signs of hypoxia. A CXR is indicated if there are signs of consolidation, hypoxia, or suspicion of neoplasm.

▶ TREATMENT

How do I manage a patient with an uncomplicated URI?

Because the illness is self-limited, treatment is nonspecific. Therapy focuses on relief of symptoms and includes rest, increasing fluid intake, and increasing environmental humidity (vaporizer and steam). Oral decongestants can relieve nasal symptoms but can have more adverse effects, which include anxiety, insomnia, palpitations, hyperglycemia, and elevation of blood pressure. Pseudoephedrine is the most common oral agent. Antihistamines have limited benefit but are often combined with decongestants. Cough suppressants are available when the cough compromises daily activities. The efficacy for zinc and echinacea is inconclusive. Large dose vitamin C has shown to modestly reduce symptoms. When bronchospasm is present, a β-agonist inhaler can be tried. Postinfectious cough can be treated with an inhaled β-agonist or steroid.

When are antibiotics indicated?

Antibiotics have no place in the treatment of the simple cold and most bronchitis. Indiscriminate use of antibiotics increases the risk of side effects and the number of resistant organisms. Antibiotics are prescribed when bacterial infections such as pneumonia and prolonged sinusitis are suspected. Antibiotic choice is based on the most frequently encountered organisms.

The same organisms cause community-acquired pneumonia, sinusitis, and bronchitis. The most common are *Streptococcus pneumoniae, Haemophilus influenzae, Mycoplasma pneumoniae, Moraxella catarrhalis,* and viruses. *Chlamydia pneumoniae, Staphylococcus aureus, Legionella pneumophila,* and gram-negative bacilli are less commonly found. Empiric antibiotics should be aimed at the most likely bacteria. Macrolides (especially azithromycin and clarithromycin), fluroquinolones, cephalosporins, and amoxicillin/clavulanate can be considered.

KEY POINTS

- URI symptoms include rhinorrhea, sneezing, nasal congestion, sore throat, cough, fever, headache, and myalgia.
- Most URIs are caused by viruses and resolve without intervention.
- The patient with prolonged URI symptoms should be evaluated for underlying sinusitis.
- The source of a cough can be at any point along the respiratory tract.
- GERD, CHF, asthma, occupational illnesses, HIV, TB, and side effects of ACE inhibitors may not be apparent during the initial evaluation of a patient with a cough.

CASE 18–1. A 50-year-old man presents with a cough after a three-day history of runny nose, nasal congestion, and slight sore throat. He has been smoking one pack of cigarettes per day for 35 years. Vital signs are blood pressure 135/80, pulse 100, respirations 24, temperature 38°C. Lung auscultation reveals wheezing, but no rales or rhonchi.

A. What is your differential diagnosis?
B. What additional testing should be performed?
C. How would you treat this patient?

CASE 18–2. A 15-year-old girl presents with chronic nasal congestion. She has a one-year history of recurrent stuffy nose, yellow nasal discharge, and itchy eyes. She is not exposed to tobacco products. Vital signs are blood pressure 110/50, pulse 80, respirations 14, temperature 37°C. Conjunctiva is injected. Nares reveal pale, boggy mucosa and a yellow discharge. There is no sinus tenderness. Throat is slightly erythematous. Lungs are clear.

A. What is the most likely diagnosis?
B. What additional evaluation could be performed if the diagnosis is in doubt?

REFERENCES

Bauman KA: The family physician's reasonable approach to upper respiratory tract infection care for this century. Arch Fam Med 9(7):596–597, 2000.

Gonzales R, Bartlett JG, Besser RE, et al.: Principles of appropriate antibiotic use for treatment of nonspecific upper respiratory tract infections in adults: Background. Ann Intern Med 134(6):490–494, 2001.

Irwin RS, Madison JM: Primary care: The diagnosis and treatment of cough. N Engl J Med 343(23):1715–1721, 2000.

Murray PR, Rosenthal KS, Kobayashi GS, Pfaller MA (eds): Medical Microbiology, 4th ed. St. Louis, Mo: Mosby, 2002, p 620.

Stein JH, Klippel JH, Reynolds HY, et al. (eds): Internal Medicine, 5th ed. St. Louis, Mo: Mosby, 1998, p 1391.

West JV: Acute upper airway infections. Br Med Bull 61:215–230, 2002.

USEFUL WEBSITE

Primary Care Practice Guidelines—Respiratory System—University of California, San Francisco. Available at *http://medicine.ucsf.edu/resources/guidelines/guide8.html.*

19

Diarrhea

▶ ETIOLOGY

How should I evaluate diarrhea?

Acute diarrhea is the sudden onset of three or more frequent loose stools a day. The duration is usually several days and less than two weeks. When evaluating patients with diarrhea, ask about severity (fever, blood, pus, number of stools per day or if there are any nocturnal stools, pain) and duration. Has there been vomiting, recent travel, an outbreak of illness in the family or community, or ingestion of a suspect meal? Is the patient immunocompromised? What medications are they taking (especially recent antibiotics, new, and over-the-counter drugs)? Determine their water source and sexual orientation. Ask if the diarrhea is related to exercise (runner's diarrhea).

For chronic diarrhea (four or more loose stools per day for over a month) also inquire about lactose, sorbitol, fructose, and fiber intake. Is the stool oily and foul smelling (pancreatic etiology)? Is there midabdominal cramping with bloating and borborygmi (small bowel cause) or frequent small stools with a sense of incomplete emptying (colonic-rectal etiology)? Are there extraintestinal signs of inflammatory bowel disease? Did it begin following a cholecystectomy (bile salt induced)? If the diarrhea alternates with constipation, consider irritable bowel syndrome.

What are the infectious causes of diarrhea?

Intestinal pathogens or their toxins usually cause acute diarrhea. Transmission is commonly fecal-oral and outbreaks are often within families or groups. If the diarrhea is watery and without signs of inflammation or fever, consider noninvasive pathogens such as food poisoning by staphylococci, enterotoxigenic *E. coli*, *Bacillus cereus,* or clostridia, or viruses such as Rotavirus or Norwalk agent, *Giardia lamblia, Cryptosporidium,* and *Cyclospora.* Inflammatory diarrheas with fever, abdominal pain, and small-volume bloody or mucus-containing stools suggests *Shigella, Salmonella, Campylobacter,* invasive *E. coli, Yersinia,* and rarely *E. histolytica.* Consider sexually transmitted infection in a person who engages in anal-receptive intercourse. HIV-infected patients may have unusual pathogens.

What drugs and foods can cause diarrhea?

New medicines are often the culprit, especially metformin, proton-pump inhibitors causing bacterial overgrowth, and antibiotics with or without *C. difficile* infection. Large amounts of sorbitol in sugarless gum, candy, or diabetic foods; lactose-containing milk products; fructose in fruit juices or soda; and caffeine are possible causes.

▶ EVALUATION

What should I look for during the patient's examination?

Consider volume status (mucous membranes and orthostatic changes in vital signs) and abdominal findings, and do a rectal exam to rule out fecal impaction and incontinence. Look for extra-intestinal signs of inflammatory bowel disease (arthritis, apthous ulcers, iridis, anal fistulas).

When do I need laboratory tests?

Patients with mild symptoms do not require laboratory evaluation. Exceptions include those with high fever, dysentery, chronic diarrhea, and the immunocompromised. If an invasive pathogen is suspected, culture the stool; obtain a *C. difficile* antigen if there was recent antibiotic use, and obtain a *Giardia* antigen; test stool specimen for *Cryptosproidia* and *Cyclospora,* if the history suggests exposure and the diarrhea is prolonged. Testing the stool for ova and parasites is seldom useful except in select populations such as recent immigrants or international travelers. Stool for white cells or lactoferrin is not helpful. Irritable bowel syndrome is a diagnosis of exclusion in those under age 50. For chronic diarrhea, weight loss, and iron deficient anemia, evaluate for celiac disease. For oily, hard-to-flush stools, a 72-hour stool for fat will assess for malabsorption.

▶ TREATMENT

How do I treat uncomplicated diarrhea?

Unless the patient is very young, old and frail, very ill, or has serious concomitant illness, simple oral fluids and loperamide 2–4mg as frequently as four times a day is adequate care for a patient with uncomplicated diarrhea. Suspected *E. coli* 0157:H7 is a contraindication to loperamide and antibiotics. With suspected invasive diarrhea—while laboratory studies are underway—empiric treatment for *C. difficile* is warranted (metronidazole 250–500mg three times a day). Give ciprofloxacin 500 mg orally twice a day or norfloxacin 400 mg orally twice a day for suspected infectious diarrhea. When culture results are available the antibiotic choice and duration of therapy can be determined. It may be helpful to minimize fatty foods, milk products, and caffeine.

What are the take-home instructions for patients?

Patients should return if vomiting or diarrhea becomes severe and dehydration occurs, or if there is blood in the stool, persistent fever, or increasing abdominal pain. Symptoms should improve in two to three days; if they don't, patients should return.

KEY POINTS

- **Always do a rectal examination and check for blood.**
- **Postural vital signs should be obtained in many patients.**
- **Irritable bowel syndrome is the most common cause of chronic diarrhea that alternates with constipation.**
- **Acute diarrhea is usually infectious. When accompanied by vomiting, consider food poisoning.**
- **Remember the public health aspects of the illness and report outbreaks promptly.**

CASE 19–1. A 70-year-old woman, previously in good health except for mild diabetes mellitus type II, has been placed in a nursing home to rehabilitate from a fractured right hip. Two days after her admission she begins to have small diarrheal stools and you are notified by the nurse two days after that. Her viral signs are normal and she is afebrile. She is on a stable dose of metformin 500 mg twice a day.

A. What is your differential diagnosis?
B. What questions do you have for the nurse?
C. You should consider ordering what tests and therapy?
D. The patient fails to improve and now develops abdominal bloating. What is your next step?

CASE 19–2. **A 12-year-old girl and her 16-year-old sister are brought to the clinic with a two-day history of bloody diarrhea, fever up to 39°C, mild abdominal cramping, nausea without vomiting, and malaise. They are passing 10 to 15 stools per day. Both children are otherwise healthy, as is their mother, who accompanies them to the office.**

A. What is your differential diagnosis?
B. What specific history should be sought out?
C. How should you treat these patients?
D. You prescribe erythromycin because you believe that *Campylobacter* is the etiological agent. The culture proves you right. What should you do now that you have the culture report?

REFERENCES

Hay DW: Acute diarrhea and chronic diarrhea. In Gastrointestinal and Liver Disease. Malden, MA: Blackwell Publishing, 2002, pp 19–25.
Holten KB: Irritable bowel syndrome: Minimize testing, let symptoms guide treatment. J Fam Pract 52:942–950, 2003.
Thielman NM, Guerront RL: Acute infectious diarrhea. N Engl J Med 350:38–47, 2004.

USEFUL WEBSITES

Mayo Foundation for Medical Education and Research: Digestive Center. Article on diarrhea by Mayo Clinic Staff. *www.mayoclinic.com/invoke.cfm?id=DS00292*
Centers for Disease Control and Prevention provides information on chronic and traveler's diarrhea at *http://www.cdc.gov/ncidod/dpd/parasiticpathways/diarrhea.htm.*

20

Dizziness

▶ ETIOLOGY

How do you classify dizziness?

Dizziness is a nonspecific term and it is useful to classify symptoms into four categories, which include vertigo, presyncope, disequilibrium, and light-headedness (Table 20–1). It is important to categorize dizziness because the etiologies are very different.

When is dizziness serious?

It is important to differentiate between central versus peripheral dizziness (Table 20–2). Central dizziness (vertigo) is usually more serious, accompanied by neurologic symptoms such as diplopia, dysarthria, paresthesias, or motor weakness. Acoustic neuroma (benign schwannoma of VIII nerve), vertebrobasilar ischemia, and strokes are some examples of syndromes leading to central vertigo.

What are the most common causes of vertigo?

The most common causes of vertigo include:

- A change in head position, which frequently triggers *benign positional vertigo,* in which the patient experiences sudden onset of room spinning that typically lasts less than a minute.
- Meniere's disease, which is a disorder consisting of severe vertigo with hearing loss, tinnitus, and fullness in the ear.
- Vestibular neuronitis, in which the patient experiences abrupt onset of vertigo that gradually becomes worse over the course of several hours. This is frequently preceded by upper respiratory infection. When this accompanies hearing loss it is called *acute labrynthitis.*

What are some other causes of dizziness?

Presyncope is dizziness that is associated with the feeling that one is about to pass out and may be due to reduced blood flow to the entire brain. Orthostatic hypotension, arrythmias, cardiomyopathies, aortic stenosis, valvular disease, constrictive pericarditis,

TABLE 20–1

Classification of Dizziness

Symptom	Description
Vertigo	A rotational sensation; whirling or spinning feeling
Presyncope	The perception of impending faint
Disequilibrium	The loss of balance
Light-headedness	Vague sensation of giddiness

TABLE 20–2

Characteristics of Central versus Peripheral Vertigo

Characteristic	Central	Peripheral
Nausea/vomiting	Moderate	Severe
Imbalance	Severe	Mild
Hearing loss	Rare	Common
Neurologic symptoms	Common	Rare
Aggravated by head position	Rare	Common
Compensation	Slow	Rapid
Duration	Long	Brief
Intensity	Moderate	Severe

cardiac tamponade, medication side effects, and hypoglycemia are some of the causes in this category.

Disequilibrium is the feeling of imbalance and it happens when there is uncompensated disturbance in the coordination of visual, propriocetive, vestibular, cerebellar, and neuromuscular systems. Multiple sensory deficits or presbyastasis, peripheral neuropathies, vestibular abnormalities, visual impairment, and musculoskeletal problems including weakness, osteoarthritis, and cervical spondolysis may all cause disequilibrium.

Light-headedness is the vague sensation of giddiness and is commonly associated with hyperventilation leading to hypocapnia. Depression and anxiety are the most common causes, but other disorders such as stress reaction and panic disorders may also cause this vague feeling.

What are some of the medications that can cause dizziness?

Table 20–3 lists some of the medications commonly associated with dizziness.

TABLE 20–3

Medications Commonly Associated with Dizziness

Drug	Symptoms
Alcohol	Disequilibrium, vertigo
Antiseizure: carbamazepine, phenytoin	Disequilibrium, vertigo
Antihypertensives, diuretics	Presyncope
Antidepressants: tricylic	Presyncope
Aminoglycosides, cisplatin	Disequilibrium, vertigo
Tranquilizers: benzodiazepines, barbiturates	Presyncope
Aspirin	Vertigo
Quinine	Vertigo

▶ EVALUATION

What are the important historical points in a patient with dizziness?

The most important step in evaluating a patient with dizziness is to take a detailed history to classify dizziness into one of the four categories. The history should include questions about hearing loss, tinnitus, and any neurologic symptoms such as diplopia, dysarthria, and extremity weakness. Medication history should also be taken.

What is the Dix-Hallpike test?

The Dix-Hallpike test is done to help identify the location of the problem that is causing vertigo, such as the inner ear or the central nervous system. It is done with the patient sitting on the exam table with legs extended. The doctor helps the patient to lie back quickly with head turned about 30–45 degrees to one side and observes for nystagmus and feeling of vertigo. The test is positive if these are present and the affected ear is the ear pointing toward the floor. A negative test rules out inner ear or central causes of vertigo.

When should I do a CT scan or MRI of the head?

Generally, patients should undergo imaging only if an abnormality is detected on neurologic examination, unless they are over age 60 or have risk factors for vascular disease.

TABLE 20–4

Medications for the Treatment of Vertigo

Medicine	Trade Name	Dosage	Side Effects
Antihistamines			
Dimenhyrdrinate	Dramamine	PO: 25–50 mg q4–6h	Anticholinergic symptoms*
Cyclizine	Marezine	PO: 25–50 mg q4–6h	Anticholinergic symptoms*
Meclizine	Antivert	PO: 25–50 mg q4–6h	Anticholinergic symptoms*
Promethazine	Phenergan	PO: 25 mg q6h Supp: 50 mg q12h IM: 25 mg q4–6h	Anticholinergic symptoms*
Anticholinergic			
Scopolamine	Transderm Scop	Transderm: 0.5 mg q3d	Anticholinergic symptoms*
Phenothizine			
Prochlorperazine	Compazine	PO: 10 mg q6h Supp: 25 mg q12h	Extrapyramidal symptoms†
Benzodiazepine			
Diazepam	Valium	PO: 2–10 mg q6h IM: 2–10 mg q6h IV: 1–10 mg q6h	Drowsiness

* Dry mouth, constipation and absent bowel sounds, blurred vision and elevated intraocular pressure, reduced lacrimation, tachycardia, urinary retention

† Acute dystonia, Parkinsonism, akathisia

▶ TREATMENT

What are some of the common medications used in the treatment of dizziness?

Initial focus should be on discovering the primary cause of dizziness and initiating specific treatment. Table 20–4 outlines some of the common medications used in the symptomatic treatment of dizziness.

KEY POINTS

- ▶ **Conditions causing dizziness may be benign or serious.**
- ▶ **Consider the common causes of dizziness during the evaluation of your patient.**
- ▶ **Differentiate between central and peripheral causes of dizziness.**

CASE 20–1. **A 50-year-old woman comes to your office complaining of a room-spinning sensation, which she has been experiencing for one week. It happens especially when she moves her head rapidly. She has no other medical problems.**

A. What is the most probable diagnosis?
B. What bedside test may be helpful?

CASE 20–2. **A 74-year-old woman comes in with a two-week history of light-headedness and the feeling that she may pass out. It usually is worse when she is walking and stands. She has a diagnosis of hypertension and is on multiple medications for her blood pressure control.**

A. What is the most likely cause for her dizziness?
B. What bedside test may be helpful?

REFERENCES

Baloh RW: Dizziness: Neurological emergencies. Neurol Clin North Am 16(2):305–321, 1998.
Derebery M: The diagnosis and treatment of dizziness. Med Clin North Am 83(1):163–176, 1999.
Hoffman R, et al.: Evaluating dizziness. Am J Med 107(5):468–478, 1999.
Walker J, Barnes S: The difficult diagnosis: Dizziness. Emerg Med Clin North Am 16(4):845–875, 1998.

21

Dyspepsia

▶ ETIOLOGY

What is dyspepsia?

Dyspepsia is a common gastrointestinal disorder defined as a pain or discomfort in the upper abdomen without associated stool symptoms (i.e., not irritable bowel syndrome [IBS]). It is usually associated more with an anatomic location (usually near the epigastrum) than a specific organ structure. The discomfort often is described as fullness, bloating, nausea, or a sensation of early satiety. Symptoms may or may not be associated with food and can be continuous or intermittent in nature. Dyspepsia is often vaguely described and poorly defined by patients.

Approximately 25% of the adult population experiences symptoms annually, most of whom do not seek professional medical care; however, in a typical family medicine practice, up to 5% of visits are patients with dyspepsia symptoms. There is considerable controversy whether to include heartburn as a core symptom. Heartburn is the cardinal symptom of gastroesophageal reflux disease (GERD), which is usually not included under the umbrella of dyspepsia.

▶ EVALUATION

What is the differential diagnosis?

Most cases of dyspepsia arise from an underlying stomach or upper intestinal condition. Causes can be separated into either structural or nonstructural etiologies. The more serious conditions tend to be structural, either gastroduodenal ulcers or gastric cancer.

Studies using endoscopy found that peptic ulcers are causative in 15% to 25% of cases. The most common symptom of an ulcer is abdominal pain or burning that worsens when stomach acid is secreted, especially in the absence of food. Heartburn, more typical of GERD, also is reported frequently. Late night discomfort is also very common when stomach acid secretion is naturally higher. Often patients will have a waxing and waning pattern of symptoms where the discomfort will cyclically disappear then reappear for weeks or months.

Gastroesophageal cancer is a rare but serious cause of dyspepsia. Fortunately, most patients with cancer will have "red-flag" symptoms that can clue the clinician to pursue further work-up. Symptoms to be concerned about include bleeding, anemia, dysphagia, weight loss, and vomiting. Age is also an important factor. Gastric cancers are more common in individuals older than 45 or 50 years of age. Cancer is rare in younger individuals without red-flag symptoms.

Functional dyspepsia, also known as non-ulcer dyspepsia, is by far the most common form, occurring in approximately 75% of cases. Its etiology is often multifactorial with gastrointestinal hypersensitivity, hypomotility, acid hypersecretion, psychosocial stressors, and *Helicobacter pylori* infection all implicated. The diagnosis is considered when other causes for an individual's symptoms have been reasonably excluded.

How is the diagnosis made?

The most important step in making an accurate diagnosis is obtaining a detailed medical history. Although there is not one item from the history that determines the diagnosis, there are characteristic symptom patterns. Patients who complain of heartburn with relief from proton pump inhibitors, H_2-blockers, or antacids are more likely to have GERD. Individuals with ulcers are more likely to have significant pain with relief from food or antacids, while those with cancer are more likely to have weight loss. Other symptoms like pain location or nausea are nonspecific in forming a diagnosis since there is much overlap with other conditions. The physical exam is often disappointing in helping to determine a diagnosis. Although it can be useful in localizing where a patient's complaint is originating from, it is not specific in distinguishing between benign conditions (gastritis, functional dyspepsia) and more serious ones (ulcers, cancers).

Diagnostic testing is often useful or necessary if a patient is not responding to treatment or has red-flag symptoms. Esophagogastroduodenoscopy (EGD) is the best tool to image the stomach mucosa directly. Although it is more expensive and has a slightly higher incidence of complications, endoscopy is more sensitive at diagnosing small ulcers than a barium upper gastrointestinal (UGI) series. Endoscopy also is better at distinguishing between an ulcer and cancer and has the additional advantage of being able to biopsy a suspicious lesion. Other diagnostic studies, including plain abdominal radiography, abdominal ultrasonography, and gastric emptying studies, are not useful in most cases of dyspepsia work-up. All have relatively poor specificity in determining an etiology for dyspeptic pain.

What is the role of testing for *Helicobacter pylori*?

The association between *H. pylori* and the development of peptic ulcers has been well established. This bacteria has been shown to be present in up to 95% of GI ulcers and occurs in up to 40% of patients without ulcers. Eradication of *H. pylori* is beneficial because the incidence of ulcer recurrence is much lower once the bacteria is eliminated. There are four main ways to test for the presence of *H. pylori*:

- Direct mucosal biopsy under endoscopy
- Serum antibody test
- Urea breath test
- Stool antigen test

The serum antibody test is most commonly used because it is the easiest to obtain. Once seroconverting, the test can stay positive since IgG antibodies remain after successful treatment for active infection. Therefore, interpreting a positive test after a patient has already been treated is not reliable. The role of *H. pylori* treatment in non-ulcer dyspepsia is more controversial. Most guidelines recommend evaluating and treating if the bacteria is present since *H. pylori* is implicated in a higher risk of gastric cancers. Whether treatment for symptoms in non-ulcer dyspepsia is helpful is unclear.

▶ TREATMENT

Describe the treatment of ulcers.

If a patient has peptic ulcer disease and is *H. pylori* positive, treatment should commence with one of the many regimens available. Triple and quadruple drug regimens have an eradication rate approaching 90%. For patients with non–*H. pylori* ulcers, antisecretory treatment with H_2-blockers, sucralfate, or proton-pump inhibitors (PPIs) are all effective, with PPIs having a higher cure rate. Follow-up endoscopy for duodenal ulcers is not usually needed. There is controversy over whether repeat endoscopy is needed for gastric ulcers out of concern for missed stomach cancers. If a patient had negative biopsies with initial endoscopy and clinically improves with antisecretory medication, repeat EGD is probably not cost-effective.

Describe the treatment of functional dyspepsia.

Treatment of patients with functional dyspepsia is less straightforward than if a peptic ulcer is present. There are a variety of treatment options, all with success rates of less than 50%. H_2-blockers seem to have the best data supporting their use. An initial trial with either an over-the-counter or prescription product is a reasonable first step. H_2-blockers appear to relieve symptoms better than PPIs at less cost. Metoclopramide, a prokinetic agent, can be effective; however, it has significant anticholinergic side effects limiting its long-term use, especially in the elderly. Antidepressants have shown some symptomatic relief but mainly in patients with cramping or stool complaints (i.e., symptoms suggestive of IBS). Lastly, patients who use tobacco and alcohol, and those taking certain medications (e.g., NSAIDs), should be counseled to avoid these substances if they are aggravating symptoms.

KEY POINTS

- **GERD is differentiated from dyspepsia if the main symptom is heartburn.**
- **"Red-flag" symptoms include vomiting, weight loss, bleeding, dysphagia, and anemia.**
- **Gastric cancer is unlikely without red-flag symptoms if the patient is under 45 to 50 years old.**
- **Endoscopy is the preferred imaging modality.**
- **Triple or quadruple medication therapy is recommended for *H. pylori* eradication.**
- **Optimal treatment of functional dyspepsia is patient specific.**

CASE 21–1. A 52-year-old construction worker presents with a six-month history of upper abdominal burning and bloating. He has been self-treating with calcium carbonate tablets two or three times daily with sporadic relief. He takes an ASA, 81 mg daily, for a family history of early CAD. You prescribe famotidine, which gives the patient excellent relief.

A. What is the most likely diagnosis?
B. Should anything else be done at this time?

CASE 21–2. A 39-year-old patient presents with a 4-month history of daily unrelieved epigastric pain. Endoscopy reveals a gastric ulcer. *H. pylori* testing is negative. You order the correct treatment, which provides good relief.

A. What are the treatment options?
B. Is any follow-up monitoring needed?

REFERENCES

Meurer L: Treatment of peptic ulcer disease and non-ulcer dyspepsia. J Fam Pract 50:614, 2001.

Smucny J: Evaluation of the patient with dyspepsia. J Fam Pract 50:538, 2001.

Tally NJ, Siverstein MD, Agreus L, et al.: AGA technical review: Evaluation of dyspepsia. Gastroenterology 114:582, 1998.

USEFUL WEBSITE

UpToDate is a subscription-based clinical information resource, written by physicians for physicians. *http://www.uptodate.com*

22

Dyspnea

▶ ETIOLOGY

What is dyspnea?

Dyspnea is a symptom that is described as shortness of breath (SOB), an inability to "catch one's breath," a feeling of "air hunger." Dyspnea may be defined as acute (lasting hours or days) or chronic (lasting weeks, months, or years).

What are the most common causes of dyspnea?

The serious causes of acute dyspnea are listed in Table 22–1. The causes of chronic dyspnea are listed in Table 22–2.

▶ EVALUATION

What are the important clinical points to remember when evaluating patients with dyspnea?

All that wheezes is not asthma. Occasionally, patients with pulmonary edema of both cardiac and noncardiac etiology will present with bronchospasm and wheezing rather than inspiratory crackles. For those with a cardiac etiology, jugular venous distention and peripheral edema may be evident. A chest x-ray should help differentiate those with noncardiogenic pulmonary edema because they will have diffuse alveolar infiltrates, bilaterally.

Pulse oximetry can reliably tell you about oxygenation but is not helpful in determining respiratory failure since this requires an evaluation of CO_2 levels found in arterial blood gases.

Infants and children tolerate tachypnea better than adults. Look for cyanosis, nasal flaring, and retraction of the rib cage for signs of respiratory distress in infants and children.

A "quiet" chest in a patient with dyspnea may be the result of severe bronchospasm; you must have air movement to have wheezing. Thus a "quiet" chest can be an ominous finding in a patient with dyspnea. Box 22–1 lists the physical and arterial blood gas findings in patients with acute respiratory failure.

TABLE 22–1

Serious Acute Causes of Dyspnea

Diagnosis	History	Physical Findings	Diagnostic Studies
Pulmonary embolus	Acute onset of SOB, chest pain. May have deep venous thrombosis.	Usually tachypnea tachycardia. Lung exam typically normal, may be cyanotic.	Sa02, ABG: hypoxic CXR: usually normal D-dimer: elevated VQ scan: intermediate or high probability
Airway obstruction	FB Aspiration (peds) Sudden onset	Tachypnea, stridor wheezing (often unilateral), cyanosis, tachycardia	Sa02, ABG: +/– hypoxia, CXR: FB bronchiectisis, mediasteinal shift
Pulmonary edema	Progressive DOE SOB, PND, peripheral edema (cardiac), none in noncardiac	Tachypnea, cyanosis tachycardia, bilateral inspiratory crackles, infiltrates, elevated +/– pedal edema, S3 displaced PMI	Sa02, ABG hypoxic CXR: bilateral BNP (cardiac)
Myocardial infarction	Chest pain w/SOB, nausea, diaphoresis	Tachycardia, tachypnea, S4	EKG ischemic ST depression, injury ST elevation, Q waves, elevated cardiac enzymes
Obstructive pulmonary disease/Asthma w/respiratory failure	Dyspnea, wheezing tightness, fatigue	Initial tachypnea, followed by progressive hypoventilation paradoxical breathing cyanosis pulsus paradoxus, wheezing, decreased breath sounds	Hypercapnea, hypoxia, reduced expiratory force

ABG = arterial blood gas, BNP = brain natriuretic peptide, CXR = chest x-ray, DOE = dyspnea on exertion, FB = foreign body, PND = paroxysmal nocturnal dyspnea, SOB = shortness of breath

▶ TREATMENT

What is the treatment for acute dyspnea?

The goals of treating a patient with acute dyspnea are to assure patency of the airway, maintain oxygenation, and reduce the work of breathing. Unless contraindicated, position the patient in an upright, sitting position, loosen restrictive clothing, apply oxygen at 2–4 L/min by mask or nasal prongs, secure intravenous access if needed, and begin your physical evaluation including vital signs

TABLE 22-2

Common Causes of Chronic Dyspnea

Diagnosis	History	Physical Findings	Diagnostic Studies
Congestive heart failure	DOE, PND-dependent edema	JVD, HJR, S3 inspiratory crackles, pedal edema	CXR: cardiomegaly pulmonary vascular congestion, infiltrates Elevated BNP, Echocardiogram: decreased EF; systolic, diastolic dysfunction
Asthma	Intermittent dyspnea associated with wheezing, often allergies	Expiratory wheezing during attack	Pulmonary function: obstructive pattern, reversible with bronchodilation
COPD	Progressive DOE, smoking, cough often productive	Increased AP diameter chest, insp/exp wheezing, blue bloater/pink puffer	Pulmonary function: obstructive pattern, not entirely reversible with bronchodilation CXR: over expansion Flattened diaphragm
Obesity physical deconditioning	Progressive DOE DOE	BMI > 30 Normal lung exam none	Improves with exercise

BMI = body mass index, BNP = brain natriuretic peptide, COPD = chronic obstructive pulmonary disease, CXR = chest x-ray, DOE = dyspnea on exertion, HJR = hepatojugular reflex, JVD = jugular venous distention, PND = paroxysmal nocturnal dyspnea

BOX 22-1

Signs of Acute Respiratory Failure

- Acute dyspnea
- Arterial oxygen partial pressure (PaO_2) <50 mmHg at room air
- Arterial carbon dioxide partial pressure ($PaCO_2$) >50 mmHg
- Significant respiratory acidemia
- Cyanosis
- Pulsus paradoxus inspiratory fall in systolic blood pressure >10 mmHg
- Paradoxical breathing (Normally during inspiration the diaphragm moves down, pushing the abdomen out. Prolonged dyspnea and respiratory muscle fatigue may cause a loss of coordination between the diaphragm and the chest muscles, resulting in the abdomen moving in rather than out during inspiration.)

and an examination of the respiratory and cardiovascular system. Begin arrangements for appropriate transfer to a facility where the patient can receive necessary treatments, if needed.

What is the treatment for chronic dyspnea?

- Reduce the work of breathing.
  - Energy conservation (efficiency in activity)
  - Position (sitting forward)
  - Reduce weight (if obese)
  - Improve nutrition (if malnourished)
  - Inspiratory muscle exercise
  - Breathing strategies (pursed-lip breathing)
  - Respiratory muscle rest (nasal ventilation, transtracheal oxygen)
- Decrease respiratory drive.
  - Oxygen
  - Opiates and sedatives
  - Exercise conditioning
- Employ psychological interventions (e.g., coping strategies, psychotherapy, group support).
- Prescribe exercise training.
- Start pulmonary rehabilitation.

See these disease-specific chapters for additional information on etiologies of and treatments for dyspnea: Chapter 41, Asthma/COPD, and Chapter 45, Heart Failure.

KEY POINTS

- **Dyspnea is a medical urgency.**
- **Dyspnea can be either acute or chronic.**
- **The most important factor in evaluating a patient with dyspnea is determining whether the patient is stable or unstable. Unstable patients need to be cared for in environments where they can receive appropriate treatment.**

CASE 22–1. **A 68-year-old woman presents with a chief complaint of a sudden onset of shortness of breath associated with sharp, pleuritic chest pain on the left side. There is no cough, fever, or chills. She has a past medical history of hypertension and type II diabetes. Medications include HCTZ 25 mg four times a day, metformin 500 mg twice a day, premarin 0.625 mg daily. Vital signs: temperature 38°C, pulse 112, respirations 30, blood pressure 148/92. Physical exam reveals lungs clear to auscultation; heart has regular rate and rhythm, and S1, S2 are normal. Exam is otherwise normal. EKG reveals sinus tachycardia, otherwise normal. Chest x-ray is normal.**

A. What is the most appropriate test to order next?
B. An ABG returns with the following results: pH 7.48, pCO_2 28, pO_2 52, and HCO_3 28. Which is the most likely explanation for her condition and how would you confirm this suspicion?

CASE 22–2. **Mr. Jones is a 42-year-old man with a long history of alcoholism. He looks quite a bit older than his stated age. He presents with a history of dyspnea on exertion over the past six months that has gotten progressively worse, such that now he cannot walk to the mailbox at the end of his driveway without having to stop and rest. The patient describes increasing pedal edema and weight gain. He admits to drinking 12 to 18 beers daily and he smokes half a pack of cigarettes daily. He denies chest pain, fever, cough, or chills. Examination reveals the following:**

Vital signs: temperature 37°C, respirations 28, pulse 100, blood pressure 100/68
HEENT: JVD to 4 cm at 30 degrees
Lungs: bibasilar inspiratory crackles
Heart: PMI displaced laterally, S1, S2 normal, S3 gallop present
Abdomen: reveals some protuberance, positive fluid wave, spleen palpable, liver palpated 5 cm below right costal margin
Extremities: 2–3 + pitting edema
Skin: multiple spider angiomas, palmer erythema
Chest x-ray: cardiomegaly, cephalization of pulmonary vasculature, and bilateral scant pulmonary infiltrates

A. What is the most appropriate next test to order?
B. An echocardiogram reveals generalized hypokinesis, with an enlarged left ventricle, and an ejection fraction of 12%. What is the most likely diagnosis that explains this patient's complaints? How should treatment commence?

REFERENCES

Mahler DA, Fierro-Carrion G, Baird JC: Evaluation of dyspnea in the elderly. Clin Geriatr Med 19(1):19–33, 2003.

Udobi KF: Acute respiratory distress syndrome. Am Fam Physician 67(2):315–324, 2003.

Zoorob RJ, Cambell JS: Acute dyspnea in the office. Am Fam 68(9):1803–1813, 2003.

USEFUL WEBSITES

The American Thoracic Society has useful links to explicit guidelines and management algorithms, and online learning materials. *http://www.thoracic.org*

The American College of Cardiology has up-to-date summaries of research, controversies in care, and CME programs. *http://www.acc.org*

23

Dysuria

▶ ETIOLOGY

What does dysuria mean?

Dysuria is defined as the sensation of pain or burning on urination.

What causes dysuria?

The causes of dysuria can vary between men and women. In men, common causes include infection (including prostate), obstruction, malignancy (bladder cancer is more common in smokers), stone disease, and the spondyloarthropathies. In women, considerations include infection (including vagina), obstruction, malignancy (bladder cancer is more common in smokers), stone disease, interstitial cystitis, and atrophic vaginitis. Urinary tract infection (UTI) is the most common cause of dysuria.

How common is dysuria?

Estimates suggest that urinary tract symptoms significant enough to cause persons to seek medical attention occur in 0.6% of women per year and 0.1% of men per year.

▶ EVALUATION

How should dysuria be evaluated?

History, physical exam, and some low-cost laboratory tests will most often point to a diagnosis. If not, further evaluation with more labs and imaging or referral to a urologist may be considered.

What is important in the history?

It is important to establish the timing, frequency, severity, and location of dysuria. For men, pain at the start of urination, especially in the distal penis, points to a urethral cause, while pain over the suprapubic area upon completion of urination suggests bladder inflammation. For women, external dysuria, meaning pain as the urine passes over the inflamed vaginal labia, suggests vaginal infection or inflammation, while a history of internal dysuria, meaning pain felt inside the body, suggests bacterial cystitis or urethritis. Also consider that pain at the start of urination points to a urethral cause while pain over the suprapubic area upon completion of urination suggests bladder inflammation. Other key historical questions include the presence of a discharge, the presence of other irritative symptoms such as urgency, frequency, and nocturia, obstructive symptoms such as weak stream, hesitancy, intermittency, and dribbling, and recent sexual history. Don't forget to ask about medications and herbal supplements; dysuria is a side effect of many drugs.

What is important in the physical exam?

General condition and vitals are important. Perform palpation and percussion of the abdomen (to gain insight into kidney, ureter, or bladder inflammation, malignancy, or distention) and percussion at the costovertebral angle (tenderness can indicate pyelonephritis or stone disease). Men should have a penile examination (discharge, trauma, infective lesion) and a digital rectal exam (to assess the prostate for obstruction or infection). Women do not necessarily need a pelvic examination unless vaginal irritation and discharge are present.

What laboratory tests are commonly ordered? What do the results mean?

Occasionally, a physician may treat or decide not to treat a patient without getting the following lab tests if the history and physical exam rule in or out, respectively, an infection. Remember, UTI is the most common cause of dysuria.

Urinalysis is the gold standard in evaluating dysuria. It is absolutely necessary to order a "clean-catch midstream" urine sample. The most sensitive laboratory indicator for urinary tract infections is pyuria. Pyuria can be screened for with a leukocyte esterase dipstick test, which is 75% to 95% sensitive in detecting infective pyuria. The urine nitrite can be tested; however, it is greater than 90% specific but only 30% sensitive, so a negative test does not rule out an infection (*Enterococcus sp.* and others may be nitrite negative). White blood cell casts suggest acute pyelonephritis. Pyuria or hematuria greater than 3–5 WBCs or RBCs, respectively, per high-power field can indicate infection (malignancy and stones are associated with hematuria). The presence of hematuria with no associated pyuria suggests the consideration for cystoscopy to assess for bladder cancer, especially if the patient smokes.

Urine cultures are generally recommended for pregnant women, immunodeficient patients, and males with suspected UTIs; otherwise, urine cultures may be deferred when dysuria is described as largely external and a probable urethral or vaginal cause is identified. A count greater than 10^2–10^3 colony-forming units (CFUs) per mL of urine is significant if there are associated symptoms. If there are no symptoms, a count of greater than 10^5 CFUs per mL is considered significant. This test is highly specific but has a low sensitivity. Culture of urethral discharge is the gold standard for diagnosing *Neisseria gonorrhoeae or Chlamydia trachomatis* infections.

Potassium hydroxide and normal saline vaginal smears may reveal trichomonads. Gram staining of urethral discharge may detect *N. gonorrhoeae or C. trachomatis* infections although currently DNA probe testing or rapid antigen testing is frequently used.

What associated signs and symptoms can guide the diagnosis for men?

From History. Obstructive symptoms (benign prostatic hyperplasia [BPH], urethral stricture, bladder dysfunction), rectal pain (prostatitis), pain during intercourse or ejaculation (cystitis, STD urethritis), recent unprotected sex (STD urethritis or cystitis), irritative symptoms (cystitis, pyelonephritis, urethritis), internal pain (cystitis, urethritis), urethral discharge (STD), systemic symptoms such as fever, chills, nausea, and vomiting (pyelonephritis), systemic symptoms such as arthralgias, ocular symptoms, oral ulcers (spondyloarthropathy such as Reiter's syndrome).

From Physical Exam. Penile discharge or meatal inflammation (urethritis, STD, candidiasis), vesicles, rashes, ulcers, tender lymphadenopathy (genital herpes, chancroid, neoplasm, dermatologic condition), testicular or epididymal swelling (epididymo-orchitis), tender and boggy prostate (prostatitis), large prostate without nodules (BPH), large prostate with nodules (neoplasm), flank tenderness (renal tumor or cyst, cystitis, subclinical pyelonephritis, urinary retention).

What associated signs and symptoms can guide the diagnosis for women?

From History. Postmenopausal without hormones (hypoestrogen-induced vaginitis), cyclic pain with menses (endometriosis), external pain (STD: *Chlamydia trachomatis* with watery mucoid discharge, *Neisseria gonorrhoeae* with yellow or gray thick discharge, fungus with thick, curdlike, white, pruritic discharge), abnormal vaginal bleeding (cervicitis), postcoital vaginal bleeding (atrophic vaginitis), painful intercourse (cystitis, cervicitis, vaginitis), recent unprotected sex (STD urethritis or cystitis), irritative symptoms (cystitis, pyelonephritis, urethritis), internal pain (cystitis, urethritis), urethral discharge (STD), obstructive symptoms (urethral stricture, bladder dysfunction), systemic symptoms such as fever, chills, nausea, and vomiting (pyelonephritis), systemic symptoms such as arthralgias, ocular symptoms, and oral ulcers (spondyloarthropathy such as systemic lupus erythematosis).

From Physical Exam. Vesicles, ulcers, tender inguinal lymphadenopathy (genital herpes), vaginal satellite pustules (candidiasis), vaginal discharge (candidiasis, STD, hypoestrogenism vaginitis), vaginal atrophy (hypoestrogenism), cervical erythema and discharge (STD), cervical motion tenderness and adnexal tenderness in association with lower abdominal tenderness (pelvic inflammatory disease, endometriosis), mass on kidney palpation (renal tumor or cyst), suprapubic tenderness (cystitis, subclinical pyelonephritis), bladder distention (urinary retention).

▶ TREATMENT

How do I treat dysuria?

To cure dysuria, the physician must determine the cause and treat it. Azole preparations such as pyridium can provide symptomatic relief. Remember, urinary tract infections are the most common causes of dysuria.

How do I treat urinary tract infections?

Depending on whether the infection is in the kidneys (pyelonephritis), bladder (cystitis), or urethra (urethritis), appropriate antibiotics are prescribed. Treatment will vary if there are complicating factors such as structural abnormalities or recurrent infections. Trimethoprim-sulfamethoxazole (one double-strength tab twice a day for three days), nitrofurantoin (100 mg twice a day for seven days), and the quinilones (ciprofloxacin 250 mg twice a day for three days) are often used.

KEY POINTS

- **Urinary tract infection is the most common cause of dysuria.**
- **Urinalysis is the gold standard test for dysuria, but must be a midstream clean catch.**
- **Pregnant patients with dysuria should have a urine culture performed.**

CASE 23–1. A 17-year-old sexually active girl presents with burning upon urination and some discharge.

A. What is important in the history and physical exam?
B. What laboratory tests should be ordered?
C. What is the most likely cause?

CASE 23–2. A 22-year-old woman presents with high fevers, shaking chills, and painful urination.

A. What is important in the history and physical exam?
B. What laboratory tests should be ordered?
C. What is the most likely cause?

REFERENCES

Bremnor J: Evaluation of dysuria in adults. Am Fam Physician 65(8):1589–1596, 2002.
Kurowski K: The woman with dysuria. Am Fam Physician 57(9): 2155–2164, 2169–2170, 1998.
Roberts R, Hartlaub P: Evaluation of dysuria in men. Am Fam Physician 60(3):865–872, 1999.

24

Earache

▶ ETIOLOGY

What are the most common causes of ear pain?

Acute otitis media (OM) and otitis externa (OE) are the most common causes of ear pain. Acute OM is an infected middle ear effusion and is seen most commonly in pediatric patients. OE is an infection of the external auditory canal and is often caused by repeated water exposure (hence it is known as swimmer's ear). Appropriate evaluation is critical: in young children, persistent ear infection or effusion may decrease hearing and delay speech and language development. Conversely, treating ear pain with antibiotics when inappropriate can lead to increased bacterial resistance.

Why is ear pain so much more common in the pediatric population?

OM is much more common in patients younger than 5 years old because their cranium is not fully developed. The eustachian tube is responsible for drainage of the middle ear space. In young children this tube is more horizontal in orientation and smaller in caliber than in older people; it therefore does not drain the space as well.

What is different about ear pain in adults?

An adult with ongoing ear pain must be evaluated further with a thorough head and neck exam. Cancers or other pathology of the neck may refer pain to the ear, and cancers of the nasopharynx may occlude the eustachian tube and cause recurrent OM.

What is otitis media?

Acute OM is an infection of an effusion in the middle ear. It usually occurs following a viral upper respiratory infection (respiratory syncytial virus, rhinovirus) that washes nasal secretions up an immature eustachian tube. Normal nasal flora (*Streptococcus pneumoniae, Hemophilus influenzae,* or *Moraxella catarrhalis*) proliferate in the effusion. Smoking exposure enhances pathogen attachment and further impairs eustachian tube function; increased smoke exposure significantly prolongs duration of OM.

What is otitis externa? Who is susceptible to it?

OE is an inflammation or infection of the skin inside the ear canal. It is usually caused by *Pseudomonas aerguinosa* or *Staphylococcus aureus*. Cerumen is both acidic and hydrophobic and makes the canal a hostile place for bacteria to grow. Aggressive swabbing or swimming circumvents this defense, and otitis externa may result.

► EVALUATION

What is the difference between acute OM and OM with effusion?

Acute OM usually presents with signs of acute illness including ear pain, fever, irritability, and rhinorrhea. OM with effusion is not an infection and does not present with fever, pain, or irritability. It may impart changes in hearing or a sensation of fullness that can cause children to pull their ears.

What characteristics of the eardrum should I examine with my otoscope?

It is important to check mobility of the tympanic membrane (TM) with your otoscope to assess for effusion. Also look for retraction of TM bulges and TM translucency, and note color. Acute OM will feature a TM with decreased mobility that is bulging, opaque, and red or amber colored. Redness of the TM is the least reliable sign, since it may be caused by fever, crying, or attempts at cerumen removal.

What are the symptoms and signs of otitis externa?

The patient with OE will usually complain of ear pain or otorrhea and occasionally of pruritis. On physical exam, the patient will have a reddened ear canal and pain when the examiner manipulates the tragus. While exam of the canal is critical, curettage for diagnosis is discouraged because this may exacerbate the irritation of the canal.

► TREATMENT

How should a patient with acute otitis media be treated?

Patients should be treated with high-dose amoxicillin (90 mg/kg/d). This dose cures 98% of acute OM cases. If a patient has received antibiotics in the last three months, proceed to second-line treatment (see next paragraph). Keep in mind, though, that 50% to 80% of acute OM resolves spontaneously. Ceftriaxone (50 mg/kg, one dose IM) is an alternative first-line treatment.

What if the symptoms don't improve with antibiotics within 72 hours?

The patient should be reexamined, and if the exam results have not changed, switch to a second-line antibiotic such as amoxicillin/clavulanic acid or ceftriaxone IM once daily for three days. If the symptoms persist another 72 hours, the practitioner should perform tympanocentesis for pain relief and send the effusion for culture and sensitivity.

What follow-up should be requested for a patient with acute OM?

Every patient diagnosed with acute OM should be reevaluated between three and six weeks. Although persistence of an effusion is within the natural course of the disease, its disappearance is important to regaining normal hearing. The effusion should be examined monthly. Persistence of effusion at three months with hearing loss or speech delay is an indication for tympanostomy tube placement.

What are my treatment options when I diagnose a patient with OE?

First, it is essential to remove the irritating, exfoliated squamous material. Then the patient should receive an antibiotic/anti-inflammatory drop such as the floroquinolones (Cipro, Cipro HC, or Ciprodex). An inexpensive treatment option is drops composed of a 1:1 mixture of white vinegar and 70% alcohol, used every four hours. This will dry the canal and return it to the normal bacteriocidal acidity usually provided by the earwax. This mixture is effective, but it may be irritating.

What can the patient do to prevent OE from recurring?

The patient should not swim for 10 days following diagnosis. Later, the patient should take care to dry ears well following swimming. The canal should be irritated as little as possible with less swabbing, leaving some earwax behind.

KEY POINTS

- **Ear pain may be caused by inflammation of the outer or middle ear, or may be referred from elsewhere in the pharynx.**
- **Otitis externa is caused by a disruption in normal defenses, and may be treated by correcting the imbalance and ending the offending cause.**
- **A good evaluation of acute otitis media must include a thorough examination of the tympanic membrane, including pneumatic otoscopy to assess for mobility and effusion.**
- **Acute otitis media must be followed closely to ensure antibiotic efficacy, remission of effusion, and normal hearing and speech development.**

CASE 24–1. **A 7-month-old boy has been pulling at his left ear for two days. He hasn't had a fever, but his mother says he has a runny nose and hasn't been eating well. He attends day care, and his mother's boyfriend smokes in the house. In the exam room, the boy appears happy and playful.**

A. What is the differential diagnosis?
B. What points are most important from his history?
C. What is important to do on physical exam?
D. What follow-up does this boy need?

CASE 24–2. **On a July day, a mother brings her 5-year-old boy into the clinic because he has yellow-white drainage from his right ear. The boy says the ear is very tender and is reluctant to let you examine it. He has been going swimming with the older kids at his day care.**

A. What is the differential diagnosis?
B. What do you need to do to obtain an appropriate examination?
C. What are your treatment options?

REFERENCES

Rothman R, et al.: Does this child have acute otitis media? JAMA 290:1633–1640, 2003.

Sander R: Otitis externa. Am Fam Physician 63:927–936, 2001.

USEFUL WEBSITE

American Academy of Pediatrics Online Learning in Otitis Media. *http://www.aap.org/otitismedia*

25

Fatigue

▶ ETIOLOGY

What is fatigue?

Fatigue is a state characterized by a lessened capacity for work and reduced efficiency of accomplishment, usually accompanied by weariness, sleepiness, or irritability. Fatigue is often classified as acute or chronic, but may also be classified as having peripheral or central origin. Central fatigue refers to abnormalities of neurotransmitters within the central nervous system (CNS), whereas peripheral fatigue involves abnormalities in the peripheral nervous system.

Chronic fatigue typically has been present for more than six months, often has multiple or unknown causes, is generally not related to exertion, and is poorly relieved by rest. It has been recognized for centuries that fatigue usually occurs with chronic disease. However, the degree of fatigue does not correlate with the severity of the illness. Both chronic and central fatigue are often accompanied by psychological complaints such as anxiety or depression.

What are common causes of fatigue?

Common etiologies include allergic rhinitis, anemia, cancer, deconditioning, depression, infection, job demands, and sleep disorders. Although fatigue can be a side effect of many medications, the most common medications causing fatigue are sedatives, first-generation antihistamines, β-blockers, and diuretics.

Is there a difference between chronic fatigue syndrome and fibromyalgia?

Although there is some overlap in symptoms, specific criteria identify chronic fatigue syndrome and fibromyalgia. Fibromyalgia involves: (1) widespread pain in all four quadrants of the body for a minimum of three months and (2) at least 11 of 18 specified tender points (which are clustered around the neck, upper back, hips, and knees). Chronic fatigue syndrome involves: (1) severe fatigue that is not relieved by rest for at least six months and (2) at least four of the following eight symptoms: impaired memory or concentration; tender cervical or axillary lymph nodes; sore throat; muscle pains; multijoint pain (not due to arthritis); new-onset headaches; unrefreshing sleep; postexertional malaise.

▶ EVALUATION

How can I take a good history quickly?

Start with open-ended questions and then ask for more specifics as needed. Listening to what the patient says is very important.

What does the patient mean by "tired"?

Is he sleepy or feeling slowed down? Does she feel rested when she first wakes up? Does the tiredness worsen as the day progresses? Often a patient struggling with depression or a sleep disorder will not feel rested on awakening. If the person is doing a very physically demanding job or is physically out of shape due to obesity or smoking, he will tire as the day progresses. If allergic rhinitis is a problem, determine whether the patient is struggling with the disease itself or side effects of medication. If side effects are the issue, could the patient be taking a medication at the wrong time (e.g., diuretic at bedtime)?

How long has the patient felt tired?

With an acute infection or acute anemia, tiredness will have been present only for a few days or weeks. The tiredness that accompanies seasonal allergic rhinitis occurs during the symptomatic season. In the other conditions (see common causes, in the previous section) the tiredness will have been present for weeks to months to years.

Why has the patient decided to mention this concern now?

Usually this topic is raised because the fatigue has begun to interfere with work or social activities. Did the patient come of his own volition or because a family member or friend urged him to get evaluated? Is a family member frustrated with the patient's snoring at night?

How well is the patient sleeping?

People with sleep apnea have significant difficulty staying awake during the day. Concurrently, the bed partner sleeps poorly due to disturbance from the snoring or actual cessation of breathing.

BOX 25–1

Depression Screen

- **S**leep disturbance
- **I**nterest loss
- **G**uilt
- **E**nergy loss
- **C**oncentration difficulties
- **A**ppetite disturbance
- **P**sychomotor depression or agitation
- **S**uicidal thoughts

Another cause of poor sleep, and hence fatigue, is pain. Complaints of sleep disturbance are very common in patients with chronic illness, especially multiple sclerosis, lupus, and rheumatoid arthritis.

What effect has the fatigue had on psychosocial issues?

Determine whether psychosocial issues are the cause or result of fatigue. Inquire about psychosocial stressors including financial concerns, family dynamics, and work schedule, and ask whether the person enjoys her lifestyle. If the history suggests depression, use the acronym *SIGECAPS* (Box 25–1) or a screening questionnaire to confirm. Remember to assess whether the person is suicidal.

What tests should be obtained?

Lab studies are ordered to identify physical causes of fatigue. Anemia is initially identified on CBC with a low hemoglobin and/or abnormal MCV. Tests such as percent iron saturation, iron-binding capacity, vitamin B_{12} level, RBC folate level, and hemoglobin electrophoresis can be used to determine whether the anemia is due to iron deficiency or another condition, including the anemia of chronic disease. Check TSH and free T4 to determine whether the patient has hypothyroidism or hyperthyroidism. Electrolytes and BUN/creatinine help identify renal failure or hypokalemia from a diuretic. Sleep apnea should be evaluated with a sleep study because this provides information about the diagnosis and treatment options.

▶ TREATMENT

What modalities are useful in acute fatigue?

Be sure to treat any underlying disease condition such as anemia, thyroid imbalance, or electrolyte imbalance. Peripheral fatigue can be alleviated by such modalities as rest, analgesia, muscle relaxants, massage, heat, and ice.

What can be done to treat the (frustrating) condition of chronic fatigue?

Remember that this condition is frustrating to the patient as well as to the healthcare provider! A multifaceted approach is needed. It is very important to treat any coexistent mood disorder, especially depression. Cognitive behavior therapy has been somewhat helpful in patients with chronic fatigue syndrome and rheumatoid arthritis. It helps the patients identify their beliefs about the illness (cognition) and how they cope (behavior). It then encourages them to identify self-help techniques to offset the fatigue.

Is exercise useful in treating chronic fatigue?

The patient needs to establish a reasonable balance between activity and rest. Excessive rest actually makes people feel more tired. Conversely, these patients tend to be overactive when they are feeling good, which then exacerbates the fatigue. Recommend a graded aerobic physical exercise program.

What is involved in sleep hygiene?

Inquire as to how quickly the patient falls asleep and how long he stays asleep. If there is difficulty falling asleep, the patient should avoid stimulants such as caffeine or exercise shortly before bedtime. Also, he should turn off distractions such as television. If he is awake for more than half an hour, he should get up and read or write until he gets sleepy, rather than lying in bed fuming about it. Some people find that tryptophan (e.g., a component of milk) helps them go to sleep.

If the patient wakes after just a few hours, determine the cause. If his mind is racing, he may benefit from an antianxiety agent. If he is hurting, analgesia may be helpful. Perimenopausal women may be struggling with hot flashes, which may respond to hormone replacement therapy or possibly selective serotonin re-uptake inhibitors (SSRIs) or gabapentin (Neurontin). Nocturia is a frequent problem in the elderly. This may improve with oxybutinin for women and saw palmetto for men.

Routine use of benzodiazepines and diphenhydramine is discouraged because of their effect on sleep architecture, but they may be useful on an intermittent basis. Sleep patterns also improve as depression is treated.

KEY POINTS

- It is important to identify and correct treatable causes of fatigue, such as anemia, hypothyroidism, medication side effects, depression, and sleep apnea.
- The hallmark of chronic fatigue syndrome is fatigue, while the main complaint in fibromyalgia is pain.
- Any patient dealing with a chronic pain or fatigue syndrome needs to learn to pace himself in order to stay as physically active as possible without overdoing.

CASE 25–1. A 52-year-old woman presents with the complaint of "being tired all the time." She has been out of work due to a back injury two years ago. The case is in litigation, so she has multiple unpaid medical bills. Ibuprofen upsets her stomach, and acetaminophen does not help her pain. For the past six months she has been waking up at least four times per night due to pain, hot flashes, and/or nocturia. Her last menstrual period was eight months ago. There is no family history of breast cancer.

A. Which type of medication would be appropriate first-line treatment for this patient?

CASE 25–2. A 57-year-old man complains that he always gets sleepy in the early afternoon, and a 30-minute nap refreshes him. He is also having difficulty with remembering instructions he was told a few minutes earlier. He reports that he has gained 50 pounds in the past two years. His wife started sleeping in a different bedroom one year ago because of his snoring.

A. What is the most likely diagnosis?
B. What are treatment options for this patient?

REFERENCE

Swain MG: Fatigue in chronic disease. Clin Sci (London) 99(1):1–8, 2000.

USEFUL WEBSITES

A chronic fatigue syndrome/myalgic encephalomyelitis site created and maintained by a CFS patient. Includes news sources, discussion groups, and more. *www.cfs-news.org*

Fibromyalgia Network. Offers educational materials on fibromyalgia syndrome (FMS) and chronic fatigue syndrome (CFS), also a quarterly *Fibromyalgia Network* newsletter. *www.fmnetnews.com*

26

Gastrointestinal Bleeding

▶ ETIOLOGY

How is gastrointestinal (GI) bleeding classified?

GI bleeds can be classified into two main groups determined by the source of the bleed: upper and lower GI bleeding. The landmark for this distinction is the ligament of Treitz. Therefore, upper GI bleeding has a source above (proximal to) the ligament of Treitz and manifests as melena or hematemesis. Lower GI bleeds have a source below (distal to) the ligament of Treitz and manifest as hematochezia.

What are the main causes of upper GI bleeding?

The main etiologies of upper GI bleeds are Mallory-Weiss tears, peptic ulcer disease, gastritis (often due to alcohol ingestion, portal hypertension, and use of anti-inflammatory medications such as aspirin and ibuprofen), and variceal bleeding secondary to portal hypertension. All of these etiologies cause mucosal erosions, resulting in hemorrhage of branches of the celiac and superior mesenteric arteries.

Neoplasms of the foregut, arteriosclerotic aortic aneurysms, and angiodysplasia can also cause GI bleeding.

What is the morbidity and mortality of upper GI bleeding?

There are approximately 350,000 annual admissions in the United States related to upper GI bleeding. There is a mortality rate of 10% associated with upper GI bleeds, although the mortality rate may reflect the underlying illnesses and related comorbidities.

What is the clinical presentation of upper GI bleeds?

Hematemesis and melena are the most common causes of upper GI bleeds; however, clinical presentation is heavily dependent on the rate and duration of the bleed. If there is rapid blood loss, hematochezia may occur. A nasogastric (NG) tube passed into the stomach can distinguish between the two. If blood is aspirated from the NG tube, then an upper GI bleed is likely (aspiration of the blood also prepares the gut for endoscopy, which will be discussed later). Typically, there must be a blood loss of at least 500 mL before the appearance of nonspecific systemic symptoms such as tachycardia, nausea, chest pain, fatigue, and diaphoresis occurs. If there is a large amount of blood loss, shock (syncope, hypotension) may occur.

What are the main causes of lower GI bleeds?

The differential diagnoses of lower GI bleeds include diverticulosis (most common cause—responsible for 60% of lower GI bleeds), angiodysplasia, colitis (secondary to infection, ischemia, or radiation), colon carcinoma, inflammatory bowel disease, polyps, and Meckel's diverticulum. Hemorrhoids and anorectal fissures also cause lower GI bleeds, but the diagnosis and treatment are usually straightforward in these cases.

Helpful hint: Remember that angiodysplasia (responsible for 1–2% of GI bleeds) is associated with the following systemic diseases: aortic stenosis, von Willebrand disease, chronic obstructive pulmonary disease (COPD), chronic renal disease, and collagen vascular diseases.

Describe the clinical presentation of lower GI bleeds.

Presentation varies greatly depending on rate and duration of the bleeding. Hematochezia occurs in an acute setting, but the blood loss can also be occult. In severe cases, there may be hemodynamic instability and a falling hemoglobin. In these instances, transfusion is necessary.

Define occult GI bleeding.

Occult blood loss is not visibly detectable in the stool and is usually discovered by fecal occult blood testing (FOBT). Normal daily blood loss from the GI tract is 0.5–1.5mL. The appearance of melena requires loss of 150 mL of blood from the GI tract. Tests for occult blood loss ideally test positive for amount of blood loss between these amounts. Half of patients with GI bleeding do not have an obvious source, and the cause of bleeding must be pursued.

▶ EVALUATION

What is a useful approach to evaluating GI bleeds?

The patient's age and symptoms should guide the differential diagnosis. A thorough history and physical exam is a necessary part of the initial evaluation. History should be focused on risk factors: use of NSAIDs and aspirin, alcohol abuse, and/or liver disease. In the acute setting, categorize the patient as having an upper or a lower GI bleed.

What is the initial evaluation in an upper GI bleed?

Always follow the ABCs (airway, breathing, circulation). Make sure that the patient is hemodynamically stable. Tachycardia and orthostasis occurs with a greater than 15% blood loss. Hypotension begins at a 40% blood loss. Immediately order a type and cross and begin large-bore intravenous lines to replenish the volume loss. Once the patient is stable, an NG tube is passed into the stomach to confirm that the hemorrhage is from an upper GI source. Saline irrigation will estimate the amount of bleeding and prepare the stomach for endoscopy. Upper endoscopy is the initial procedure of choice. Endoscopy can identify the source of bleeding and provide therapeutic options.

Does endoscopy always reveal the source of bleeding?

No test is perfect, and 10% of cases are nondiagnostic. In these instances, angiography can be used. Angiography is advantageous because it can identify the source of hemorrhage with bleeding rates of at least 0.5 mL/min. It can also be therapeutic.

What is the initial evaluation of lower GI bleeds?

The priority is to be certain that the patient is stable. Once a lower source has been confirmed, colonoscopy is generally the procedure of choice. However, for massive bleeding, angiography should be used.

What will lab values show in GI bleeds?

Hemodilution and equilibration with extravascular fluid cause initial lab values to be normal in acute cases of GI bleeding. Within six hours, mild leukocytosis and thrombocytosis occur, and the hemoglobin may begin to drop. Blood urea nitrogen is increased because of digestion of blood proteins by bacteria in the gut.

▶ TREATMENT

What is a general approach to treatment of GI bleeds?

The treatment plan depends on the acuteness of the situation. Again, always start with the ABCs for patients in acute situations, order a type and cross, and start large-bore IVs. Rapidly assess how much blood has been lost with clinical exam. Determine if the source is from the upper or lower GI tract. Next, the etiology of the problem will dictate if the treatment is endoscopic, medical, surgical, or angiographic. Although most GI bleeds will halt without intervention, most patients with GI bleeds will need to be admitted. In severe cases, the patient should be admitted to the ICU.

What are the treatment options of endoscopy?

Polypectomy can be performed during colonoscopy. Esophagogastroduodenoscopy (EGD) has several therapeutic options for upper GI bleeds. Thermal ablation is the most common technique used by this method. Injection sclerotherapy, in which vasopressin or embolization material is injected into vessels, is another option. Laser coagulation and banding are also used. Choice of treatment depends on the patient's comorbidities, whether there has been recurrence of the bleed, and operator experience with the techniques. A combination of these modalities has been shown to be more effective than any of them alone.

How does vasopressin work to treat GI bleeding?

Vasopressin, used in upper and lower GI bleeds, causes arteries, arterioles and capillaries to vasoconstrict. Vasopressin will be successful in stopping bleeding 70% to 90% of the time. Recurrence of bleeding is around 22%. Major side effects of vasopressin therapy in these situations are myocardial ischemia and infarction, arrhythmia, hypertension, bowel and peripheral vascular ischemia, and antidiuretic effects.

How does embolization work to treat GI bleeding?

Embolization is also used for both upper and lower GI bleeds. The arterial flow is decreased by the procedure, which lowers the pressure at the hemorrhaging site and allows for clot formation. Microcoils, polyvinyl alcohol, and Gelfoam are the options available for this technique. Microcoils are usually used in combination with one of the other substances. Side effects include ischemia and infarction of tissues secondary to devascularization.

What are some examples of medicinal treatment of GI bleeds?

Octreotide is a somatostatin analogue used for variceal hemorrhage that can be infused even before endoscopy. Octreotide is considered to be superior to vasopressin because of the systemic side effects of the latter. Octreotide exerts its effect by decreasing splanchnic blood flow; it is often used in combination with endoscopy to treat varices.

Arterial–venous malformations are treated with combined estrogen and progesterone. Anytime a systemic medication is given, there will be systemic side effects of which the patient should be warned. In these cases, side effects are from the hormonal consequences on the remainder of the body.

What about refractory upper GI bleeding from varices?

For uncontrolled bleeding from varices despite endoscopic and medical therapy (octreotide), balloon tamponade with a Sengstaken-Blakemore tube (esophagogastric) or Linton tube (gastric) may be used.

If the variceal hemorrhage is recurrent despite multiple endoscopic trials, the use of transjugular intrahepatic portosystemic shunts (TIPS) is preferred over other surgical methods. A nonspecific β-blocker titrated to reduce the pulse by 25% is thought to decrease rates of rebleeding.

How is angiography used in treating GI bleeds?

Although a disadvantage of angiography as a diagnostic tool is the invasive nature of the procedure, the advantage is that it can immediately be used for treatment. Embolization material is used to halt the bleeding. This method is useful in an unstable patient because no preparation is needed and immediate treatment is available.

What role does surgery play in management of GI bleeds?

With current technology, surgery should be used as a last resort or when other treatment options have failed. For example, recurring variceal bleeds will often be treated by surgical insertion of TIPS.

When is no treatment required?

Most often, acute GI bleeding will halt with conservative measures. For example, 80% of Mallory-Weiss tears will stop bleeding upon observation. The rebleeding rate in these patients is only 2% to 5%. The decision to treat is made based on clinical assessment of the patient, the patient's related morbidities, and experience and judgment of the gastroenterologist. Major blood loss that requires therapeutic action can be measured by pulse greater than 110 beats per minute, systolic blood pressure less than 100 mmHg, orthostatic drop in systolic blood pressure of at least 16 mmHg, oliguria, cold and clammy extremities, and mental status changes.

KEY POINTS

- **GI bleeding must be differentiated by location of its source (upper versus lower).**
- **Do not forget to screen appropriate patients annually for occult GI bleeding. Evaluate for colon cancer if FOBT is positive.**
- **Evaluation always should start with an initial clinical assessment of the patient. Do not forget the ABCs of patient care.**
- **Endoscopy (colonoscopy versus EGD) is usually the initial evaluation in GI bleeding.**
- **Diagnosis and treatment of the GI bleed can often be simultaneous.**
- **Treatment depends on the etiology of the GI bleed and can be endoscopic, medical, surgical, or angiographic.**

CASE 26–1. A 55-year-old alcoholic woman presents to the acute care clinic vomiting bright red blood. The patient reports binge-drinking the preceding evening, followed by vomiting and retching throughout the night.

A. What are the initial steps to take?
B. Is this patient's bleeding from an upper GI source or a lower GI source?
C. What evaluation is needed?
D. What is the most appropriate treatment for this patient?

REFERENCES

Adler DG, Baron TH: Gastrointestinal hemorrhage: Review questions. Hospital Physician, 37:25–26, 2001.

Beers MH, Berkow R: The Merck Manual of Dianosis and Therapy. Chapter 22, Section 3. Medical Services, USMEDSA, USHH. Available at http://www.merck.com/mrkshared/mmanual/section3/chapter22/22a.jsp.

Mitchell SH, Schaefer DC, Dubagunta S: A new view of occult and obscure gastrointestinal bleeding. Am Fam Physician 69:875–881, 2004.

Rana A: Lower gastrointestinal bleeding. Omaha, Nebraska, eMedicine.com, Inc., 2004. Available at http://www.emedicine.com.

Varma MK: Upper gastrointestinal bleeding. Omaha, Nebraska: eMedicine.com, Inc., 2002. Available at http://www.emedicine.com.

USEFUL WEBSITES

eMedicine: This site provides articles on upper and lower GI bleeds in more detail, as well as excellent radiological pictures. *http://www.emedicine.com*

Nuclear Medicine Imaging and Function Studies of the Gastrointestinal System. This site provides more detail about the differential diagnosis of GI bleeding and offers cases, a quiz, and links to other websites. *http://www3.sympatico.ca/lgoodin/nmgi/bleed/gi_bleed.htm*

27

Headache

▶ ETIOLOGY

How common are headaches?

More than 90% of young adults report at least one headache annually. More than 10% of both young men and women will visit a physician at some point for the symptom of headache. Headaches also have a significant social and economic impact: a 1993 survey estimated that 155 million workdays are lost and 329,000 school days are missed annually. Costs are estimated to be $50 billion annually.

How are headaches classified?

Headaches may be categorized in multiple ways; however, for the family physician it is probably most appropriate to view headaches as either primary or secondary. Primary headaches are often episodic and not associated with other illnesses whereas secondary headaches are a symptom or result of another underlying diagnosis.

What are the common primary headache diagnoses?

Primary headaches make up the vast majority of the cases that present to the family physician's outpatient office. These headaches are then subcategorized as tension-type, migraine, or cluster.

How are tension-type headaches described?

Tension-type headaches are the most common variant of primary headache. Characteristics include episodic nature, gradual onset, bilateral distribution, tightening/pressure quality, and the ability to continue with most daily activities.

What causes tension-type headaches?

Muscle contraction or tightness has often been theorized to be the cause of tension-type headaches; however, no study has been able to measure this phenomenon.

How are migraine headaches classified?

The terminology for migraine headache sufferers is changing. Previous terms included "classic migraine" and "common migraine." These are now known as migraine with and without aura, respectively. Auras are by definition temporary and fully reversible neurologic deficits. The most typical description of an aura is that of the visual fields being disturbed by flashing lights. However, they may also affect motor or speech abilities. "Complicated migraines" or migraine variants are distinguished by the persistence of the neurologic deficit.

What are the characteristics of a migraine headache?

The International Headache Society offers the following diagnostic criteria for a migraine headache:

- The headache attacks last 4–72 hours.
- The headache has at least two of the following characteristics:
  Unilateral location
  Pulsating quality
  Moderate or severe intensity
  Aggravation by routine physical activity
- The patient experiences at least one of the following during the headache:
  Nausea and/or vomiting
  Photophobia
  Phonophobia
- History, physical examination, and neurologic examination do not suggest underlying organic disease.
- Episodic, with at least five attacks fulfilling the above criteria.

What are cluster headaches?

Cluster headaches share many clinical characteristics with migraine headaches. However, cluster headaches have the following distinctions: more common in men than women, nearly exclusively unilateral and periorbital in distribution, with a severe stabbing quality; they are also associated with autonomic signs including ipsilateral rhinorrhea, nasal congestion, eyelid redness/tearing, and Horner's syndrome. The duration is approximately one hour and will occur repetitively over a short period in the individual sufferer often at the same times, most frequently night, and then spontaneously remit for months.

▶ EVALUATION

List some key "red flags" to be considered in a patient presenting to the office with headache.

Red flags that indicate a secondary cause and suggest increased risk for the patient include sudden onset, new headache over age 50, associated systemic illness, focal neurologic findings, increasing frequency or severity, and post-traumatic headaches.

What is the differential diagnosis of headache?

The differential diagnosis of headache is broad. The following discussion is by no means all-inclusive, but it covers the more emergent diagnoses that should be initially considered in a patient suffering from a headache.

A number of vascular events/diagnoses must be considered. These include subarachnoid hemorrhage, acute cerebrovascular accident, and arterial–venous malformation (AVM). Also, inflammation of the vasculature may cause a secondary headache in the form of temporal arteritis. Uncontrolled hypertension and hypertensive emergency may also manifest as headache.

Infection must also be included in the differential, especially in febrile and/or immunocompromised patients. Encephalitis and meningitis must be considered. The evaluation should also include structures near to the central nervous system such as the ears, throat, sinuses, and dentition.

Other intracranial diagnoses include tumor with its potential associated mass effect and pseudotumor cerebrii. Also, low cerebrospinal fluid pressure secondary to medical procedures and/or their complications, including lumbar puncture and epidural/spinal anesthesia, may potentiate headaches. Postconcussive headaches are also increasingly seen, as research into the sequelae of concussions in athletes continues.

Finally, primary ocular pathology may also present as a headache. This includes the relatively benign eyestrain associated with a need for refractive correction to the more ominous diagnoses of open or closed-angle glaucoma and optic neuritis.

What are key historical elements to ask about and discuss with the patient in regard to headache?

When evaluating a patient with headache, the importance of the history is paramount in narrowing down the differential diagnosis and guiding therapy. Essential questions to ask include the descriptors of pain that are common to any part of the body. Location, quality, intensity, duration, onset, and aggravating/alleviating factors must be characterized. The information will often fit the descriptions of tension-type, migraine, and cluster headaches described in the previous section. A complete review of systems will also often rule out many of the secondary causes of headaches discussed in the previous question. It is also of great concern if the patient describes a loss of consciousness or altered level of consciousness before, during, or after a headache.

Also, it is important to review the past medical/surgical history of the patient. This is often difficult because the patient is acutely uncomfortable and desires only immediate relief from pain—he or she may not see the pertinence of the history in the current setting. A medication and allergy history should include not only prescriptions but also any over-the-counter medications, vitamins, herbs, and/or supplements that the patient is or recently has been taking.

What are important physical exam findings?

The most important finding on the physical exam is included in the diagnostic criteria for primary headaches—a normal neurological exam that does not suggest any underlying organic disease. Therefore, the finding of any focal deficit or significant asymmetry on exam should prompt a search for secondary causes and is most commonly the driving force behind specific laboratory or radiologic tests. The vital signs and a careful head, ears, eyes, nose, and throat exam including inspection and palpation may also point to secondary causes of headaches. Further examination components should be guided by the history elicited from the patient and the differential diagnosis that has been formulated.

What tests are helpful, and when are they indicated?

The use of laboratory and radiology should be targeted to assist the physician in narrowing down the differential diagnosis after the history and physical is completed. This will include emergent imaging (noncontrast CT) to test for a subarachnoid hemorrhage or vascular malformation. Other tests may include a lumbar puncture for meningitis, encephalitis, or subarachnoid hemorrhage. Laboratory tests such as CBC and ESR may assist with possible infectious or vasculitic diagnoses. If a primary cause of headache is determined from the history and the exam is normal, no imaging or laboratory study has proven beneficial or cost-effective.

▶ TREATMENT

How are tension-type headaches treated?

Episodic tension-type headaches are best initially treated by over-the-counter analgesics including acetaminophen, ibuprofen, and aspirin. Increasing evidence supports the use of cognitive therapies for chronic tension-type headache sufferers; these may include biofeedback and stress reduction techniques. Physical therapy may be beneficial as well.

How are acute migraine headaches treated?

The American Academy of Neurology has established goals for successful treatment of acute migraines. If NSAIDs or aspirin/acetaminophen/caffeine combinations fail, the Academy recommends migraine-specific agents, which include the triptan family and dihydroergotamine. Also, because nausea/vomiting is a frequent characteristic of migraines this symptom should be addressed as well and medications administered via a non-oral route as needed.

What is a "rebound" headache?

Patients who suffer from headaches more than two days per week are at increased risk of drug-induced headaches caused by the recurrent use of analgesic medications. This then often creates a cycle of chronic headaches. A patient requiring more than two days of acute therapy per week should be on nonanalgesic prophylactic therapy.

What are preventive therapies for migraine headaches?

The medications most researched and found to be effective as of now for migraine prophylaxis include amitriptyline, divalproex, and propanolol/timolol. Continuing research and studies use other β-blockers, calcium-channel blockers, antidepressants, and other epilepsy drugs. Over-the-counter medications that have been evaluated include feverfew, magnesium, and vitamin B_2. Given the variability in individual responses it is important to tailor any regimen to the patient's comorbidities and monitor effectiveness via a headache journal kept by the patient.

KEY POINTS

- **Migraine therapy should be specific for migraine and aggressively treat concomitant nausea and vomiting.**
- **All encounters with patients with headaches must include a search for red-flag signs/symptoms.**

CASE 27–1. **A 45-year-old man presents to clinic for evaluation of headache of three- to four-month duration. He has had similar headaches over the past 20 years, but they have worsened with his new job. They do not prevent him from attending work, and he is not taking any prescription medications. The headache is dull and bilateral and progresses throughout the day. The patient reports increasing fatigue and stress at work. He denies any neurologic symptoms. He has been using Tylenol and generic over-the-counter headache medications on a near-daily basis. On exam he is alert and experiencing only mild discomfort. Temperature is 36.6°C, pulse 84, respirations 18, blood pressure 135/84. The exam is negative.**

A. Are any studies—either laboratory or radiologic—indicated?
B. What is your differential diagnosis?

CASE 27–2. **A 23-year-old woman presents to clinic with a severe, left temporal, throbbing headache of six-hour duration. The patient is a graduate student and has been staying up nearly all night for the past week completing her master's thesis. She states that she has been vomiting and cannot tolerate the sound of conversational-tone voices since her headache started. She anticipated her headache after seeing "flashing lights" this morning. It is similar to headaches that she has had in the past. There are no known drug allergies, and she takes oral contraceptives but no over-the-counter medications. Her vitals are temperature 36.6°C, pulse 108, respirations 20, blood pressure 138/90. On exam the patient is lying on the table in the dark in significant discomfort.**

A. What are pertinent "red-flag" findings to be looking for on exam?
B. If the exam is within normal limits, what is your diagnosis?
C. What treatment options would you consider?

REFERENCES

Bajwa Z, Wooton R: Evaluation of headache in adults. UptoDate Online. Available at http://www.uptodate.com. Accessed Dec. 1, 2003.

Clinch C: Evaluation of acute headaches in adults. Am Fam Physician 63:685, 2001.

Silberstein S: Practice parameter: evidence-based guidelines for migraine headache (an evidence-based review). U.S. Headache Consortium,* Neurology, 55:754–763, 2000.

USEFUL WEBSITE

American Academy of Neurology: Practice Guidelines. *http://www.aan.com*

* The U.S. Headache Consortium is composed of seven member organizations with an interest in improving the quality of care for people with migraine disorders: the American Academy of Neurology (AAN), the American Headache Society (AHS), the American Academy of Family Physicians (AAFP), the American College of Emergency Physicians (ACEP), American College of Physicians-American Society of Internal Medicine (ACP-ASIM), the American Osteopathic Association (AOA), and the National Headache Foundation (NHF).

28

Heartburn

► ETIOLOGY

What are the common causes of heartburn?

Gastroesophageal reflux disease (GERD), present in 20% of Americans weekly and 40% monthly, is the principal cause of heartburn. Other causes include hiatal hernia, erosive esophagitis, esophageal strictures, and adenocarcinoma. Cardiac ischemia can present as heartburn; therefore, careful evaluation of history and risk factors is crucial.

► EVALUATION

What history is important in evaluating heartburn?

Initial diagnosis of GERD is primarily based on the history. Smoking history, meal size and history (including timing), alcohol consumption, and medication use are important. Obese patients have GERD more frequently, and symptoms of heartburn are often more prevalent at night. Burning pain suggests a GI etiology, while crushing pain or pressure radiating to the jaw or left arm is suggestive of cardiac etiology. Positional pain (pain on lying down) or pain that lasts for hours suggests GI etiology. Gastrointestinal and cardiac pain can present similarly, posing a difficult diagnostic challenge. Certain foods, such as chocolate, peppermint, and spearmint, can relax the lower esophageal sphincter. Heartburn may present atypically, with symptoms of asthma, chest pain, chronic cough, globus sensation, or recurrent sore throat or laryngitis. Weight loss, early satiety, GI bleeding, and dysphagia or odynophagia are warning signs suggesting complicated GERD.

Which components of the physical exam are critical?

In most patients, the physical exam will be entirely unremarkable except perhaps for epigastric tenderness. It is useful to assess hemodynamic status (hypotension or tachycardia can result from anemia from an occult GI bleed) and to test stool for guaiac positivity.

List the medications that can cause or exacerbate heartburn.

Medications can cause heartburn by a variety of mechanisms. Always review a patient's medication list to find common offenders. Look for:

Acarbose
α-receptor blockers
Anticholinergic agents
Benzodiazepines
β-blockers
Calcium channel blockers
Codeine
Erythromycin
Iron
Metformin
NSAIDs
Potassium
Prednisone
Progestins
Theophylline

Also discuss any use of herbal products, home remedies, and dietary supplements.

When is esophagogastroduodenoscopy (EGD) or pH monitoring necessary?

There is no gold standard for diagnosing heartburn, although 24-hour pH monitoring is accepted as standard for establishing or excluding its presence. While endoscopy lacks sensitivity for identifying pathologic reflux, it is useful in assessing esophageal complications of GERD. The following warning signs and symptoms suggest complicated GERD and should prompt endoscopic evaluation: dysphagia, early satiety, weight loss, guaiac positive stool, vomiting, iron deficiency anemia, or odynophagia.

What is the role of *Helicobacter pylori* testing?

Because *H. pylori* is a common cause of heartburn, serologic testing may be appropriate. Depending on the population, degree of heartburn, and the initial response to therapy, it may be reasonable to test for *H. pylori* and treat toward eradication if the test is positive. Newer guidelines suggest that a positive *H. pylori* titre should be followed by endoscopy, prior to treatment.

▶ TREATMENT

What treatment steps are appropriate for heartburn?

Lifestyle modifications, including diet, exercise, and smoking cessation where appropriate, are always recommended. Large meals, especially those containing acidic foods, alcohol, and caffeine, are to be avoided. Dietary fat should be decreased, and it is advisable to avoid lying down within three to four hours after a meal. Elevating the head of the bed 4–8 inches can also help with nocturnal symptoms.

What about medications?

While it is advisable to begin with lifestyle modifications, many clinicians prefer to begin with medical therapy. The preferred approach is step-up therapy: Initiate treatment with an H_2 receptor antagonist (H2RA), and maintain treatment once or twice daily for eight weeks. If symptoms do not improve, change to a proton-pump inhibitor (PPI). Step-down therapy is also an acceptable option where treatment begins with a PPI; it is then titrated down to the least expensive medication type and dose. In patients with erosive esophagitis identified on endoscopy, PPI is the initial therapy of choice.

What about surgical options?

Surgery, reserved for extreme cases, aims to reduce hiatal hernia, repair diaphragmatic hernia, or strengthen the gastroesophageal junction. Referral should be made by a GERD subspecialist, for patients who have reflux esophagitis documented by EGD and normal esophageal motility as evaluated by manometry. Surgical options include open and laparoscopic Nissen fundoplication. Newer endoscopic modalities are also available. These include the Stretta procedure (radiofrequency heating of the gastroesophageal junction) and the endocinch procedure (endoscopic gastroplasty).

KEY POINTS

- **GERD and cardiac ischemia can present with similar symptoms.**
- **Lifestyle modifications should always be offered as treatment for GERD.**
- **Step-up therapy with an H_2-blocker followed by a PPI is a reasonable, cost-effective approach to treatment of GERD.**

CASE 28–1. **A 46-year-old male smoker presents with a two-month history of midsternal burning, worse at night and worse following a large greasy meal. He has tried over-the-counter antacids without effect.**

A. What other historical information is important?
B. What initial recommendations would you have?

REFERENCES

Heidelbaugh JJ, Nostrant TT, Kim C, and Van Harrison R: Management of gastroesophageal reflux disease. Am Fam Physician, 68(7):1311–1318, 2003.

University of Michigan Health System. Management of Gastroesophageal Reflux Disease (GERD). Ann Arbor, Mich: University of Michigan Health System, 2002.

29

Dyslipidemia

▶ ETIOLOGY

What are the different types of lipids?

The major classes of lipids are low-density lipoprotein cholesterol (LDL-C), high-density lipoprotein cholesterol (HDL-C), and very low–density lipoprotein (VLDL), which primarily contains triglyceride (TG). Total cholesterol (TC) consists of 60% to 70% LDL-C, 20% to 30% HDL-C, and 10% to 15% VLDL.

Why are lipids important?

Dyslipidemia is a major risk factor for cardiovascular disease (CVD), including coronary heart disease (CHD), which is the number one cause of morbidity and mortality for both men and women in the United States. Elevated LDL-C is the major factor in the development of atherosclerosis, while a high HDL-C is protective. LDL-C levels less than 100 mg/dL are optimal. However, elevated triglycerides (≥150 mg/dL) and low HDL-C levels (<40 mg/dL) are also associated with increased risk and should be addressed.

What are the risk factors for CVD other than abnormal LDL-C?

The CVD risk factors are current cigarette smoking, hypertension (≥140/90 mmHg) or current treatment of hypertension, diabetes mellitus, HDL-C lower than 40 mg/dL, family history of premature CVD (father, brother, or son before age 55 and mother, sister, or daughter before age 65), male age 45 or older, and female age 55 or older. Obesity, physical inactivity, and an atherogenic diet are also risk factors but are not included in the lipid risk assessment. HDL-C of 60 or greater is a negative risk factor.

What are CHD risk equivalents?

Forms of atherosclerosis other than CHD are CHD risk equivalents, e.g., peripheral arterial disease (PAD), carotid artery stenosis (CAS), and abdominal aortic aneurysm (AAA). Because persons with type 2 diabetes mellitus have a 10-year risk of CHD close to the risk of CHD patients without diabetes mellitus, diabetes mellitus is included in this category. Other individuals without CVD or diabetes mellitus but who have multiple risk factors with a 10-year risk above 20% are also considered CHD risk equivalents.

▶ EVALUATION

Who should be screened and how often?

The National Cholesterol Education Program's Third Report of the Expert Panel on Detection, Evaluation, and Treatment of High Blood Cholesterol in Adults (Adult Treatment Panel III, or ATP III) recommends screening every five years starting at age 20. Other organizations, including the U.S. Preventive Services Task Force, recommend screening males starting at age 35 and females at age 45. High-risk individuals with normal lipids should be screened every one to two years starting at age 20.

What tests should be used for screening?

A lipid profile that includes TC, LDL-C, HDL-C, and TG should be obtained after a 9- to 12-hour fast. LDL-C is routinely calculated from measured levels of TC, HDL-C, and TG. However, a TG level above 400 mg/dL renders the calculation of LDL-C inaccurate. Abnormal tests should be repeated.

What is non–HDL-C and why is it important?

Non–HDL-C is TC minus HDL-C and can be obtained without fasting, making it a useful office test. LDL-C and TG are both very atherogenic, and non–HDL-C equals LDL-C in its CHD predictive value. If TC is above 200 mg/dL or the HDL is below 40 mg/dL when non–HDL-C is used for screening, a fasting lipid profile should be performed. Non–HDL-C can also be used for monitoring therapy in those patients with TG above 200 mg/dL. Non–HDL-C target values are 30 points higher than those for LDL-C.

What are abnormal and desirable levels of lipids?

See Table 29–1.

What evaluation is indicated to rule out secondary causes?

The more common secondary causes of dyslipidemia include diabetes mellitus, chronic renal failure, obstructive liver disease,

TABLE 29-1

Classification of Lipid Levels (mg/dL)

LDL-C		TC		HDL-C	
<100	Optimal	<200	Desirable		
100–129	Near/above optimal	200–239	Borderline high	≥60	High/protective
130–159	Borderline high	≥240	High	<40	Low
160–189	High				
≥190	Very high				

hypothyroidism, and drugs such as progestins, corticosteroids, anabolic steroids, and protease inhibitors.

How do I assess a patient's risk?

Risk assessment is a one-step or two-step process. First, the patient is classified to one of three categories of risk: CHD or CHD equivalent, multiple (two or more) risk factors, or zero to one risk factor. Those with zero to one risk factor do not require formal risk calculation because their 10-year risk is usually less than 10%, and risk calculation is not required for those with CHD or its equivalent because they are already at highest risk. However, for those with multiple risk factors a second step is required to classify them to one of three categories based on 10-year CHD risk assessment: greater than 20% risk (CHD risk equivalent); 10% to 20% risk; or less than 10% risk. The estimate of 10-year risk is based on Framingham data (the risk calculator is found online at the ATP III website; a downloadable Excel spreadsheet and a Palm version are also available).

What is the metabolic syndrome?

Metabolic syndrome is defined as three or more of the following: waist circumference greater than 40 inches for men and greater than 35 inches for women (central/abdominal obesity); TG 150 mg/dL or higher; blood pressure of 130/85 or higher or currently being treated; fasting glucose of 110 mg/dL or higher; or HDL-C less than 40 mg/dL in men and less than 50 mg/dL in women. Metabolic syndrome is associated with insulin resistance, inflammation, atherosclerosis, and impaired fibrin breakdown, resulting in increased incidence of CVD, diabetes, and death regardless of the LDL-C level.

▶ TREATMENT

What are the LDL-C goals of treatment?

The LDL-C goal for treatment varies by risk status (Table 29–2). The two major modes of treatment include therapeutic lifestyle changes (TLC) and medications.

What are therapeutic lifestyle changes (TLC)?

TLCs include reduced dietary intake of cholesterol and saturated fat, weight reduction, regular physical activity, and dietary enhancements (plant stanols/sterols and soluble fiber). TLCs also include reduction of other risk factors, e.g., tobacco cessation and blood pressure control. TLCs are followed for six weeks and if the desired LDL-C level is not achieved, TLCs are reinforced and intensified with dietician consultation. If after another six weeks the LDL-C goal is still not achieved, drug therapy should be considered.

What are the drug therapies?

Major classes of drugs include HMG CoA reductase inhibitors (statins), bile acid sequestrants, nicotinic acid, cholesterol absorption inhibitors, and fibric acid. All classes increase HDL-C and decrease LDL-C to varying degrees, while all but bile acid sequestrants lower triglycerides. Once drug therapy is started, the LDL-C should be measured in six weeks. If the LDL-C goal is not achieved, drug therapy can be intensified by increasing the dose or adding additional agents. After an additional six weeks, if the goal is reached the patient should be followed in four to six months. If the goal is not achieved, the drug therapy is adjusted or the patient is referred to a lipid specialist.

TABLE 29–2

LDL-C Goals* and Levels to Initiate TLC and Drug Therapy (mg/dL)

Risk Category	LDL Goal	Initiate TLC	Initiate Drug Rx
CHD risk equivalents (>20% 10-year risk)	<100	≥100	≥130 (100–129 optional)
Multiple (2+) risk factors (≤20% 10-year risk)	<130	≥130	≥130 (10-year risk 10% to 20%) ≥160 (10-year risk <10%)
Low risk (0–1 risk factors)	<160	≥160	≥190 (160–189 optional)

* Target goals for non–HDL-C are 30 points above the LDL-C targets.

KEY POINTS

- **Adults age 20 and older should have a CHD risk assessment and lipid screening every five years and more often if high risk.**
- **Persons with CVD of all kinds, diabetes, or a 10-year risk above 20% are considered CHD risk equivalents and their LDL-C goal is less than 100 mg/dL.**
- **Ten-year absolute CHD risk should be determined for persons without CHD risk equivalents who have two or more CHD risk factors.**
- **Fasting lipid profile or nonfasting non–HDL-C are both suitable screening tests.**
- **Secondary causes of dyslipidemia should be ruled out prior to treatment.**

CASE 29–1. **A 39-year-old man presents to your office for the first time. His father died recently of a myocardial infarction at age 64; he also had abnormal lipid levels. The patient would like to have his cholesterol checked. Vitals: height 68 inches, weight 168 lb, pulse 80, respirations 14, and blood pressure 122/86.**

A. What other questions should you ask to complete the patient's risk assessment?
B. Assuming that no other cardiovascular risk factors are identified, what is his CHD risk category?
C. If his LDL-C is measured at 145 mg/dL, what treatment, if any, is indicated?
D. How often should he be rescreened?

CASE 29–2. **A 50-year-old woman presents to the emergency department with marked fatigue and exertional dyspnea of one-week duration. Although she denies chest pain, an EKG and subsequent lab studies indicate she is having a myocardial infarction.**

A. Her initial LDL-C upon admission is 168 mg/dL, and a week after discharge it is 108 mg/dL. Which value is most indicative of the patient's true baseline value?
B. What is her LDL-C goal?
C. She has a 22-year-old son. What advice would you give him?

CASE 29–3. **A 66-year-old obese man returns to your office for follow-up. He smokes one pack of cigarettes per day and takes a diuretic for hypertension (blood pressure today is 122/78). You obtain nonfasting lipids with the following results: TC 266 mg/dL and HDL-C 30 mg/dL. You calculate his 10-year risk at 29%.**

A. What is his non–HDL-C? Should you order fasting lipids?
B. What is his LDL-C goal? What would his LDL-C goal be if his 10-year risk is 19%?
C. Would you start drug therapy?
D. What common secondary causes of dyslipidemia should be ruled out in this patient?

CASE 29–4. **A 40-year-old woman is identified as having metabolic syndrome (three or more of the following: waist circumference greater than 35 inches, TG above 150 mg/dL, HDL-C less than 40 mg/dL, blood pressure of 130/85 or above, and fasting glucose of 110 mg/dL or above).**

A. What are the two first-line therapies for this condition?
B. This patient's LDL-C is 110 mg/dL. Does that reduce the patient's CHD risk?
C. What drug therapies would be indicated for this patient?

USEFUL WEBSITES

The National Cholesterol Education Program's (NCEP) Third Report of the Expert Panel on Detection, Evaluation, and Treatment of High Blood Cholesterol in Adults
http://www.nhlbi.nih.gov/guidelines/cholesterol/index.htm

U.S. Preventive Services Task Force, 3rd ed.
http://www.ahrq.gov/clinic/uspstfix.htm

30

Hypertension

▶ ETIOLOGY

What is hypertension?

Hypertension is a term that refers to high blood pressure. It is not a distinct disease but rather a chronic condition that confers increased risk for untoward cardiovascular events. Hypertension as defined by the Joint National Committee on the Detection, Evaluation, and Treatment of Hypertension—version 7 (JNC-7) is a blood pressure of 140 mmHg or higher systolic or 90 mmHg or higher diastolic (Table 30–1). The diagnosis is made following two confirmatory readings on two separate occasions with readings in each arm.

Hypertension is a major contributor to the development of coronary artery disease (CAD), congestive heart failure (CHF), stroke, and kidney failure. It affects approximately 50 million Americans, with 30% of them unaware of their diagnosis, 60% in treatment, and only about 35% in good control of the problem. At 55 years of age the projected lifetime risk of developing hypertension is 90%. Hypertension is the reason for nearly 10% of all primary care office visits; it is the most common reason for which people see a doctor.

What are the causes of hypertension?

Primary or essential hypertension accounts for 90% of patients and has no identifiable cause. Primary hypertension commonly occurs in the setting of specific comorbidities such as insulin resistance, lipid abnormalities, and abdominal obesity (the metabolic syndrome). An unrecognized neuroendocrine abnormality may be the root cause. In secondary hypertension (10%), a specific diagnosis can be identified as the underlying cause. These include kidney disease, renovascular disease, pheochromocytoma, disorders of cortisol (Cushing's syndrome), hyperaldosteronism, coarctation of the aorta, sleep apnea syndrome, parathyroid or thyroid disorders, and the effects of therapeutic or illicit drugs. Renovascular disease is the most common secondary cause of hypertension.

TABLE 30-1

Classification of Blood Pressure

BP Classification	Systolic BP (mmHg)		Diastolic BP (mmHg)
Normal blood pressure	<120	and	<80
Prehypertension	120–139	or	80–89
Stage 1 hypertension	140–159	or	90–99
Stage 2 hypertension	≥160	or	≥100

From the Joint National Committee on the Detection, Evaluation, and Treatment of Hypertension–version 7, 2004.

What is the pathophysiology of hypertension?

A number of complex neural and humoral pathways are involved in the regulation of blood pressure. Some of the better understood pathways include the sympathetic nervous system and the rennin–angiotensin–aldosterone system. These neurohormonal systems exert their influence on regulation of intravascular volume, vascular smooth muscle tone, and cardiac output. Individual patients often experience a combination of these factors. Medication treatments are aimed at each of these pathways.

▶ EVALUATION

What are the important components of the history and physical in hypertension?

A careful history and physical exam may identify signs and symptoms that indicate the presence of end-organ damage, comorbid diagnoses, or underlying diseases that are secondary causes of hypertension. The report of visual changes, neurologic deficits, angina, claudication, dyspnea, and lower extremity swelling could all indicate advanced neurologic and vascular complications of hypertension. Episodic pallor and palpitations suggest pheochromocytoma, whereas central weight gain, polyuria, and polydipsia could indicate new onset of diabetes or Cushing's syndrome. Use of particular prescribed or over-the-counter pharmaceuticals or illicit drugs may explain elevation of blood pressure.

The physical examination should be focused on relevant organ systems to evaluate end-organ damage, comorbid diagnoses, or underlying secondary hypertension. Areas of interest include the eyes for retinopathy or papillaedema; the cardiopulmonary system for signs of ventricular enlargement, heart failure, or atherosclerotic disease; the abdomen for aortic aneurysm or renal artery stenosis; neurologic and mental status exams for signs of encephalopathy or stroke; and general appearance for the characteristic round face, central obesity, and striae of Cushing's syndrome.

Which tests should I order to evaluate a patient with hypertension?

Initial lab tests are focused on revealing end-organ damage, secondary causes, and comorbid conditions that would benefit from treatment to lower a patient's overall risk.

Patients with an established diagnosis of hypertension need monitoring for effects of treatment and disease on target organs as well as medication side effects. Routine recommended laboratory tests include a hematocrit, serum potassium, creatinine, glucose, calcium, fasting lipid profile, urinalysis, and an electrocardiogram.

When is hypertension an emergency?

Hypertensive emergencies are defined as very high blood pressures that occur in the setting of life-threatening or organ-threatening conditions and require immediate and accurate control, perhaps with intravenous drug therapy. Stroke, pulmonary edema, myocardial ischemia, dissecting aortic aneurysm, retinal hemorrhages, and acute renal failure are examples of these conditions. Hypertensive encephalopathy is the finding of papillaedema and mental status changes in the setting of severely elevated blood pressure and is also considered a hypertensive emergency.

Patients with severely elevated blood pressure that has developed gradually over time and who are not showing signs of acute end-organ damage may actually be harmed if their blood pressure is rapidly lowered to normal levels. These patients can be started on antihypertensive medication and followed as outpatients. Studies have shown that the use of non-dihydropyridine calcium channel blockers to rapidly lower blood pressure in patients with coronary disease increases the rate of acute coronary events and death.

▶ TREATMENT

What recommendations should be given to all patients with hypertension?

While the majority of patients with hypertension require prescription medication, therapeutic lifestyle changes alone can lower blood pressure and reduce the dosage requirement for patients taking antihypertensive medication (Table 30–2). Therapeutic lifestyle changes include habitual aerobic activity for at least 30 minutes most days of the week, maintenance of body mass index (BMI) less than 25, limiting salt intake to 6 g daily (2 g of sodium), and limiting

TABLE 30-2

Initial Treatment Recommendations for Blood Pressure	
Initial Treatment for Patients without Compelling Indications	
Prehypertension	**Lifestyle Modifications**
Stage 1 hypertension	Lifestyle modifications + single drug therapy
Stage 2 hypertension	Lifestyle modifications + two-drug combination
Initial Treatment for Patients with Compelling Indications	
Prehypertension	**Lifestyle Modifications + Specific Drug**
Stage 1 hypertension	Lifestyle modifications + specific drug +/– second drug
Stage 2 hypertension	Lifestyle modifications + specific drug + second drug

From the Joint National Committee on the Detection, Evaluation, and Treatment of Hypertension–version 7, 2004.

consumption of alcohol to two equivalents daily for men and one equivalent daily for women. Additionally, patients should be educated as to the early warning signs of heart attack and stroke.

What are the goals of treating hypertension?

The ultimate goal of treating hypertension is to lower the risk of death and end-organ disease such as heart failure, coronary disease, stroke, and kidney failure. The short-term goal is to lower the risk of these adverse clinical outcomes by achieving blood pressure levels below 140/90 mmHg. In certain high-risk conditions such as diabetes and chronic renal disease, the short-term goal is to achieve an even lower blood pressure (<130/80 mmHg). "Ideal" blood pressure is lower than 120/80 mmHg. For every mmHg above that level there is a measurable increase in the risk of end-organ disease. In patients with stage 1 hypertension (SBP 140–159 mmHg and/or DBP 90–99 mmHg) and the presence of CVD or target organ damage, achieving a sustained 12 mmHg reduction in SBP over 10 years will prevent one death for every nine patients treated.

When should I prescribe medication for treating hypertension?

Patients with no additional risk factors, no evidence of end-organ damage, and JNC-7 stage 1 hypertension should try 12 months of lifestyle modifications before medication is prescribed. Patients at high risk are candidates for medications at lower blood pressure levels. Compelling risk factors include high coronary artery risk, previous myocardial infarction, CHF, diabetes, chronic renal failure, and previous stroke. Patients with compelling indications or with JNC-7 stage 2 or higher blood pressure should be considered for medication in addition to lifestyle modifications at the time of diagnosis.

Which medications are the best to use in the treatment of hypertension?

There are many studies evaluating the ability of medications to lower blood pressure and more importantly to lower the development of end-organ damage. Generally the medications fall into six categories: (1) thiazide diuretics, (2) β-adrenergic blockers, (3) angiotensin converting enzyme inhibitors (ACE-I) and the similar angiotensin receptor blockers (ARB), (4) calcium channel blockers (CCB), (5) aldosterone antagonists, and (6) α-adrenergic blockers. The largest and most enduring body of evidence demonstrating favorable effects on clinically significant endpoints exists for thiazide diuretics and β-adrenergic blockers. This has led to the recommendation to use these agents, particularly thiazide diuretics, as the first line of treatment for uncomplicated hypertension in the general population.

Certain comorbid conditions also respond favorably to specific classes of antihypertensive medications, and in these situations a single medication can be favored for first-line treatment for both. Examples include treatment of hypertension with ACE-I in diabetic nephropathy and heart failure and treatment with β-blockers in CAD. Aside from these guidelines, the best medication is the one that the patient can afford and will take regularly without experiencing unwanted adverse effects while achieving the target blood pressure goal.

What should I consider when the target blood pressure goal is not reached?

It is always important to ascertain that the patient is able to adhere to therapeutic lifestyle changes and the prescribed medication regimen before considering a change in medication. It has been well demonstrated that patients typically need to take an average of 2.7 medications to achieve blood pressure goals. Lower doses of several drugs used in combination are preferable to higher doses of a single drug. Used in this manner it has been shown that blood pressure reduction is additive while adverse effects are minimized. When a patient requires many drugs in combination at high doses, consider searching for a secondary cause of hypertension, particularly if the blood pressure goal had been achieved previously.

When should I refer a patient to a hypertension specialist?

Refer to a consultant with expertise in the management of hypertension when significant progress toward achieving treatment goal blood pressure is not made despite the use of three antihypertensive agents, prescribed in adequate doses, including a thiazide diuretic. This is known as *resistant hypertension*. However, thoroughly review appropriate adherence to prescribed lifestyle changes and drug regimens prior to a referral. When there is a strong suspicion of a secondary cause of hypertension, a specialty referral can facilitate completion of the most cost-effective evaluation and appropriate treatment plan.

KEY POINTS

- **Treating hypertension significantly reduces mortality and morbidity such as stroke, heart disease, and renal failure.**
- **Evaluation should be focused on identifying secondary causes of hypertension as well as comorbid conditions and target organ damage.**
- **Therapeutic lifestyle changes are indicated for all patients with hypertension, including those who require medications.**
- **Thiazide diuretics are the preferred first line of drug therapy for most patients. An average of 2.7 medications is required to ultimately achieve control.**
- **Patients with higher stages of hypertension or end-organ damage may require combination drug therapy initially.**
- **Consider a secondary cause of hypertension when patients require multiple medications to achieve control even if achieved previously.**

CASE 30–1. **A 45-year-old man comes in for a hand rash and is noted to have a blood pressure of 150/98 mmHg. He has no other significant medical history. He is taking no medications. Vital signs are otherwise normal. He appears well and comfortable. Skin examination reveals a mild contact dermatitis. Auscultation of the chest reveals a normal S1 and S2 with no murmur or gallop and clear lung fields bilaterally. There is no pedal edema.**

A. What is the next diagnostic step that should be undertaken?
B. What other history and physical findings would be most helpful?
C. Which tests should be ordered?
D. How will you treat this patient?

CASE 30–2. **A 55-year-old woman with a 10-year history of well-controlled hypertension comes to the office for a periodic management visit. She has no complaints. Her medication list consists of only HCTZ 25 mg daily. On exam she appears well, with blood pressure of 165/100 mmHg taken appropriately and confirmed, pulse 80, respirations 16. Heart exam reveals an S4 gallop. Lungs are clear to auscultation.**

A. What should you do next?
B. What new diagnoses should be considered to explain her elevated blood pressure?
C. What would be the next step in managing her hypertension?

REFERENCES

Furberg CD, Wright JT: The Antihypertensive and Lipid-Lowering Treatment to Prevent Heart Attack Trial (ALLHAT). JAMA 288:2981–2997, 2002.

National Institutes of Health; National Heart, Lung, and Blood Institute. The Seventh Report of the Joint National Committee on Prevention, Detection, Evaluation and Treatment of High Blood Pressure (JNC-7). 2004. Available at http://www.nhlbi.nih.gov/guidelines/hypertension.

31

Lower Extremity Pain and Swelling

▶ ETIOLOGY

What are the most common causes of leg pain?

A variety of conditions can cause leg pain; incidence varies depending on age group. Common causes of leg pain include the following:

Skin *infections* are most commonly caused by *Staphylococcus* or *Streptococcus*. Diabetics are at risk of more sinister infections, such as *Pseudomonas*. Patients who have had problems with venous stasis are at risk of recurrent cellulitis, owing to damage to the valves in the veins.

Joints damaged by *osteoarthritis* tend to fluctuate in the amount of swelling, redness, and pain exhibited. Usually the patient is more uncomfortable after unusually vigorous physical activity or with prolonged inactivity. A popliteal cyst is lined with synovial tissue and filled with fluid from the knee joint; it may appear slowly or suddenly without history of trauma.

Thrombophlebitis involves thrombus (clot) and phlebitis (inflammation). Deep vein thrombosis (DVT) should be suspected when a patient has unilateral leg swelling. Often the thrombus is accompanied by phlebitis, which causes localized pain and redness. It is imperative to determine whether the thrombus is deep or superficial because of the risk of pulmonary embolus from clots in the leg in DVT. DVT in the thigh is of concern when the clot propagates proximally.

Trauma can cause a fracture or soft-tissue injuries such as a sprain (injury to ligaments), strain (injury to tendons), or shin splints (microtears in the pretibial muscles). These are especially likely to happen in athletes and "weekend warriors." Soft-tissue injuries can be as painful and disabling as fractures. If the person does not remember a specific injury, inquire about repetitive activities, such as an activity at work, exercising, or household chores, which may be aggravating the original injury.

Primary bone *tumors* are more likely in children, while metastatic disease is much more likely in adults.

▶ EVALUATION

What are important points in the history?

Important questions to ask when evaluating lower extremity pain and swelling include: How long have the pain and swelling been present? Did the pain and swelling start simultaneously? Was the onset sudden or gradual? Was there any history of trauma before the symptoms started? What helps or aggravates the condition? What did the pain feel like initially versus now? Rate the pain on a scale of 0 to 10.

What are important features on physical exam?

Look for swelling, tenderness, discoloration, and/or warmth. If pitting edema is present, consider venous stasis, congestive heart failure, or kidney failure. If the discoloration is a result of trauma, it can range from blue (early) to green to brown. Infection generally causes red discoloration and may have a distinct border. Gangrene may be red, black, or white. Increased warmth may occur with infection or superficial phlebitis.

How is thrombophlebitis diagnosed?

DVT should be considered when there is the sudden onset of swelling in one leg and/or the patient is very tender along the saphenous or femoral vein. The presence of a positive Homan's sign (pain in the posterior calf with dorsiflexion of the ipsilateral foot) is also strongly suggestive of phlebitis. The clinical suspicion should be confirmed by a radiologic study, usually a venous ultrasound. Superficial phlebitis can occur in any vein. It often presents with localized redness and tenderness, and a negative Homan's sign.

What if there is no visible swelling or discoloration?

The fact that the patient is complaining of pain signals that something is amiss. Consider a trial of anti-inflammatory medication and reevaluate in two to four weeks. Remember that hip pathology may present as knee pain because of the distribution of L4 nerve branches. Discogenic pain from the back generally follows a nerve-root distribution and is reproducibly aggravated by certain maneuvers. Peripheral arterial disease can cause claudication in which the pain escalates in the lower extremity with physical activity and resolves with rest; peripheral pulses will be difficult to palpate.

▶ TREATMENT

What medications are appropriate?

Pain from *acute trauma* is often quite severe initially but will improve with protection of the injured area and pain control. The Cox-II nonsteroidals often provide analgesia as effective as narcotics without the side effects of narcotics (sedation and constipation) or the Cox-I agents (indigestion, GI bleeds). Acetaminophen is helpful in milder injuries or when the patient cannot tolerate other medications. If the medications are needed on a chronic basis, kidney function should be monitored with a Cox-I and liver enzymes with acetaminophen.

Anti-inflammatory medication (Cox-I or -II) is very helpful in *superficial phlebitis*. *Deep vein thrombosis* has traditionally been treated with IV heparin until the Coumadin level becomes therapeutic. The advent of low-molecular-weight heparin (such as Lovenox) has made it possible to treat patients largely on an outpatient basis. The Coumadin is continued for six weeks with the international normalized ratio (INR) maintained in the range of 2 to 2.5. Patients who have had more than one DVT (unrelated to surgery or pregnancy) should probably be on long-term anticoagulation. These people may do well with an INR of 1.5 to 2 and will have significantly less risk of a bleed from the Coumadin.

Penicillins or cephalosporins are recommended for *skin infections* caused by *Staphylococcus* or *Streptococcus*. If the patient is allergic to these medications, consider a macrolide or a quinolone with gram-positive coverage.

When should the injured site be immobilized?

It is sometimes very difficult to determine whether the injury involves only soft tissue damage or an actual fracture. In those situations it is wise to treat the injury like a broken bone for one to two weeks. If localized pain persists, consider repeating the x-rays at least 10 days later, looking for callus formation at the site of the fracture. Refer to an orthopedist as soon as possible if the fracture is accompanied by an open wound or if there is significant misalignment of the bone fragments.

What are pitfalls to avoid in treatment?

If a fracture has occurred, be sure the patient understands that he/she has a "broken bone." Tell the patient with a sprain or strain that the injury will probably take as long as a broken bone to completely heal. If pain or swelling escalates, reevaluate the situation promptly to be sure the neurovascular supply has not been compromised. Avoid extended immobilization of a soft-tissue injury; an orthopedist or a physical therapist can provide guidance on this. Ongoing use of narcotics is likely to cause dependence.

KEY POINTS

- **It is imperative to diagnose deep vein thrombosis (DVT) because of the risk of pulmonary embolus. Be especially suspicious of a DVT when there is sudden unilateral leg swelling.**
- **The diagnosis of DVT is usually confirmed by ultrasonography.**
- **Treatment of DVT involves anticoagulation with some form of heparin until the Coumadin level becomes therapeutic.**
- **Reassess if the problem does not improve as anticipated. Do not be afraid to consult!**
- **Avoid prolonged immobilization of soft-tissue injuries.**
- **Avoid prolonged use of narcotics.**

CASE 31–1. **A 42-year-old woman presents to the office with a two-day history of left lower extremity pain and swelling. She has recently returned from a business trip where she flew across the country. On exam she has erythema of the left lower leg and it measures 2 cm larger at the midcalf than the right leg. Her left calf is tender when squeezed on exam.**

A. What is the likely cause of this patient's pain and swelling?
B. What testing would be helpful?
C. How should this patient be treated?

CASE 31–2. **A 62-year-old diabetic presents with a three-day history of redness and warmth in the right lower leg. He notes that his blood sugars have been running "high" for the past week. The patient recalls scratching his leg on a bench in the park one week ago.**

A. What is the likely diagnosis?
B. How would you treat this problem?

REFERENCES

Fredericson M: Differential diagnosis of leg pain in the athlete. J Am Podiatr Med Assoc 93(4):321–324, 2003.

Hyers TM: Management of venous thromboembolism: Past, present, and future. Arch Int Med 163(7):759–768, 2003.

Nutescu EA: Hospital guidelines for use of low molecular weight heparin. Ann Pharmaco Ther 37(7–8):1072–1081, 2003.

32

Lymphadenopathy

▶ ETIOLOGY

What is lymphadenopathy?

Lymphadenopathy is enlargement of lymph nodes; the nodes are abnormal in size, consistency, or number. The body has approximately 600 lymph nodes, but only those in the cervical, axillary, or inguinal regions are palpable in healthy people as a normal finding. Lymphadenopathy may be an incidental finding on exam or may be a presenting sign or symptom to a patient's illness. Lymph nodes in children can be palpated as early as the neonatal period. With subsequent antigenic exposure, lymphoid tissue continues to enlarge through puberty. As a result, most normal children have palpable cervical, inguinal, and axillary lymphadenopathy.

The most important factor in evaluating patients with lymphadenopathy is to determine whether it is caused by a benign, self-limited condition or by a malignancy.

What is the pathogenesis of lymphadenopathy?

The following mechanisms result in lymphadenopathy:

- Lymphocyte proliferation or macrophage hyperplasia in response to an antigenic interaction
- Infiltration by metastatic malignant cells
- Neoplastic proliferation of malignant lymphocytes or phagocytes

How is lymphadenopathy classified?

Lymphadenopathy can be classified as generalized or localized:

Generalized: If lymph nodes are enlarged in two or more noncontiguous areas, it is usually the result of a systemic disease.
Localized: Only one area is involved; the enlargement is caused by local infection, tumor, or systemic disease.

What are the causes of lymphadenopathy?

See Box 32–1.

BOX 32–1

Causes of Lymphadenopathy

Infections (most common cause)

Bacterial: Group A streptococci, staphylococcus, cat scratch disease, syphilis
Mycobacterial: Tuberculosis, atypical mycobacterial infection, leprosy
Viral: Infectious mononucleosis (EBV), cytomegalovirus, HIV/AIDS, hepatitis B, measles, rubeola
Fungal: Histoplasmosis, coccidiomycosis
Parasitic: Toxoplasmosis, filariasis, trypanosomiasis
Chlamydial: Lymphogranuloma venereum

Collagen vascular disorders

Systemic lupus erythematosus, rheumatoid arthritis

Endocrine disorders

Hyperthyroidism, adrenal insufficiency, thyroiditis

Malignant disorders

Leukemia, non-Hodgkin's lymphoma, Hodgkin's disease, Waldenström's macroglobulinemia, multiple myeloma with amyloidosis, malignant histiocytosis, and metastasis (breast, lung, head and neck carcinoma, gastrointestinal malignancies)

Hypersensitivity states

Serum sickness, drug reactions (phenytoin, hydralazine, allopurinol, propylthiouracil, others)

Miscellaneous

Sarcoidosis, amyloidosis, Kawasaki disease

▶ EVALUATION

How do I evaluate lymphadenopathy?

History and physical exam play a key role in evaluation. In most cases, a careful history and physical exam will identify a readily diagnosable cause of lymphadenopathy.

What are the key questions to ask in the history?

- What is the onset, duration, and rate of growth of all palpable nodes?

- Is the node tender?
- Is there a history of recent infections and trauma?
- Are there constitutional symptoms of weight loss, night sweats, and fatigue?
- Is the patient on any medication (that could cause lymph node enlargement)?
- Has the patient been exposed to animals?
- Has there been recent travel, substance abuse, or sexual exposure?
- What is the past medical, family, and occupational history?

What type of exam should I perform?

Examination of the lymph nodes involves inspection and palpation. Large lymph nodes may be clearly visible on inspection. It is important to inspect the draining area when you discover an enlarged node for evidence of infection, skin lesion, or tumors (Table 32–1). Also examine other nodal sites to exclude the possibility of generalized lymphadenopathy. Use your fingertips to palpate the regional nodes. Feel the nodes by applying moderate pressure over the region and moving your fingers in an attempt to feel the node/nodes slipping under your fingers.

What are the common lymph nodes?

See Table 32–1.

TABLE 32–1

Lymph Nodes with Lymphatic Drainage

Nodes	Lymphatic Drainage
Preauricular nodes	Temporal region, eyelids, and conjunctiva
Postauricular	External auditory meatus, pinna scalp
Submandibular nodes	Tongue, submaxillary gland, lips, and mouth cavity
Submental	Lower lip, floor of mouth, tip of tongue, skin of cheek
Posterior cervical nodes	Scalp, neck, skin of arms and pectoralis, thorax, cervical and axillary nodes
Anterior cervical nodes	Larynx, tongue, oropharynx, anterior neck
Suboccipital nodes	Posterior scalp and neck
Supraclavicular nodes	GI tract, GU tract, pulmonary
Axillary nodes	Breast, upper extremity and thoracic wall
Epitrochlear nodes	Ulnar forearm, hand
Inguinal nodes	Lower abdomen, external genitalia, anal canal, lower one third of vagina, lower extremity

What are the characteristics to note during exam?

The nodes should be assessed for location, length, width, consistency (soft, firm, rubbery, hard, craggy), tenderness, and mobility or fixity to surrounding nodes and tissue.

Location: It is important to examine the draining area and other nodal sites to rule out generalized lymphadenopathy. (See Table 32–1.)

Size: In general, a lymph node is considered enlarged if it measures more than 1 cm in its longest diameter. There are two exceptions to this rule: Epitrochlear nodes greater than 0.5 cm in diameter are considered abnormal and, in the inguinal region only nodes greater than 1.5 cm are considered abnormal.

Consistency: In reactive lymphadenopathy, the nodes are usually discrete and rubbery. In metastatic cancer, the nodes are hard. Very firm rubbery nodes usually suggest lymphoma. In pathologic lymphadenopathy, node consistency may not be helpful in distinguishing between benign and malignant lesion.

Tenderness: Pain is usually from stretching of the capsule caused by the rapidly enlarging lymph node, and it can be caused by inflammation or hemorrhage into the necrotic center of a malignant node. Painful tender nodes usually indicate infection, which may or may not be hidden from obvious view (e.g., inguinal lymphadenopathy from infected cracks between toes and axillary lymphadenopathy from infections of the hand). In *lymphadenitis,* nodes are enlarged and tender and overlying skin may be red and inflamed. In *lymphaginitis,* superficial vessels leading to group of nodes are inflamed and channels can be seen as thin red streaks leading from a more distal side of inflammation.

Mobility and Fixity: Reactive lymph nodes are usually mobile and rubbery. Metastatic lymph nodes are matted and fixed. For example, metastatic disease, Hodgkin's disease, and tuberculosis can be associated with rock-hard nodules but can also present with soft nodes.

▶ TREATMENT

How should I treat lymphadenopathy?

Evaluation forms an important basis for treatment. Treatment is guided by careful history and diagnosis of the cause of lymphadenopathy (Figure 32–1). When the history and physical exam is diagnostic (e.g., streptococcal pharyngitis), provide treatment. If the exam is suggestive of a particular disease, perform the required diagnostic tests (e.g., RPR for syphilis or monospot for infectious mononucleosis). When exam results are negative, look for

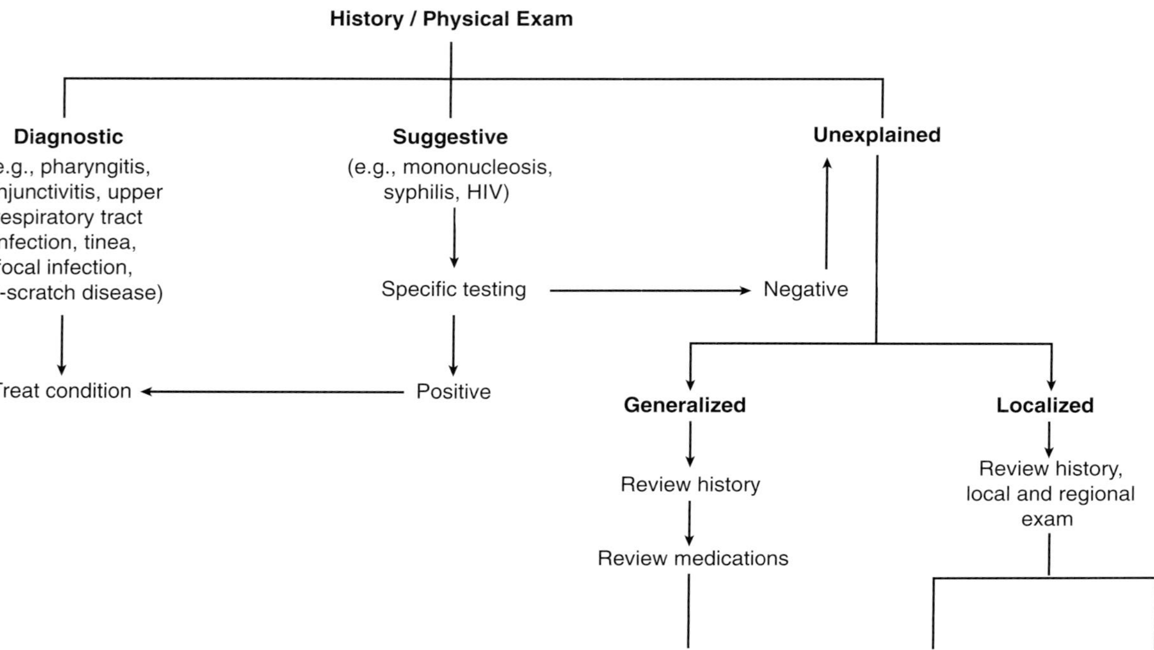
History / Physical Exam
Diagnostic
(e.g., pharyngitis, conjunctivitis, upper respiratory tract infection, tinea, focal infection, cat-scratch disease)
Suggestive
(e.g., mononucleosis, syphilis, HIV)
Unexplained
Specific testing
Negative
Treat condition
Positive
Generalized
Localized
Review history
Review history, local and regional exam
Review medications

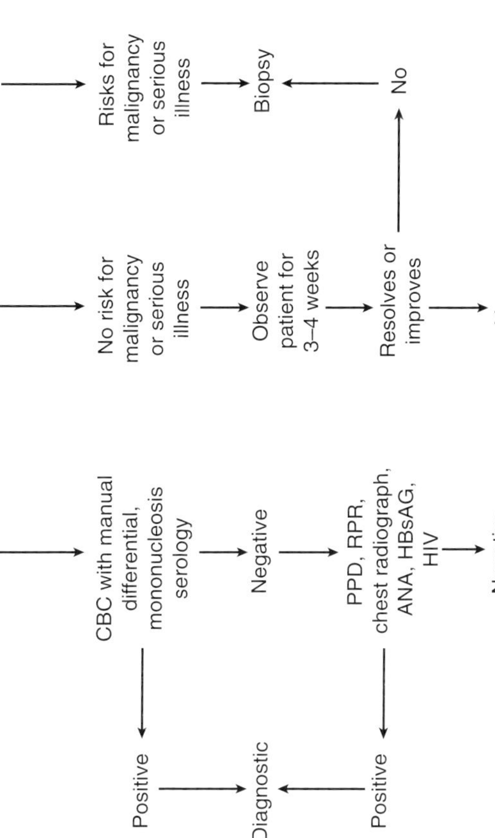

Figure 32–1. Algorithm for approach of a patient with lymphadenopathy. (From Ferrer R: Differential diagnosis and evaluation. Am Fam Physician, 58(6):1315, 1998.)

HIV = human immunodeficiency virus; CBC = complete blood count; PPD = purified protein derivative, RPR = rapid plasma regain; ANA = antinuclear body; HbsAg = hepatitis B surface antigen.

unexplained lymphadenopathy. It is prudent to observe for three to four weeks if the setting suggests a high probability of benign disease and there is no evidence to support use of a short course of antibiotics or corticosteroids.

KEY POINTS

- **Although the prevalence of malignancy in patients presenting with lymphadenopathy in the primary care setting is very low, careful history and physical are vital for evaluation of lymphadenopathy.**
- **Key risk factors for malignancy are duration greater than two weeks, age, firm fixed nodes, and supraclavicular presentation.**
- **Supraclavicular lymphadenopathy has the highest risk of malignancy.**
- **Excisional biopsy is the initial diagnostic procedure of choice.**
- **When the clinical case suggests a benign unexplained cause of lymphadenopathy, it is prudent to observe for three to four weeks.**

CASE 32–1. **A 20-year-old man has a two-day history of fever, headache, sore throat, and lumps in his neck. On exam, he is alert. His vitals are temperature 38.8°C, respirations 16, pulse 110, and blood pressure 110/80. Examination of the patient's neck reveals bilateral anterior cervical lymphadenopathy. His posterior pharynx is erythematous with tonsillar exudate.**

A. What is your diagnosis?
B. What would you do next?

CASE 32–2. **A 16-year-old boy is in your office with his father for a history of significant swelling in the left supraclavicular area that has been present for approximately three to four months. The patient denies any significant change in size over time. He denies history of fever, chills, nausea, vomiting, fatigue or malaise, weight loss, or other symptoms. On exam, the abdomen is soft with no enlarged liver or spleen. A mass measuring 2.5 cm by 1.5 cm is felt attached to the area above the left clavicle. Examination of other lymph nodes does not show any significant enlargement.**

A. What is the first step in evaluation of this patient?
B. What is the most likely diagnosis?

REFERENCE

Ferrer R: Lymphadenopathy: Differential diagnosis and evaluation. Am Fam Physician 58:1315, 1998.

Uphold CR, Graham MV: Clinical Guidelines in Family Practice, 3rd Edition. Gainesville, Florida: Barmarrae Books, 1999.

USEFUL WEBSITE

American Academy of Family Physicians. *http://www.aafp.com*

33

Rashes

▶ ETIOLOGY

What are the most common causes of acute skin rashes?

Most acute skin rashes are caused by allergies, infections, or acne-related disorders. Allergies may lead to atopic dermatitis, contact dermatitis, drug reactions, eczema, and urticaria. Infections can be divided into viral, bacterial, and fungal infections. Viral-induced rashes can be exanthems such as measles and rubella or be actual viral skin infections such as herpes simplex or chickenpox. Bacterial skin infections are usually caused by *Streptococcus pyogenes* or *Staphylococcus aureus*. Fungal infections can literally cause infections from head to toe and include ringworm (tinea) and athlete's foot (tinea pedis). Infestations include lice or scabies. Acne and related conditions include rosacea and hidradenitis suppurativa (recurrent inflammatory nodules in the axilla and groin).

Give some descriptive examples of acute rashes.

Atopic dermatitis is a type of eczematous eruption that is itchy, recurrent, symmetric, and often found on flexural surfaces. It can appear as an acute rash when it first starts or when an exacerbation occurs. Patients with this condition often have either a personal or a family history of asthma, allergic rhinitis, or conjunctivitis. In infancy, atopic dermatitis often appears on the face. After infancy, the dry, scaling, and red lesions are found in flexural areas such as the antecubital or popliteal fossa.

Contact dermatitis is an allergic response to an allergen such as a chemical found in the poison ivy or poison oak plant (rhus dermatitis). These lesions are often linear and vesicular (Figure 33–1). Other contact allergens include nickel in jewelry and belt buckles and chemicals in deodorants.

Urticaria is the medical term for hives. A hive or wheal is an erythematous, skin-colored or white, nonpitting, edematous plaque that changes in size and shape by peripheral extension or regression during a few hours or days that the individual lesion exists. These wheals are usually pruritic but do not have to itch. Urticaria can be found anywhere on the body and is often on the trunk and extremities (Figure 33–2). Acute urticaria is defined as urticaria lasting

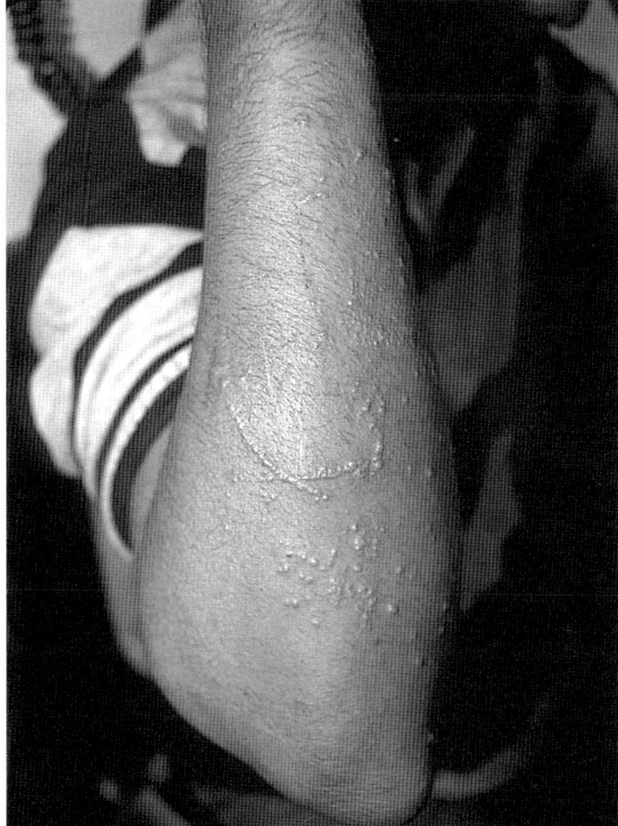

Figure 33–1. Poison oak on the arm with vesicles following a linear pattern.

less than six weeks. Occasionally a person will continue to have urticaria for many years.

What are the serious causes of rashes that I should not miss?

Fortunately most skin conditions are not life threatening. However, *necrotizing fasciitis* (flesh-eating bacteria) can be both life- and limb-threatening. Patients with necrotizing fasciitis usually appear quite ill and have fever and pain in the affected area. There is often diffuse swelling of the arm or leg, which may be followed by bullae with clear fluid that becomes violaceous in color. This may lead to cutaneous gangrene, myonecrosis, and shock. Necrotizing fasciitis

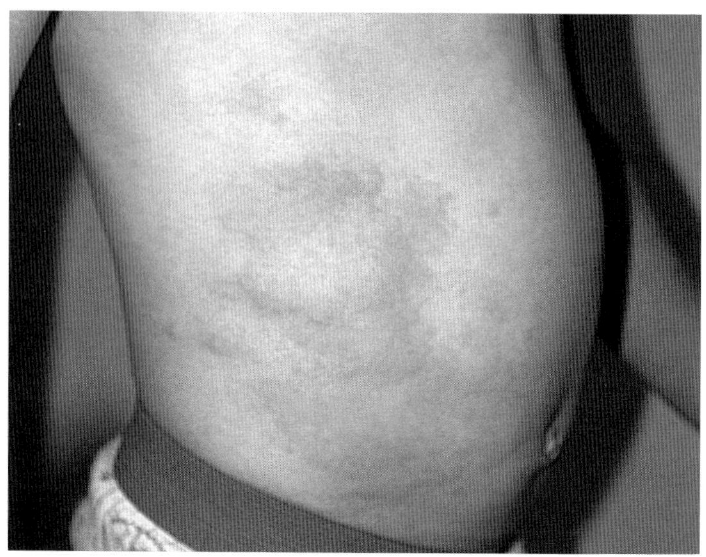

Figure 33–2. Uticaria (hives) on the trunk of a young boy.

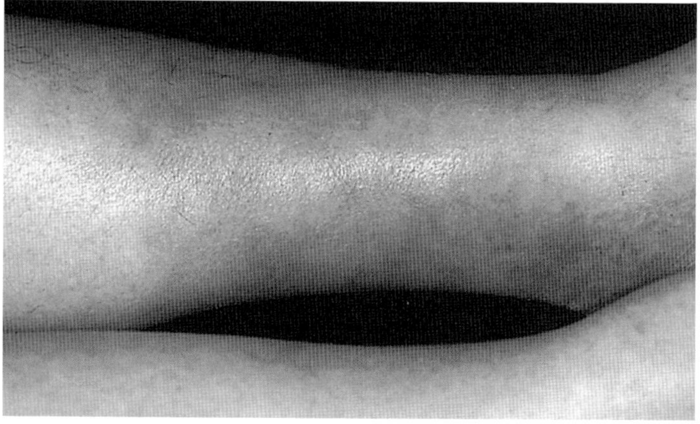

Figure 33–3. Cellulitis on the lower leg.

may look like cellulitis at first but necrotizing fasciitis requires surgical debridement along with antibiotics. Even *cellulitis* should not be missed and can be dangerous. Cellulitis can be well treated with oral or parenteral antibiotics (Figure 33–3).

Erythema multiforme (EM) major is a dangerous type of allergic hypersensitivity reaction that occurs in response to medications, infections, or illness. It occurs primarily in children and young adults. EM minor may present with a classic "target lesion" with or without systemic symptoms. EM major (Stevens-Johnson syndrome) is characterized by involvement of the mucous membranes, multiple body areas, and severe systemic symptoms. Patients may need hospitalization for fluids and support.

Other potentially dangerous conditions include skin cancers, pustular psoriasis, disseminated zoster, angioedema, and pemphigus vulgaris. Also do not miss the diagnosis of STDs such as syphilis or gonorrhea, which may present with a rash.

Give some examples of chronic rashes.

Psoriasis is a chronic condition characterized by epidermal proliferation and inflammation. The lesions are well-circumscribed, red, scaling patches, with white thickened scales. Areas affected can include the scalp, nails, and extensor surfaces of limbs, elbows, knees, the sacral region, and the genitalia. Psoriasis lesions may also be guttate as in water drops, inverse when found in intertriginous areas such as the inguinal and intergluteal folds, or volar when found on the palms or soles (Figure 33–4).

Seborrhea is a superficial inflammatory dermatitis that can be chronic and recurrent. It is a common condition that is characterized by patches of erythema and scaling (Figure 33–5). The typical distribution of seborrhea includes the scalp (dandruff), eyebrows, eyelids, nasolabial creases, behind the ears, eyebrows, forehead, cheeks, around the nose, under the beard or mustache, over the

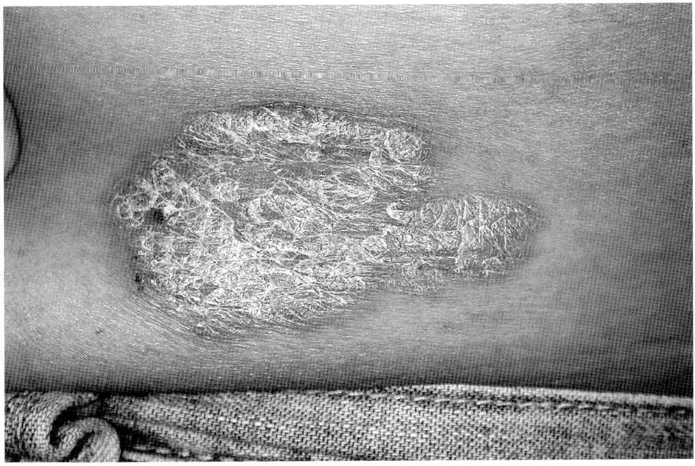

Figure 33–4. Psoriatic plaque with silvery scale on the abdodemen above the waistline.

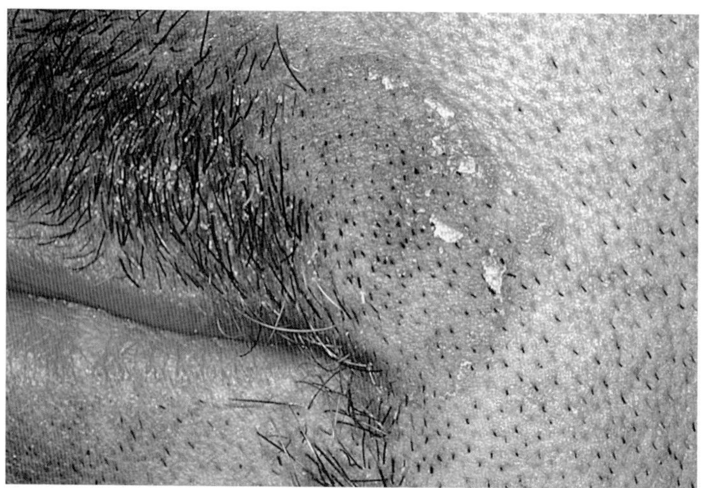

Figure 33–5. Seborrheic dermatitis under and around the mustache with erythema and scale.

sternum, axillae, submammary folds, umbilicus, groin, and the gluteal creases. These areas are the regions with the greatest number of pilosebaceous units producing sebum.

What are the common causes of chronic or recurrent rashes?

See Table 33–1.

▶ EVALUATION

How do I describe the rash using morphology terms?

Much of the diagnostic process involves pattern recognition. You will be able to learn the patterns of the rashes better once you have learned the basic terms and patterns of the primary and secondary skin morphologic lesions (Table 33–2). This will give you the proper vocabulary and conceptual model to observe and describe what you are seeing.

What questions should I ask in the history?

Your history is best taken while looking directly at the rash or skin. Once you have started to look at the skin, your history will be more focused on the correct diagnosis. The list on page 184 will help you make a diagnosis and plan the treatment.

TABLE 33–1

Common Causes of Chronic Rashes

Chronic Rashes	Cause
Atopic dermatitis	Allergic or inflammatory
Eczema	
Seborrhea	
Psoriasis	
Chronically superinfected dermatitis	Infectious
Syphilis	
Herpes simplex–recurrent	
Tinea versicolor	
Acne	Acneiform
Rosacea	
Hidradenitis suppurativa	
Basal cell carcinoma	Skin cancers
Squamous cell carcinoma	
Melanoma	
Lupus	Immunologic
Vasculitis	

TABLE 33–2

Primary and Secondary Skin Lesions

Lesion Type	Description
Primary (basic) lesions	
Macule	Circumscribed flat discoloration
Papule	Elevated solid lesion (up to 5 mm)
Plaque	Circumscribed, superficially elevated solid lesion (0.5 mm; often, a confluence of papules)
Nodule	Palpable solid (round) lesion, deeper than a papule
Wheal (hive)	Pale-red edematous plaque—round or flat-topped and transient
Pustule	Elevated collection of purulence
Vesicle	Circumscribed elevated collection of fluid (up to 5 mm in diameter)
Bulla	Circumscribed elevated collection of fluid (0.5 mm in diameter)
Secondary lesions (complications or progression of primary lesions)	
Scale	Excess dead epidermal cells (desquamation)
Crusts	A collection of dried serum, blood, or purulence
Erosion	Superficial loss of epidermis
Ulcer	Focal loss of epidermis and dermis
Fissure	Linear loss of epidermis and dermis
Atrophy	Depression in the skin from thinning of epidermis and/or dermis
Excoriation	Erosion caused by scratching
Lichenification	Thickened epidermis with prominent skin lines (induced by scratching)

- Onset and duration of skin lesions—acute, continuous, or intermittent?
- Pattern of eruption: Where did it start? How has it changed?
- Any known precipitants, such as exposure to medication (prescription and over-the-counter), foods, plants, sun, topical agents, chemicals (occupation and hobbies)?
- Skin symptoms: itching, pain, paresthesia.
- Systemic symptoms: fever, chills, night sweats, fatigue, weakness, weight-loss.
- Underlying illnesses: diabetes, HIV/AIDS.
- Family history: acne, atopic dermatitis, psoriasis, skin cancers, dysplastic nevi.

What tests will help me determine the cause of the rash?

The most important laboratory tests in the diagnosis of a rash are:

- Microscopy: in diagnosing a fungal infection, scrape some of the scale onto a microscope slide, add 10% KOH with DMSO, and look for the hyphae of dermatophytes or the pseudohyphae of yeast forms of *Candida* or *Pityrosporum* species.
- Cultures: may be useful for some suspected bacterial, viral, or fungal infections.
- RPR or VDRL: if syphilis is suspected. Primary syphilis presents with an ulcer but secondary syphilis may cause a generalized rash with macules on the palms and soles.
- ANA (antinuclear antibody): helpful in determining the etiology of unknown skin lesion such as a butterfly rash that might be lupus erythematosus.
- Wood's light examination: helpful in diagnosing tinea capitis and erythrasma. Tinea capitis caused by *Microsporum* species produce green fluorescence, but *Trichophyton* species do not fluoresce. Erythrasma, a bacterial infection, has a coral red fluorescence.
- Surgical biopsy: can be used as a diagnostic and treatment tool. Having a good differential diagnosis will help you choose the appropriate type of biopsy. A punch biopsy will usually work well for most skin cancers and inflammatory or infiltrative disorders. Superficial skin cancers such as squamous cell carcinoma (SCC) and nodular basal cell carcinoma (BCC) can be biopsied with a shave biopsy.

In most cases, these laboratory tests are used to confirm your clinical diagnosis based on history and physical examination.

Can I use therapeutic trials to diagnose and treat rashes?

Treatment in dermatology can be divided into two categories: medical and surgical. Medical treatments include topical and systemic steroids, antibiotics, antifungal, antiviral, and antiacne agents.

Topical corticosteroids can be beneficial in the treatment of many inflammatory conditions. It is better to know what you are treating than to indiscriminately prescribe steroids. If a condition appears to be seborrhea, eczema, atopic dermatitis, or psoriasis it will often respond to a topical steroid. There are also other efficacious topical treatments for these conditions, which all tend to be chronic and relapsing. Because topical steroids may cause skin atrophy over time, it is better to determine the exact diagnosis of the rash and use more targeted therapy than using empiric steroids alone. Topical steroids when applied to a fungal rash may make it better temporarily and then allow the fungal infection to become worse.

A therapeutic trial of a topical antifungal agent may be appropriate for a superficial fungal infection. It is still best to make the diagnosis first with microscopy, but it is possible to have a false negative KOH preparation. Topical over-the-counter preparations of clotrimazole, miconazole, or terbinafine should eliminate small areas of superficial fungal infection. Tinea capitis (ringworm of the scalp) will require oral antifungal agents for cure.

When the etiology of a rash is unknown, it is best to have a more experienced clinician or specialist help make the diagnosis rather than using "shot-gun" treatment with a topical preparation. Even the experienced clinician may need a biopsy to make the diagnosis.

When is a biopsy needed?

Many skin biopsies are done to diagnose suspected skin cancer. While skin cancers are not exactly rashes, they can look like other nonmalignant rashes. When a lesion looks like a BCC, SCC, or melanoma, it should be biopsied to determine if it is truly a cancer.

The most common skin cancers and their percentage of total skin cancer incidence are:

- Basal cell carcinoma 80% (Figure 33–6)
- Squamous cell carcinoma 16%
- Melanoma 4% (Figure 33–7)

A biopsy can be used to make the diagnosis of inflammatory rashes that are of unknown etiology or when the etiology is uncertain because the rash is not responding to treatment. Inflammatory (psoriasis, lupus erythematosus) or infiltrative rashes (sarcoidosis) can be diagnosed with a simple punch biopsy.

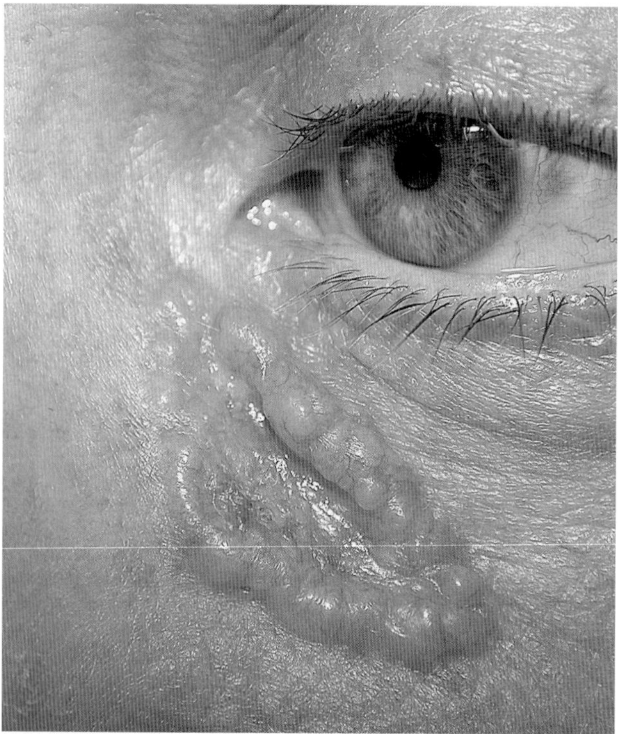

Figure 33–6. Nodular basal cell carcinoma with pearly border and telangiectasias.

Describe biopsy methods.

Biopsy methods include shave, punch, and elliptical excisions. A shave biopsy is done with a scalpel or a sharp shaving blade. This biopsy type is usually superficial and no sutures need to be placed. A punch biopsy is done with a round cookie-cutter type punch instrument that ranges from 2 to 9 mm in diameter. These biopsies are full-thickness and often require one or two sutures to close the defect. The elliptical biopsy is the largest and most difficult to perform. It involves using a scalpel or electrosurgical instrument to cut an elliptically shaped segment of skin out around the lesion. The defect is cut so that the long axis follows the skin lines. These biopsies always need suturing and may even require a two-layer closure.

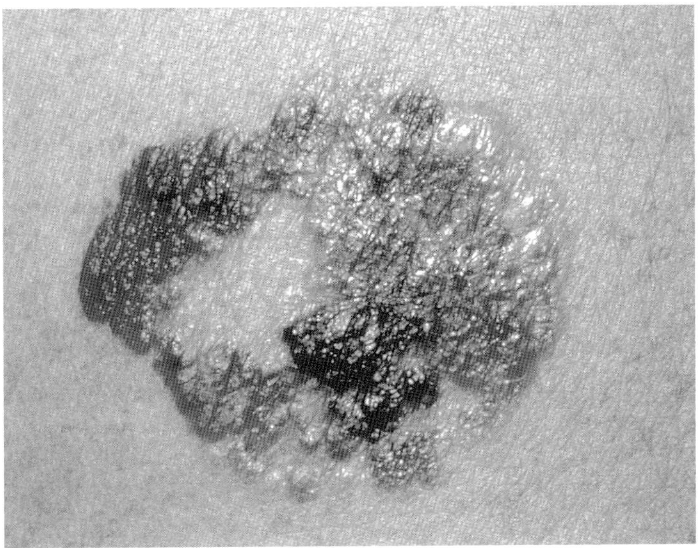

Figure 33–7. Melanoma with asymmetry, irregular border, and variations in color. (Courtesy of the Skin Care Foundation)

How many types of basal cell carcinoma are there?

There are three major morphologic types for the BCC: nodular, superficial, and sclerosing. The typical nodular BCC is pearly and raised with telangiectasias. As it expands, its center may ulcerate and bleed and become crusted. Superficial BCC looks like SCC: pink, flat, scaling plaques that may have erosions or crusts. A fine, raised, pearly "thready border" around the superficial BCC may distinguish it from a SCC. Sclerosing BCC is rare (1% of BCC), flat, and scarlike. SCC can look like a superficial BCC or can be more elevated and nodular. SCC is frequently hyperkeratotic and bleeds easily. The rash of eczema and atopic dermatitis can resemble some of the scaly nonmelanoma skin cancers. (See Box 33–1.)

What are the benign rashes and growths that can be confused with skin cancers?

You should learn to recognize the most common benign skin growths so that you can differentiate them from melanoma and other skin cancers. Some benign pigmented lesions that may be confused with melanoma include nevi, congenital nevi, seborrheic keratoses, dermatofibromas, and lentigines. Seborrheic keratosis may mimic melanoma when they are dark with irregular borders. Although they usually are verrucous and have a stuck-on

BOX 33–1

The ABCDE Guidelines for Diagnosis of Malignant Melanoma

Asymmetry: Benign nevi are symmetric; melanomas tend to have pronounced asymmetry.
Border: Benign lesions usually have smooth borders; melanomas tend to have notched, irregular outlines.
Color: Benign lesions usually contain only one color; melanomas frequently have a variety of colors.
Diameter: Melanoma is usually larger than 6 mm in diameter.
Elevation: Malignant melanoma is almost always elevated, at least in part, so that it is palpable.
or
Enlarging: A pigmented lesion that is enlarging is more suspicious for melanoma.

appearance, they can be flat and irregular. When uncertain as to the diagnosis, get a consult or do a biopsy. Any growths that are suspicious for melanoma should receive a full-depth biopsy (punch or ellipse) to make a definitive diagnosis.

Sebaceous hyperplasia and nonpigmented intradermal nevi on the face may look like basal cell carcinoma. These benign lesions are raised and can have pearly borders and telangiectasias like a nodular BCC. When you are uncertain of the diagnosis, a shave biopsy can remove the lesion and determine whether it is malignant. Completely benign-appearing sebaceous hyperplasia is a cosmetic issue that can be treated electively if desired.

► TREATMENT

How do I manage rashes?

Once you have diagnosed the rash, management can be looked up in any good dermatology textbook (see References). There are also good online references that will help you determine the appropriate treatment.

Acne and Related Disorders. Acne, rosacea, and hidradenitis suppurativa often respond well to oral tetracyclines. Mild acne can be treated with topical over-the-counter benzoyl peroxide and prescription retinoids (Retin-A and Differin Gel). Mild rosacea often responds to topical metronidazole preparations. More severe inflammatory acne often requires oral antibiotics in combination with topical retinoids and benzoyl peroxide. If this fails and acne is scarring, consider isotretinoin (Accutane).

Dermatitis. The following treatment strategies apply for all types of dermatitis (atopic, contact, and eczema):

- Teach the patient to avoid skin irritants such as drying soaps and bathing in water that is too hot or for too long.
- Encourage the use of emollients or moisturizers to moisten the skin, especially to be applied after bathing.
- Treat the inflammation with a topical steroid, choosing the strength and vehicle based on diagnosis, chronicity, and location.
- Consider treating the itching to stop the scratch-itch cycle. The oral sedating antihistamines work well to stop itching, especially at night.
- Look for signs of a secondary bacterial infection, such as weeping or crusting. If present, treat with an antibiotic such as oral cephalexin to cover group A *Streptococcus* and *Staphylococcus aureus*.

Drug Allergies. Stop the medication and treat the symptoms, which are most often pruritus.

Infections. Viral rashes from measles and rubella are very rare now that we administer two MMR immunizations before school. We still see viral rashes from the herpes virus family. Herpes simplex, varicella, and herpes zoster can all be treated with antiviral medications in the acyclovir family. These include acyclovir, famciclovir, and valacyclovir.

Bacterial skin infections can be superficial as in impetigo, deeper as in cellulitis, or deeper still as seen in an abscess below the skin. Because all of these infections are usually caused by *Streptococcus pyogenes* or *Staphylococcus aureus*, antistaphylococcal antibiotics (cephalexin, dicloxacillin, and erythromycin) are the treatment of choice for impetigo and cellulitis. Cellulitis may require parenteral antibiotics for higher tissue levels of the antibiotic. Incision and drainage is the treatment of choice for most types of abscesses. Learning to recognize the few skin infections caused by pseudomonas or haemophilus influenza will help avoid using the wrong antibiotic in these more rare circumstances. It is crucial to not miss necrotizing fasciitis because it is life- and limb-threatening and requires surgical debridement along with intravenous antibiotics.

Fungal infections on the skin and not in the hair or nails should respond to topical over-the-counter antifungals (miconazole, clotrimazole, terbinafine). When large areas of the skin, hair/scalp, or nails are involved, the infection may require treatment with oral antifungals (griseofulvin, terbinafine, itraconazole) for weeks to months.

Infestations with *lice or scabies* are best treated with permethrin-containing preparations (Nix for lice and Elimite for scabies). Other agents exist but have greater risks of toxicity. It is also essential to clean the clothing and bedclothes to avoid getting reinfested.

Seborrhea. The cause of seborrhea is an inflammatory hypersensitivity to *Pityrosporum ovale* on the skin. Although this yeast can be a normal skin inhabitant, persons who have seborrhea appear to respond to its presence with an inflammatory reaction. The treatment of seborrhea should be directed at the inflammation and the *Pityrosporum.* Seborrhea is highly responsive to topical steroids, so a low-potency steroid is usually adequate. To avoid atrophy, it is especially important to use a low-potency steroid for the treatment of seborrhea on the face; 1% hydrocortisone cream or lotion works well. Prescribe lotion for seborrhea in hair-covered areas because it is easier and less messy to apply than a cream. If scalp seborrhea is severe, you may prescribe a higher-potency steroid solution such as fluocinonide (Lidex) solution or clobetasol propionate (Temovate) scalp application, because the risk of atrophy on the scalp is less than on the face.

To reduce the profusion of *Pityrosporum,* direct the patient to apply antifungals to the affected areas. For seborrhea of the scalp, the antifungal shampoos that are most effective contain selenium sulfide, zinc pyrithione, or ketoconazole. For seborrhea of the skin, ketoconazole cream is the most effective antifungal preparation.

Psoriasis. Treatment options for psoriasis include emollients, topical steroids, topical vitamin D, anthralin, topical tar and tar shampoo, intralesional steroids, ultraviolet light, methotrexate, and retinoids. The most common treatment of psoriasis involves topical steroids, with strong ointments being the most effective. Combination therapy with topical vitamin D and a high-potency steroid can be a valuable safe treatment. More severe psoriasis should be referred for systemic and/or light therapy.

Urticaria. The H1 antihistamines are the first-line of therapy for urticaria. The first generation antihistamines such as diphenhydramine, chlorpheniramine, and hydroxyzine can be very effective, especially in the acute case. These first generation antihistamines can be sedating during the day. The sedation may be a benefit in reducing the pruritus but can be dangerous to persons that are driving or operating machinery. The second generation H1 antihistamines cause less sedation and are better tolerated in the daytime for chronic use. While these are more expensive, they play a large role in the management of chronic urticaria.

What medications can be used to treat the itching that goes along with many rashes?

Topical steroids can be used to treat localized areas of pruritus. Oral steroids are often used to treat a bad case of urticaria or contact dermatitis. Oral antihistamines can be valuable to treat all kinds of itching but have not been shown to change the course of atopic dermatitis. The older generic sedating antihistamines are more powerful for pruritus but run the risk of making the patient drowsy. Patients who drive or run machines at work must be particularly careful to avoid taking medications that cause drowsiness.

When should I refer?

As a medical student, you will need to review all the cases you see with your faculty supervisor. There are some cases that should prompt immediate referral from the family physician to a specialist. Necrotizing fasciitis will need to be referred for surgical debridement along with antibiotics. Even cellulitis should not be missed; the patient may need hospitalization.

Patients with erythema multiforme, pustular psoriasis, disseminated zoster, angioedema, or pemphigus vulgaris may need hospitalization for fluids and support.

Many simple nonmelanoma skin cancers can be diagnosed and treated by the family physician. However, there are five principal situations that should prompt a referral for skin surgery:

1. Aggressive skin cancer
2. A large lesion
3. A lesion located in a sensitive area (cosmetic or functional)
4. A lesion is beyond the scope of one's skills.
5. The patient has a higher chance than normal of having a complication or may require close monitoring during or after surgery.

KEY POINTS

- ▶ **Follow a systematic approach when evaluating and describing skin rashes.**
- ▶ **When the diagnosis of a skin lesion is in doubt, consider a skin biopsy.**
- ▶ **Learn the clinical characteristics of melanoma and common skin cancers.**

CASE 33–1. **A 47-year-old man walks into your office with severe itching that started yesterday and kept him up at night. The patient has wheals all over his arms and chest area (Figure 33–8). He denies previous skin problems and has no known allergies. He also has no fever, pain, or malaise. Upon further questioning, you discover that he had started taking one trimethoprim-sulfamethoxazole DS tablet twice a day one month ago for chronic prostatitis. He was told that he would need to keep taking it for a total of three months in order to fully treat his prostate problem. Aside from his prostatitis, he has no other medical problems and is not on any other medications.**

A. What is the most likely diagnosis?
B. What is the best course of management?

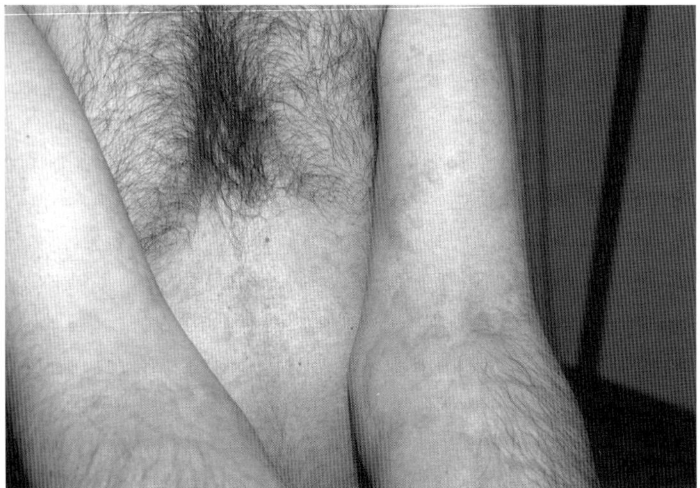

Figure 33–8. Pink raised pruritic eruption on the arms and trunk.

CASE 33–2. **A 2-year-old girl is brought to your office by her mom with a new widespread rash on her arms, abdomen, and behind both knees (Figure 33–9). The rash is of two-week duration. The girl is scratching while sitting in the office, and the mother states that it is interfering with her sleep. The family history is positive for asthma and allergic rhinitis. On exam you discover that the rash is particularly severe in the popliteal fossa. It is a fine papular rash with some slight scale and prominent erythema. She is afebrile and not taking any medications. There are no crusts or exudate on physical exam.**

A. What is the differential diagnosis?
B. What is the best course of management?

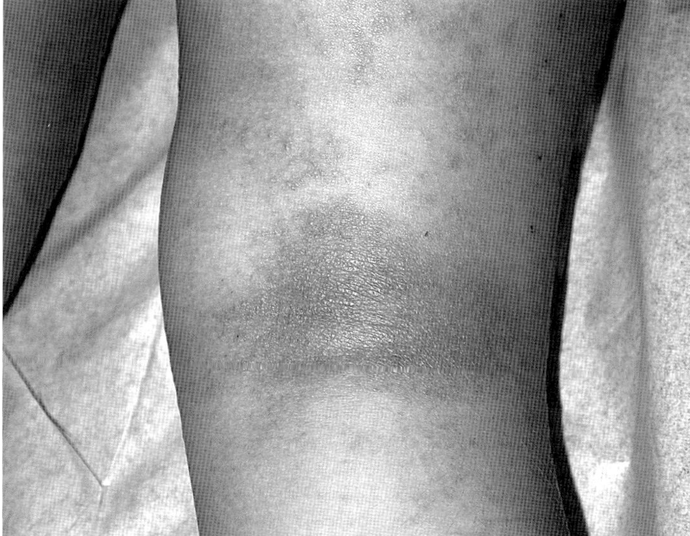

Figure 33–9. Red fine papular rash in the popliteal fossa of a 2-year-old girl.

REFERENCES

Habif T: Clinical Dermatology: A Color Guide to Diagnosis and Therapy, 4th ed. St. Louis, Mo: Mosby, 2003.

Milgrom E, Usatine R, Tan R, Spector S: Practical Allergy. St. Louis, Mo: Mosby, 2003, pp 39–96.

Fitzpatrick TB, Johnson R, Wolff K, Suurmond R: Synopsis of Clinical Dermatology. New York: McGraw-Hill Professional, 2000.

Usatine R, Moy R, Tobinick E, Siegel D: Skin Surgery: A Practical Guide. St. Louis, Mo: Mosby-Year Book, Inc., 1998.

USEFUL WEBSITES

Dermatology Online Atlas has more than 4500 images. *http://dermis.multimedica.de/index_e.htm*

eMedicine contains an excellent dermatology section. *http://www.emedicine.com*

Over fifty interactive dermatology cases simulate the diagnosis and treatment of a real patient with immediate feedback at *http://fm.mednet.ucla.edu/derm2*. A reference section includes video segments of skin surgery procedures. The atlas contains more than 1000 photographs, a sophisticated search tool, and a fun quiz mode.

Dermatology Image Atlas with over 6800 images and 240 contributors. *http://dermatlas.org*

34

Sleep Problems

▶ ETIOLOGY

What is the biology of "normal" sleep?

Sleep is a necessary biological phenomenon as a period of restoration and consolidation of learning, composed of several distinct stages with characteristic EEG changes and behaviors. Broadly, sleep is classified into either rapid eye movement (REM) or non-REM sleep. Non-REM sleep is divided into four stages, with each progressive stage representing deeper sleep.

How does sleep change with age?

Newborn infants spend most of the day (16 to 20 hours) asleep. As children mature, there is an accompanying decrease in total sleep time (primarily in REM sleep time). Upon becoming adults, people often sleep about 7 to 8 hours a day, but normal sleep intervals range from 4 to10 hours per day. As individuals age, there is decreasing REM sleep and a corresponding increase in the lighter stages of non-REM sleep. Accordingly, elderly people are prone to more transient arousals.

What is insomnia?

Insomnia often becomes the focus of clinic visits. Insomnia is not a clinically useful diagnosis because it can mean trouble falling asleep, trouble staying asleep, or waking feeling unrefreshed. Each symptom represents unique differentials; therefore, fleshing out the exact complaints of the patient is important. Acute insomnia, lasting less than four weeks, is often tolerated by the patient without involving the physician. It is useful to inquire during all visits about the patient's sleep, regardless of his or her age.

What are some of the specific sleep disturbances that clinicians may diagnose?

Primary care clinicians should differentiate patients' complaints relating to falling asleep, which may be a consequence of restless leg syndrome or circadian rhythm disturbances, from complaints associated with sleeping too much, as in narcolepsy. These conditions also should be differentiated from those disorders that can cause arousal from sleep or excessive daytime sleepiness, such as periodic limb movements or sleep apnea. Medical conditions, medications, poor sleep hygiene, and psychiatric disorders should be eliminated as possible causes of the patient's insomnia.

What is sleep apnea?

Sleep apnea is a disorder that consists of either total (apnea is the cessation of airflow for greater than 10 seconds) or partial (hypopnea) episodes of pharyngeal tissue obstruction during sleep. This syndrome consists of daytime sleepiness and excessive snoring at night, and can lead to right-sided heart failure. Partners of the patient are useful historians, identifying increased episodes of snoring followed by 20 to 30 seconds of silence, followed by either gasping or arousal and the restarting of breathing. Obesity, alcohol, and sedative medications can all exacerbate this condition secondary to increased flaccidity of the pharyngeal tissues. The typical adult patient is middle-aged with a large neck circumference and truncal obesity. Children can develop sleep apnea secondary to adenoid-tonsillar hypertrophy, for which surgery is curative.

What is restless leg syndrome?

Patients with restless leg syndrome (RLS) complain of funny sensations in their lower extremities such as "pins and needles" or "crawling sensations," usually at night. Accompanying these sensations is an almost irresistible urge to move the legs in an attempt to get relief. RLS is a relatively common problem, occurring in up to 15% of the population. A familial pattern suggests a genetic component. RLS can also be caused by low iron levels, uremia, medications, and pregnancy.

What are circadian rhythm disturbances?

Circadian rhythm disturbances most often affect people who have shift work or are frequent travelers. These activities can interfere with the natural sleep rhythm, causing insomnia. All patients should be asked about work hours, travel, and ingestion of stimulants like caffeine and nicotine.

What are periodic limb movements?

Periodic limb movements are bilateral, repeated, rhythmic jerking or twitching movements of small amplitude. They usually occur in the lower extremities, as often as every 90 seconds. The movements usually do not awaken the patient; the bed partner usually gives the history. The condition is treated with dopaminergic medications such as Sinemet.

What is narcolepsy?

Narcolepsy is a relatively uncommon sleep disorder consisting of excessive daytime sleepiness and a tendency to involuntarily fall asleep. These sudden sleeping spells can put the patient at risk for harm when they occur during activities such as operating machinery or driving. Narcoleptic patients often have cataplexy, which is a sudden loss of muscle tone brought on by emotional experiences involving laughing or surprise. Behavioral therapy targeted at improving sleep hygiene and taking scheduled daytime naps is used. Additionally, stimulant medications such as methylphenidate (Ritalin), dextroamphetamine (Dexedrine), and modafinil (Provigil) have all been used.

What are common medical conditions that interfere with sleep?

Difficulty sleeping is often a manifestation of some underlying medical condition. Patients with heartburn or gastroesophageal reflux disease (GERD) will often notice an exacerbation of their symptoms when lying down flat at night (especially if eating shortly before bed). Cardiac patients may experience orthopnea or paroxysmal nocturnal dyspnea with resulting interference with sleep. Additionally, patients with poorly controlled diabetes, any form of chronic pain, vasomotor symptoms of menopause, or any condition that causes urinary symptoms can present initially with insomnia.

What are common medications that interfere with sleep?

Alcohol, which is often self-prescribed by patients to assist with their sleeping difficulty, can cause insomnia itself. Additionally, both caffeine and nicotine are stimulants and can produce enough arousal to disrupt sleep. Finally, almost all medications prescribed by physicians can affect sleep and thus should be carefully scrutinized when dealing with an insomnia complaint.

▶ EVALUATION

Which questions are important on the history?

Insomnia is a symptom and not a diagnosis itself. The examiner has to press the patient to be more specific about the type of sleep problem experienced. The exact times, duration, and types of sleeping difficulty are diagnostically important. Key questions should cover whether the patient has: (1) difficulty in falling asleep, (2) multiple periods of awakening during the night, (3) early morning awakening, (4) normal sleep pattern but still feeling tired in the morning, (5) duration of insomnia, (6) transient problems that are environmental in nature, (7) medications, (8) medical history including medication, (10) psychological stress, (11) psychiatric problems such as depression and anxiety.

What should I look for during the physical exam?

Many medical problems present as insomnia. Specific attention should be paid to the oropharynx and neck, looking for signs of obstruction such as in sleep apnea, and to the cardiovascular system, looking for signs of heart failure. A thorough mental status exam should be completed, because 30% of all chronic insomnia patients have underlying psychiatric disease.

What is a sleep study?

A sleep study is often conducted at a center designed for this purpose. It usually involves checking in to the center after work and spending the night hooked up to monitors. Standard measures include an EEG, an EKG, continuous pulseoximetry, peripheral muscle activity, and body temperature. The sleep lab is also equipped for a trial of continuous positive airway pressure (CPAP).

When should I order a sleep study?

A sleep study is used to evaluate cases of sleep apnea and movement disorders such as periodic limb movements or sleepwalking. With a reliable history (especially from the patient's partner), a sleep diary, and a physical exam, almost all sleep problems can be diagnosed without relying on a sleep study.

How does a patient keep a sleep diary?

A sleep diary is useful for diagnostic purposes by more clearly identifying and monitoring the problem. Forms are available commercially or on the Internet but can easily be constructed by the patient. Information to be collected includes date and day of week, habits before going to bed, activities before turning in, how long until the patient went to sleep, quality of sleep, any dreams/snoring/unusual movements, what time the patient woke up, sense of restfulness, and whether the patient took any daytime naps.

▶ TREATMENT

List behaviors that constitute good sleep hygiene.

Examining a patient's sleep hygiene is a useful exercise for both revealing potential problems and educating patients about sleep hygiene. Some of the important topics to be covered include:

- Avoiding naps during the day
- Increasing exercise during the day but avoiding it within six hours before bedtime
- Going to bed and waking up at the same time each day
- Eliminating alcohol/nicotine/caffeine before bed
- Using the bedroom only for sleeping or sex
- Controlling the environment in the bedroom to make it comfortable

Are there nonpharmacological treatments for sleep problems?

Any treatment should be tailored to help with the target problem. A program may include relaxation techniques, progressive muscle relaxation, guided imagery, and hypnosis. These may be taught by the practitioner or by referral. Improving the patient's sleep hygiene is also a useful intervention. Shift workers and travelers may find relief through the use of light therapy.

What medications are useful for sleep problems?

A class of medications referred to as hypnotics is most often used for sleep problems (Table 34–1). Some of the drug families in this class include the benzodiazepines, the benzodiazepine receptor antagonists, and several over-the-counter medications. The sleep induced by all of these medications is an artificial pharmacological one and thus many patients will still complain of daytime fatigue. Many of the medications are addicting (especially the benzodiazepines). Oversedation may lead to injuries or accidents. This factor suggests that these medications are appropriate for only short-term usage and thus have a small role in the treatment of chronic insomnia. The use of these medications can make some sleep-related problems, such as sleep apnea, worse. Movement-related sleep disorders are usually treated using the dopamine-based medication for Parkinson's disease. There are no medications currently available to treat obstructive sleep apnea (see next question).

TABLE 34–1

Medications Used in Treatment of Acute Insomnia

Class	Drug	Duration of Action	Half-life (hr)	Usual Daily Dose (mg)
BNZ receptor antagonist	Zaleplon (Sonata)	Ultrashort	1	5–10
BNZ receptor anatagonist	Zolpidem (Ambien)	Short	2.5	5–10
Benzodiazepene	Triazolam (Halcion)	Short	1.5–5.5	0.125–0.5
Benzodiazepene	Estazolam (ProSom)	Intermediate	10–24	1–2
Benzodiazepene	Temazepam (Restoril)	Intermediate	9–15	7.5–30
Benzodiazepene	Flurazepam (Dalmane)	Long	47–100	15–30
Benzodiazepene	Quazepam (Doral)	Long	41	7.5–15.0
OTC	Diphenhydramine (Nytol)	Intermediate	3–10	25–50
OTC	Doxylamine (Unisom)	Intermediate	10	25
OTC	Melatonin	Short	< 1	1–2

BNZ = benzodiazepine, OTC = over the counter

What are the therapies for sleep apnea?

Patients in whom sleep apnea has been diagnosed need education about the condition and potentially serious health consequences. Patients should be encouraged to modify their diet and exercise level with the goal of a 10% reduction in body weight. The next line of therapy involves CPAP. This is administered via a mask-like device that is strapped to the patient's face overnight. The air blown through it and the resulting pressure is sufficient to keep the airway open and prevent apnea. Although somewhat uncomfortable initially, many patients feel so much better that they take their CPAP machines with them on all trips.

KEY POINTS

- Insomnia is a common symptom, but many patients have not discussed their concerns with their physician.
- Accurate diagnosis can usually be made based on history.
- A short course of pharmacological therapy is the primary means of treating acute insomnia.
- Behavioral therapy approaches are more efficacious and preferable to pharmacological therapy for chronic insomnia, with the exception of the movement-related disorders.
- Medical problems, poor sleep hygiene, medication use, drug or alcohol use, and underlying psychiatric illness cause most cases of chronic insomnia. These are usually correctable.

CASE 34–1. **A husband and wife come to your clinic complaining of sleeping problems. She is 52 years old, mildly obese, and takes medication for hypertenson, diabetes type II, arthritis, and menopause. Her husband is 58 years old and moderately obese. You are currently treating him for prostate enlargement, "seasonal allergies," hypertension, and increased cholesterol. The wife states that her husband snores loudly, which keeps her awake at night. Her husband quickly offers that she tosses and turns all night, often kicking him in the process, such that he feels tired during the day as if he had not slept the night before. They are at the point of obtaining single beds and want your advice.**

A. What is the differential diagnosis for the couple's insomnia?
B. How would you proceed with the work-up for their situation?
C. What are some of the preliminary treatment options?

CASE 34–2. **During your nursing home rounds you encounter a new patient who is requesting a sleeping pill. She is 83 years old and moved into the nursing home approximately one year ago when her husband died. She has had difficultly falling asleep for the past few months. Most of her day is spent in her room because she is "just too tired" to participate in any of the activities despite once being an active bridge player. On exam she is afebrile and appears tired; her pulse is 70, respirations 18, blood pressure 120/70. She weighs 130 lb, which is a 15-lb increase from her admission weight. The only past medical history you gather is GERD and chronic obstructive pulmonary disease (COPD) for which she takes some medication, but she can't remember what it is. She continues to smoke a half pack of cigarettes per day.**

A. What are some of the risk factors in this patient's history and physical exam for insomnia?
B. Provide a list of laboratory investigations or tests you would order.
C. What are the pharmacological and nonpharmacological treatment options?

REFERENCES

Chesson AL, Milligan SA: Current trends in the management of insomnia. Emergency Med 4:11–20, 2002.

Johnson TA, Deckert JJ: Care of the patient with a sleep disorder. In Taylor RB (ed): Family Medicine Principles and Practice, 6th ed. Portland, Or: Springer, 2003, pp 470–475.

Neubauer DN: Sleep problems in the elderly. Am Fam Physician 59:2551–2559, 1999.

Thiedke CC: Sleep disorders and sleep problems in childhood. Am Fam Physician 63:277–284, 2001.

USEFUL WEBSITES

American Academy of Sleep Medicine. *http://www.aasmnet.org/home.htm*

National Institutes of Health; National Heart, Lung, and Blood Institute. Sleep Disorders Information. *http://www.nhlbi.nih.gov/health/public/sleep/index.htm*

35

Sore Throat

▶ ETIOLOGY

What are the most common causes of sore throat?

Most sore throats (about 60%) are caused by the "common cold," which is often an infection caused by rhinovirus, coronovirus, or parainfluenza virus. Other common and uncommon causes of sore throat have distinctly different presentations, such as "strep throat" (caused by group A strep, which includes *Streptococcus pyogenes*), mononucleosis (caused by Epstein-Barr virus), or allergic rhinitis with postnasal drip. Clinical findings do not differentiate between these cold viruses, but the astute clinician should be able to distinguish important etiologies.

What are some other causes of sore throat that may be considered?

Other causes of acute sore throat include diptheria, which presents with a gray pseudomembrane in nonimmunized people, and gonorrhea, which may present in persons who have a history of oral sex with infected partners. Simply breathing cold, dry air at night gives some people sore throats in the morning; these may improve through the day. Gastroesophageal reflux disease (GERD) and postnasal drip from allergic rhinitis may also cause sore throat. Acute retroviral syndrome presents three to five weeks after a patient has acquired HIV; patients with this syndrome can have a nonexudative pharynx, fever, enlarged lymph nodes, arthralgias, and myalgias.

▶ EVALUATION

What complications can come from group A strep (GAS) infections?

Complications of GAS infections may be suppurative or nonsuppurative. Suppurative complications include local extension to peritonsillar or retropharyngeal areas, sinusitis, otitis media, meningitis, bacteremia, and endocarditis. Nonsuppurative complications are caused by *Streptococcus* toxins, not the bacteria itself.

Nonsuppurative complications include scarlet fever and rheumatic fever; the latter is diagnosed clinically and includes carditis and polyarthritis.

What history and physical exam findings are important in diagnosing a sore throat?

From the patient's history, determine the duration of the illness and history of fevers or chills. Does the patient drool, have a stiff neck, or have difficulty breathing? Are there associated symptoms such as cough, conjunctivitis, or runny nose? Has the patient been exposed to anyone with a diagnosed viral or strep sore throat? While doing your physical exam, first note the vital signs, especially temperature and pulse rate. It is important to do a thorough head and neck exam, including checking the tympanic membranes, nasal mucosa, and cervical lymph nodes. In the mouth and pharynx, look for erythema or petechiae, tonsillar enlargement and exudates, and ensure patency of the airway.

What signs and symptoms differentiate cold viruses from mononucleosis and strep?

If a patient has a recent cough, conjunctivitis, coryza, or diarrhea, he/she most likely has the common cold. Mononucleosis usually has a prodrome of fevers, which progresses into a sore throat with fever and generalized lymphadenopathy. Over the course of weeks, the sore throat will recede and a generalized fatigue will remain.

The following five criteria are useful in the diagnosis of strep throat:

- Temperature above 38.3°C
- Exposure to diagnosed strep
- Tonsillar exudates
- Enlarged cervical lymph nodes
- Absence of coughing

When should I obtain further tests? How do I perform a throat swab?

When two or three of the above strep throat criteria are positive, a rapid antigen strep test should be performed. Use a Dacron swab, and obtain mucous samples from both posterior tonsils and the retropharyngeal mucosa. Because the rapid strep sensitivity is only 80%, negative results should be confirmed by culturing the sampled mucous. If a sore throat is not improved in 10 days, a Mono-spot test is useful to diagnose mononucleosis.

▶ TREATMENT

What common causes of sore throat need to be treated?

Although most cases of strep throat will resolve without any treatment, antibiotic therapy is important to reduce the small risk of complications. It is also important to identify and quickly manage a patient with severe sore throat, toxic presentation, or airway compromise. This patient may have epiglottitis, or peritonsillar or retropharyngeal abcess, and otolaryngologic consult should be quickly obtained. If epiglottitis is suspected (rapid onset, high fever, drooling), *do not* attempt an oral physical exam.

How do I manage patients with sore throat?

Any patient with a sore throat may benefit from increased fluid intake, gargling with warm salt water, or throat lozenges. NSAIDs may provide analgesic and antipyretic relief. If a patient has four or five of the five strep criteria, or fewer with positive rapid strep or culture, you should treat with antibiotics. Antibiotic options include penicillin (oral or IM) or erythromycin.

When should consultation be made for tonsillectomy?

A tonsillectomy may be considered in a patient with more than seven episodes of group A strep pharyngitis in one year, or ten in two years. The infections should all be documented in the physician's progress notes and should each have positive culture or rapid strep. In this patient, a tonsillectomy should provide a significant reduction in the frequency of pharyngitis for two to three years. Tonsil size by itself is not an indication for tonsillectomy, but the procedure may be considered for problems other than sore throats, such as sleep apnea or swallowing disorders.

KEY POINTS

- **Most sore throats are caused by common cold viruses, and avoiding antibiotic treatment will save the patient from side effects and reduced bacterial resistance.**
- **Evaluate the following five criteria for strep throat: temperature above 38.3°C, exposure to diagnosed strep, tonsillar exudates, enlarged cervical lymph nodes, and absence of coughing.**
- **Penicillin is still the best antibiotic for strep throat. It may be administered IM if patient compliance is questionable.**

CASE 35–1. **A 4-year-old boy is brought to your clinic with a sore throat and decreased appetite of four-day duration. He attends day care, and he cannot return until he is healthy. On physical exam, he has a fever of 38°C. He has normal TMs and his posterior oropharynx is red with enlarged, nonexudative tonsils. He does not have cervical lymphadenopathy. There is no cough.**

A. What causes are in your differential diagnosis?
B. Is it appropriate to order further laboratory tests? If so, what?
C. Should you send this child home with antibiotics?

CASE 35–2. **A 19-year-old college freshman presents with a seven-day history of sore throat. She has felt feverish and hasn't been attending class. She doesn't think any of her close contacts have had similar symptoms.**

A. What further history and exam do you want to obtain to differentiate causes of sore throat?
B. Are laboratory tests required?
C. What can she tell her roommates and professors about the likely course of her disease?

REFERENCE

Bisno A: Acute pharyngitis. New Engl J Med 344:205–211, 2001.

USEFUL WEBSITE

Kazzi AA, Wills J: Pharyngitis. eMedicine.com, Inc. *http://www.emedicine.com/EMERG/topic419.htm*

36

Syncope

▶ ETIOLOGY

What is syncope?

Syncope is defined as a transient loss of consciousness accompanied by loss of postural tone followed by spontaneous recovery after a few seconds to minutes. Patients may use the word to actually describe presyncope (the impending feeling of loss of consciousness), dizziness without the loss of consciousness, tinnitus, or even the feeling of nausea and vomiting. The significance of this word may be associated with embarrassment, a feeling of loss of control or impending disability, or a harbinger of something worse. Syncope is responsible for 3% of accidents and emergency room visits and 1% to 6% of hospital admissions annually.

What are the most common causes of syncope?

Decreased cerebral perfusion is caused by either a transient decrease of systemic blood pressure or an increase of cerebrovascular resistance. Studies of causation are difficult because of various definitions and classification systems. In a third of the cases, no cause is identified. Decreased systemic blood pressure can be caused by cardiac dysrhythmia (atrial fibrillation, ventricular tachycardia, sick sinus syndrome, atrioventricular block), altered peripheral vasculature (arterial vasodilation or increased venous pooling), or a cardiopulmonary obstruction (pulmonary embolus, aortic stenosis, hypertrophic obstructive cardiomyopathy). Vasovagal syncope is caused by the venous relaxation that occurs through carotid sinus baroreceptor stimulation from activities such as micturition, defecation, eating, or quickly standing; this venous relaxation can result in hypotension and syncope. Increased cerebrovascular resistance can be caused by hyperventilation, panic attacks, cerebral vasoconstriction, and chronic atherosclerosis.

When is syncope indicative of a serious problem?

Any episode of true syncope should be a matter of concern. Those causes that are associated with focal neurologic findings, seizures, or cardiac symptoms are most indicative of serious problems, which can include arrhythmias, valvular heart or cardiomyopathy, acute myocardial infarction, pulmonary embolus, or aortic dissection.

▶ EVALUATION

What historical features need to be considered?

In up to 50% of cases, the history can identify the probable cause of syncope. Ask the patient about activities just prior to the episode (eating, exercise, cough, micturition) and any prodromal symptoms (dizziness, palpitations, chest pain). A review of medications and administration times is important to identify adverse reactions. A complete list of comorbid conditions (especially heart disease, diabetes, hypertension, neurologic disease) is also important. Underlying psychiatric conditions should be investigated in the patient with frequent episodes of unexplained presyncope (i.e., no loss of consciousness).

Which parts of the physical examination should I especially focus on?

The physical examination must include measurements of vital signs in lying, sitting, and standing positions. Orthostatic hypotension is identified with a fall of systolic blood pressure and rise of pulse. A careful cardiovascular exam—to identify arrhythmia, murmurs, bruits, and alterations of pulses—and a complete neurologic exam are indicated. Carotid sinus massage may be useful in elderly patients, but should not be performed by the primary care physician if the patient has a history of ventricular tachycardia, carotid bruits, or recent stroke or myocardial infarction.

How helpful are basic laboratory studies in the evaluation of syncope?

While an abnormal blood composition (anemia, hypocarbia, hypoglycemia, hypoxemia) may be in the differential diagnosis of syncope, blood tests should be ordered based on suspected causes from history and physical examination. An electrocardiogram (EKG) can be very helpful in identifying ongoing arrhythmia, ischemia, or infarction.

What additional studies should I consider ordering?

Depending on suspected diagnosis, lab studies could include CBC, metabolic panel, chemistry profile, toxicology screens, therapeutic drug levels, and pregnancy test. Further cardiac evaluation can include echocardiography or stress testing. Cardiac event monitoring and a Holter monitor are useful in identifying irregular heart rhythms, both chronic and intermittent.

What is a tilt-table test? How can it help me?

A tilt-table test is recommended in patients with unexplained, recurrent syncope when cardiac causes, including arrhythmias, have been excluded. It is a positive test if the patient's symptoms are reproduced when he or she lies on a table that is then tilted to 60 degrees for up to 45 minutes. In men older than 45 or women older than 55, an exercise treadmill test is recommended first.

▶ TREATMENT

How is vasovagal syncope managed?

Vasovagal symptoms frequently improve over time. The patient should avoid precipitating factors such as prolonged standing or sitting, excess alcohol intake, or exercise after large meals or in hot environments. Salt and fluid intake should be increased to support intravascular status. Culprit medications that cause vasodilation, venous pooling, or dehydration should be minimized or withdrawn. The use of compression hose may also help in improving lower extremity tone.

How do medications affect syncope?

Many types of drugs have side effects that include syncope; some common culprits are antihypertensive agents, antidepressants, antianginal drugs, and analgesics. Any drug that depresses the central nervous system can also be a problem. Careful drug regimen review and reduction should be tried. Some medications that have been used to treat vasovagal symptoms include fludrocortisone, midodrine, scopolamine, theophylline, as well as β-blockers, ACE inhibitors, and selective serotonin re-uptake inhibitors. Permanent cardiac pacing may also be indicated.

KEY POINTS

- History, physical examination, and EKG are the core of the work-up for patients with syncope.
- It is important to rule out orthostatic hypotension as a cause of syncope.
- Cardiac evaluation may include Holter monitor or loop event records. If exercise tolerance testing is considered, echocardiography should be done for those patients with exertional syncope first.
- Reserve neurologic testing should be used for patients who have neurologic signs or symptoms or carotid bruits.
- Include psychiatric evaluation for patients with normal cardiac findings and frequent episodes of syncope.

CASE 36–1. **A 28-year-old woman is beginning a new sales job following an uncomplicated maternity leave. She presents with four episodes in the past week of feeling like she is going to pass out. She describes a numbness and tingling sensation in her lips and fingertips. Coworkers report that she is red in the face and diaphoretic. She has no chest pain or palpitations and has no previous cardiac, pulmonary, or neurologic conditions. She is on no medications.**

A. Does this patient have syncope?
B. What management options would you consider?

CASE 36–2. **A 50-year-old man with longstanding hypertension presents after an episode of passing out over the weekend. He was doing heavy yardwork at the time and recalls some chest aching whenever he exerted himself. He recently had his blood pressure medications adjusted.**

A. What are the most worrisome features of this case?
B. What studies would you prioritize in the evaluation of this patient?

REFERENCES

Kapoor WN: Syncope. New Engl J Med 343:1856–1862, 2000.
Linzer MD, Yang EH, Estes M, et al.: Diagnosing syncope: Part 1: Value of history, physical examination and electrocardiography. Ann Intern Med 126:989–996, 1997.
Linzer MD, Yang EH, Estes M, et al.: Diagnosing syncope: Part 2: Unexplained syncope. Ann Intern Med 127:76–86, 1997.

USEFUL WEBSITES

Rumm Morag, D Barry Brenner. Syncope. eMedicine.com, Inc. 2004*http://www.emedicine.com/emerg/topic876.htm*
American Heart Association. Syncope. 2004. *http://www.americanheart.org/presenter.jhtml?identifier=4749*
National Institute of Neurological Disorders and Stroke, National Institutes of Health, Bethesda, Maryland. 2002. *http://www.ninds.nih.gov/health_and_medical/disorders/syncope_doc.htm*

37

Vaginal Bleeding

▶ ETIOLOGY

What is abnormal vaginal bleeding?

Bleeding can occur from the vaginal mucosa or, more often, from the uterus. Bleeding from the vagina is usually caused by trauma or tumor and is always abnormal. Abnormal uterine bleeding has different causes based on the patient's clinical setting. Normal, or functional, vaginal bleeding (menses) will not be discussed in this chapter.

What are the terms used to describe abnormal bleeding?

Oligomenorrhea is the term for menstrual cycles that occur more than 35 days apart, while *polymenorrhea* describes cycles that occur less than 24 days apart. *Menorrhagia* describes cycles of normal intervals, but with excessive flow and length of bleeding time. *Metrorrhagia* is the term for menses that occur at irregular intervals and include heavy flow and longer bleeding.

What are the causes of abnormal vaginal bleeding?

In patients of childbearing age, pregnancy is usually the first concern. Then consideration is given to medications that the patient may be taking, including anticoagulants, antipsychotics, hormones, SSRIs, and steroids. Overall health of the patient is assessed because it can impact uterine bleeding caused by systemic concerns such as weight loss, exercise addiction, or liver, kidney, endocrine, or thyroid disease. Polycystic ovary syndrome is a frequent cause of infrequent, irregular periods.

The presence or absence of pain before or during a cycle further helps to differentiate between causes of vaginal bleeding. Endometriosis frequently gives pain before menstruation that ceases when the period ends. Pelvic fullness, urinary tract symptoms, or painful intercourse are frequently reported with ovarian or uterine pathology.

Excessive hair growth and obesity may be clues to the diagnosis of polycystic ovary syndrome. A history of bruising may be present in patients with coagulopathy.

Endometrial cancer is a concern in many women with abnormal vaginal bleeding. The incidence increases with age. Other risk factors are a history of unopposed estrogen use, not having had children, and being obese or diabetic.

In postmenopausal women, abnormal bleeding is more worrisome; the causes are usually of more serious etiology. Postmenopausal bleeding is defined as bleeding that occurs more than one year after periods have ceased. In this group of patients, including those on hormone replacement therapy, it is important to evaluate the endometrium for premalignant or malignant changes. Bleeding caused by lack of ovulation, or anovulatory cycles, is a diagnosis of exclusion, made after other evaluation is negative.

▶ EVALUATION

What questions should be asked when obtaining the history in a patient with vaginal bleeding?

Questions regarding last menstrual period, sexual activity, nausea, weight gain, change in sexual partners, vaginal discharge, pelvic pain, and dyspareunia will address the possibilities of pregnancy, miscarriage, infection, and trauma. To evaluate for thyroid disorders, ask about changes in weight, constipation, palpitations, fatigue, and sweating. Symptoms of bruising and bleeding, jaundice, and history of hepatitis will address liver diseases and coagulopathies. A history of headaches and galactorrhea may assist in diagnosis of a pituitary adenoma or hyperprolactinemia. A recent history of weight loss, stress, and excessive exercise might lead to a diagnosis of hypothalamic suppression.

What are the key points of the physical examination?

An examination of the genital tract is performed, including a Pap smear and pelvic exam, checking for cervical inflammation or neoplasm, uterine enlargement caused by fibroids, or ovarian pathology. Examine the skin for bruises, jaundice, and edema. Palpate the thyroid and the liver. Auscultate the heart for tachycardia or ectopic beats. Note the body habitus, and whether the patient has acne or hirsutism (an obese patient with these findings may have polycystic ovary syndrome).

What tests should be done?

Testing depends on the age of the patient (Table 37–1).

Suspicious vaginal lesions should be biopsied. Pregnancy tests should be performed if there is any possibility of pregnancy. The American College of Obstetricians and Gynecologists recommends

TABLE 37-1

Common Diagnosis for Abnormal Vaginal Bleeding Based on Patient Age

Prepubertal	Trauma
Menarche through age 20	Anovulatory cycles, pregnancy or complications of pregnancy, infection
Age 20–35	Pregnancy, complications of pregnancy such as miscarriage, infection, medications
Age 35–menopause	Hyperplasia, pregnancy, dysplasia, cancer, medications
Postmenopausal	Cancer, hyperplasia, medications

endometrial evaluation in women over the age of 35 with abnormal bleeding.

Worrisome uterine bleeding warrants evaluation by diagnostic ultrasound or biopsy. An endometrial biopsy can be performed in the office to evaluate for carcinoma. In an endometrial biopsy, a small catheter is placed into the uterine cavity with suction extraction of cells for microscopic evaluation. Ultrasound, using the transvaginal technique, will demonstrate leiomyoma, thickening of the endometrium, and polyps. Ultrasound may be done with saline-infusion technique (injection of 5 to 10 mL of saline into the endometrial cavity to define intracavitary lesions) in postmenopausal women, where there is little variability in a normal endometrial strip thickness. An endometrial strip less than 5-mm thick is normal. An endometrial strip thickness of 5 to 8 mm may be clinically significant, and a strip more than 8-mm thick demands sampling via a biopsy or dilatation and curettage (D&C) because of concerns about endometrial carcinoma. Blood work including complete blood count (anemia screen), TSH, glucose, and serum pregnancy test begins the laboratory evaluation of abnormal bleeding.

▶ TREATMENT

What treatment is available to young women with abnormal vaginal bleeding?

For premenopausal women, patients at low risk for endometrial cancer are initially managed medically with hormone therapy. Should that regimen fail, an ultrasound is performed with consideration of an endometrial biopsy. If hyperplasia is found, the patient is cycled with progestins and repeat biopsy in three months. If pathology is found on biopsy or ultrasound, it should be treated appropriately.

In premenopausal women at high risk for endometrial cancer, treatment is begun only after an endometrial biopsy is performed. Patients with hyperplasia are cycled with progestins and biopsied again in three to six months. Patients with a normal endometrial biopsy with bleeding are further evaluated with a diagnostic hysteroscopy or saline-infusion ultrasound, and the identified pathology is treated.

Menorrhagia, or heavy cyclical menses, is treated with nonsteroidals or hormonal therapy, including progestins, which may be delivered through an intrauterine system (IUD).

In premenopausal women, irregular menses owing to lack of ovulation are treated with combination oral contraceptives. Acute bleeding is treated with a 35 mcg ethinyl estradiol with progestin pill two to four times daily until bleeding has stopped (then finish package) or with conjugated estrogens 25 mg IV every four to six hours.

Surgical management for abnormal bleeding includes operative hysteroscopy (diagnosis and removal of polyps), myomectomy (removal of fibroids laparoscopically or using an open technique), endometrial ablation (thermal balloon destruction of the lining of the uterus), and hysterectomy. Hysterectomy is used after less invasive treatment plans have failed.

How does the treatment differ if the patient is postmenopausal?

If it has been longer than 12 months since menopause *or* since the patient started hormone replacement therapy, it is time to offer her dilatation and curettage for diagnostic purposes. If the patient is a poor candidate for general anesthesia, transvaginal ultrasound or saline sonography along with endometrial biopsy may be considered. If these results are normal, an adjustment to hormonal therapy may be made. If abnormal, however, refer the patient to gynecology for further care.

KEY POINTS

- **Evaluation and treatment for patients with abnormal vaginal bleeding is age dependent.**
- **A thorough history and physical examination can provide the diagnosis for most patients with abnormal vaginal bleeding.**
- **Perimenopausal and postmenopausal vaginal bleeding should be thoroughly evaluated.**

CASE 37–1. **A 23-year-old woman presents to the office with a history of irregular cycles. She states that her periods only come every three to five months and are heavy. In addition, she complains of excessive hair growth on her face and abdomen. She has difficulty losing weight.**

A. What should you consider?
B. What other medical concerns will face this patient?

CASE 37–2. **A 54-year-old woman presents with what she describes as a normal period. She last had a period two years ago.**

A. What additional history is important?
B. What test should be performed?

REFERENCES

Albers JR, Hull SK, Wesley RM: Abnormal uterine bleeding. Am Fam Physician 69(8):1915–1926, 2004.

Speroff L, Glass RH, Kase NG: Dysfunctional uterine bleeding. In Mitchell C (ed): Clinical Gynecologic Endocrinology and Infertility, 6th ed. Philadelphia, Pa: Lippincott Williams & Wilkins, 1999, pp 575–587.

Vilos GA, Lefebvre G, Graves GR: Guidelines for the management of abnormal uterine bleeding. J Obstet Gynaecol Can 23(8):704–709, 2001.

USEFUL WEBSITES

Women's Health Information: *http://www.womens-health.co.uk*

OBGYN.net, designed by obstetricians and gynecologists and monitored by advisory board. *http://www.obgyn.net*

Healthcommunities.com, Inc., developed and monitored by physicians. *http://www.womenshealthchannel.com/dub/index.shtml*

38

Vaginal Discharge

▶ ETIOLOGY

What are the most common causes of vaginal discharge?

Abnormal vaginal discharge is primarily a complaint of adult women. A small amount of discharge is often normal and will vary throughout the menstrual cycle, but it should not have an odor. An abnormality of the vaginal mucosa or cervix can lead to discharge. Table 38–1 lists pathologic causes of vaginal discharge by age. The office diagnosis can usually be confirmed by simple laboratory tests. Up to 20% of patients have two coexistent infections. Infection, including sexually transmitted diseases (STDs), may be present without causing any symptoms. Prepubertal vaginal discharge requires an investigation including careful examination and laboratory studies.

What is bacterial vaginosis (BV)?

BV is an imbalance of the vaginal flora, with a decrease in lactobacilli and overgrowth of bacteria such as *Gardnerella vaginalis, Mycoplasma hominis, Ureaplasma urealyticum,* and anaerobes. There is usually little true inflammation, but BV can cause symptoms of excess discharge and odor. Although BV in pregnancy has been linked to preterm birth, randomized, controlled trials treating asymptomatic BV in pregnant women have failed to decrease preterm deliveries.

Compare and contrast some of the disorders that cause vaginal discharge.

See Table 38–2.

▶ EVALUATION

What historical points and exam findings are important?

Ask about prior infections, new sexual partners, use of condoms, last menstrual period, unusual vaginal bleeding, recent antibiotics

TABLE 38–1

Causes of Vaginal Discharge by Age

Age	Common Causes	Less Common Causes
Prepubertal	Foreign body, allergic or irritant vulvovaginitis	STD due to abuse
Adult	*Candida*, *Trichomonas*, BV, cervicitis	HSV, fistula, allergic
Postmenopausal	Atrophic vaginitis, *Candida*, *Trichomonas*, BV	Leukoplakia, ulcer, fistula

BV = bacterial vaginosis, HSV = herpes simplex virus, STD = sexually transmitted disease

TABLE 38–2

Characteristics of Bacterial Vaginosis, Trichomoniasis, and Candidiasis

	Normal	BV	Trichomoniasis	Candidiasis
Patient complaint	None	Discharge, bad odor, itching may be present	Excessive discharge, bad odor, itching, dysuria	Discharge, itching or burning
Vaginal pH	3.8–4.2	>4.5	>4.5	≤4.5
Discharge	Scant to thin, white	Thin, gray, adherent	Yellow or green, frothy, adherent	White, curdy or thick
Amine odor KOH "whiff" test	Absent	Present (fishy)	May be present (fishy)	Absent
Microscopic	Lactobacilli, normal epithelial cells	"Clue" cells with adherent coccoid bacteria, few WBCs	Moving Trichomonads, WBCs > 10/hpf	Budding yeast, hyphae or pseudohyphae (KOH prep)

or oral contraceptive use, and use of over-the-counter treatments. Uncontrolled diabetes predisposes to recurrent *Candida* vaginitis. Dyspareunia (pain with intercourse), fever, or new genital lesions may indicate cervicitis or upper genital track infection. Dysuria is common with vaginal infections, but may be an indication of a urinary tract infection.

Carefully inspect the external genitalia for any dermal or mucosal lesion, and check for inguinal adenopathy. On speculum examination, note the appearance of the discharge along with any odor. Atrophic vaginitis usually produces a pale, smooth mucosa with loss of rugal folds. Observe for cervical friability, bleeding with light touch of a swab. Pain on lateral motion of the cervix or adnexal tenderness suggests pelvic inflammatory disease.

Which laboratory tests should be performed in the office? What specimens should be obtained for outside laboratory testing?

Routine history and office pelvic examination are not sufficient for determining the cause of vaginal discharge. If pH paper is available, test the discharge directly. Use a swab to collect a sample of the discharge from the vaginal wall. If the cervix is friable, obtain a sample from above the cervix to avoid blood contamination. The swab must remain moist to preserve any *Trichomonas.* Prepare saline and KOH slides immediately, or place the swab in a test tube with 0.5 mL normal saline and prepare slides in the laboratory. It is a good idea to swab the discharge onto two areas of a single slide. Add a single drop of KOH to one area, noting any odor produced. Cover both areas separately with cover slips, and observe each area under the microscope.

Samples for detection of *Chlamydia* and/or gonorrhea should be obtained from the cervical os. Purulent discharge from the cervical os can be gram-stained to look for polys and intracellular gram-negative diplococci. Some labs may use a DNA-based test using urine. This should be a "dirty" collection to collect urethral organisms. Pap test collection is discouraged during a visit for vaginal discharge, since an infection can cause false positives requiring follow-up. Any ulcers suspicious for HSV should be swabbed for culture. If a sexually transmitted disease is diagnosed, consider additional testing for syphilis, hepatitis B or C, and HIV.

▶ TREATMENT

How do I treat candidal vaginitis?

Topical antifungals (clotrimazole, miconazole, butoconazole, tioconazole, econazole, or terconazole) are all quite effective in treating candidal vaginitis when used for three to seven days. Oral fluconazole, 150-mg single dose, is also effective. Recurrent vulvovaginal candidiasis may require maintenance regimens such as clotrimazole vaginal suppositories once weekly.

How do I treat *Trichomonas* vaginitis?

Metronidazole, 2-g single dose, is effective for treatment of *Trichomonas* vaginitis. Alternative dosing is 250 mg three times a day for seven days or 500 mg twice daily for seven days. Tinidazole, 2-g single dose, is a newly approved alternative. Partners must be treated to avoid reinfection.

How do I treat bacterial vaginosis?

Metronidazole provides bacterial vaginosis cure rates of 80% to 90%. Orally, it may be given as a 2-g single dose, 500 mg twice daily for seven days, or 750 mg extended release once daily for seven days. Topical treatment with metronidazole 0.75% vaginal gel twice daily for five days is an alternative. Clindamycin orally or topically is also effective. Partners do not need to be treated.

How do I treat atrophic vaginitis?

Replacement topical or intravaginal estrogen is often used to treat atrophic vaginitis. Oral or transdermal estrogen can also be given. If the patient has a uterus and estrogen is given for more than a short course, progesterone must be added.

KEY POINTS

- **Always perform microscopic examination to confirm the diagnosis.**
- **The most common causes of vaginal discharge are yeast, *Trichomonas*, and bacterial vaginosis.**

CASE 38–1. **A 25-year-old woman presents with one week of vaginal itching and discharge. She has had "yeast infections" in the past, so she used over-the-counter miconazole ("Monistat") from the pharmacy starting four days ago without relief of symptoms. She has a new sexual partner in the past month and does not use condoms consistently. On exam, she is afebrile, and the abdominal exam is benign. On speculum exam, her cervix appears erythematous, and there is a malodorous greenish discharge with a pH of 5. There is no tenderness on bimanual exam.**

A. What are possible etiologies of her vaginal discharge?
B. What is the most likely finding on wet mount exam?
C. What will you advise her to tell her sexual partner(s)?

CASE 38–2. **A 43-year-old woman presents to your office for the second time in two weeks. Last week, you treated her empirically for a UTI with trimethoprim-sulfa. Three days later, her urine culture grew out *Escherichia coli*, sensitive to trimox. She is now here with a one-week history of vaginal discharge and burning. She has no history of STD and denies recent sexual activity. On exam, she is afebrile. Her abdomen and back are normal, with no CVA tenderness. There is vulvar erythema. Speculum exam shows normal cervix, with some white discharge. There is no tenderness on bimanual exam.**

A. What is the most likely finding on wet mount exam?
B. What are your treatment options?

REFERENCES

Egan ME, Lipsky MS: Vaginitis. Am Fam Physician 62:1095–1104, 2000. Available at *http://www.aafp.org/afp/20000901/1095.html.*

Nasraty S: Infections of the female genital tract. Primary Care; Clinics in Office Practice 30(1):193–203, 2003.

Workowski KA, Levine WC: Sexually Transmitted Diseases Treatment Guidelines 2002. MMWR Morb Mortal Wkly Rep 51 (RR-6):1–78, 2002.

USEFUL WEBSITES

National Guideline Clearinghouse, sponsored by the Agency for Healthcare Research and Quality, U.S. Department of Health and Human Services. *http://www.guideline.gov*

Centers for Disease Control guidelines for STD treatment. *http://www.cdc.gov/STD/treatment*

39

Vomiting

▶ ETIOLOGY

What are the most common causes of vomiting?

Most commonly, acute episodes of vomiting occur when various viral infections or forms of food poisoning cause irritation and inflammation of the GI tract; the condition is better known as gastroenteritis. However, vomiting can be a warning sign of more serious conditions, which differ somewhat depending on the patient's age group. (See Boxes 39–1 and 39–2.)

▶ EVALUATION

Why are the history and physical exam so important in a patient who is vomiting?

The causes of vomiting are endless, ranging from emotional distress and indigestion to life-threatening infections and surgical emergencies requiring immediate diagnosis and treatment. The diagnosis can be accomplished by a thorough history and physical exam that includes exploring for pertinent positive findings of certain "red flag" diagnoses, such as those in Table 39–1.

▶ TREATMENT

How do I manage a vomiting patient?

Many cases of gastroenteritis are self-limiting and require only supportive treatment with attention placed on slow rehydration as the patient can tolerate fluids. Severely dehydrated patients who are unable to tolerate oral fluids may, however, require inpatient treatment. Antibiotics are not necessary unless indicated by a specific infectious organism. Symptomatic relief of nausea may be provided with antihistamines such as promethazine or serotonin antagonists such as ondansetron.

BOX 39–1

Common Causes of Vomiting

Gastroenteritis (viral, bacterial, parasitic)
Indigestion
Motion Sickness
Vertigo
Medications, often chemotherapeutic agents or postanesthesia
Alcohol ("hangover" effect)
Early pregnancy
Stress/anxiety
Migraine headaches
Eating disorders (anorexia or bulimia)
Inflammatory bowel disease
Cholecystitis
Appendicitis
Pancreatitis
Diabetic ketoacidosis
Meningitis
Pyloric obstruction
Brain tumors
Hydrocephalus
Hepatitis
Peptic ulcer disease

BOX 39–2

Important Causes of Vomiting in Infants

Gastroenteritis
Lactose intolerance
Formula intolerance
Milk allergy
Pyloric stenosis
Diabetic ketoacidosis
Intussusception
Strangulated hernia
Urinary tract infection

TABLE 39–1

Important History and Exam Findings in a Vomiting Patient

Cause	History	Exam
Early pregnancy	Missed menstrual periods, breast tenderness/enlargement, fatigue, nausea often occurring in the morning, aversions to certain foods/odors	Fetal heart tones, enlarging abdomen
Meningitis	Headache, drowsiness/lethargy	Stiff neck, photophobia, rash (if meningococcal), fever
Increased ICP (Hydrocephalus, tumor)	Headache, nausea occurring in am, behavioral changes, past cancer history, seizures	Increased blood pressure, papilledema, focal neurologic deficits
Appendicitis	Epigastric, then RUQ pain, loss of appetite	Fever, abdominal guarding/ rigidity

ICP = intracranial pressure, RUQ = right upper quadrant

KEY POINTS

- **A thorough history and physical examination is essential to rule out life-threatening causes of vomiting.**
- **The most common side effect of vomiting is dehydration, and patients who cannot tolerate oral fluids may require inpatient treatment.**
- **Antiemetics may provide symptomatic relief and aid in facilitating oral rehydration.**

CASE 39–1. **A 22-year-old woman comes in with a two-week history of nausea and vomiting that gradually improves throughout the day. On average she vomits one to two times per day and can only eat bland foods. Her nausea is often triggered by strong odors. She denies fevers or any recent family history of similar symptoms. Vital signs are temperature 37. 2°C, blood pressure 102/45, respirations 20, pulse 112. Physical exam is significant for bilateral breast tenderness.**

A. What is this patient's differential diagnosis?
B. What additional history would be most helpful?
C. Should any tests be ordered? If so, which ones?

CASE 39–2. **A mother brings in her 6-year-old son because, three days prior, he began to complain of pain around his "belly button" with a gradually decreasing appetite. This morning he had two episodes of emesis and now appears very uncomfortable, clutching his right side. Vital signs are temperature 39.6°C, blood pressure 130/81, respirations 28, pulse 124. Physical exam is significant for involuntary guarding, rebound tenderness, and pain on percussion. The patient is unable to tolerate hyperextension of his right hip secondary to pain.**

A. What must be ruled out on your differential diagnosis?
B. Which lab tests and imaging studies should be ordered?

CASE 39–3. **A 26-year-old man is experiencing watery diarrhea and numerous bouts of vomiting about an hour after attending a church picnic. He also complains of abdominal cramping and retching in between episodes of emesis. His girlfriend, who also attended the picnic, is experiencing similar symptoms.**

A. What are the most common organisms to consider as possibly associated with these symptoms?

REFERENCES

Fauci A, et al. (eds): Harrison's Principles of Internal Medicine, 14th ed. New York: McGraw-Hill, 1998, pp 230–232.
Hasler WL, Chey WD: Nausea and vomiting. Gastroenterology 125:1860–1867, 2003.
Quigley EMM, et al.: AGA technical review on nausea and vomiting. Gastroenterology 120:263–286, 2001.
Rudolph AM, Kamei RK: Rudolph's Fundamentals of Pediatrics, 3rd ed., New York: McGraw-Hill, 1994, pp 466–467, 485, 489–490.

USEFUL WEBSITES

Family Practice Notebook. *www.fpnotebook.com*
WebMD Corporation. *www.webmd.com*
Centers for Disease Control provides information on infectious causes of gastroenteritis. *www.cdc.gov*

SECTION 3

Patients Presenting with a Known Condition

40

Family Violence

▶ ETIOLOGY

What is family violence?

Family violence refers to any behavior directed toward one family member by another family member or caregiver that threatens or impairs physical or emotional health. Victims include children, adult partners, and the elderly. Family violence is a problem of epidemic proportions in the United States, affecting more than 7 million people each year.

What are the forms of family violence?

Child abuse includes four major categories: physical abuse, sexual abuse, neglect, and emotional abuse. Physical abuse is the physical act of harm against a child by a caregiver. Sexual abuse refers to any contact or interaction between a child and another person in which a child is sexually exploited for the gratification of the perpetrator. Neglect is a condition in which the caregiver either deliberately or inattentively fails to meet a child's basic needs. Emotional abuse relates to an act or an omission on the part of the caregiver that has caused or could cause a serious behavioral, cognitive, emotional, or mental disorder in a child.

There are three major types of *partner abuse*. Physical abuse involves actions that may result in pain, injury, and/or impairment. Sexual abuse is a form of violence in which sex is used to hurt, degrade, humiliate, or gain power over the victim. Psychological abuse refers to threats or actions that result in mental anguish, anxiety, or depression.

The four most common forms of *elder abuse* are physical abuse, psychological abuse, financial abuse, and neglect. Physical and psychological abuse of the elderly parallels that of victims of partner abuse. Financial abuse pertains to the misuse of an elderly person's income or resources for the personal gain of the caregiver, or the failure to use available funds or resources necessary to maintain or restore the well-being of the elderly. Neglect relates to the failure of the caregiver to provide the goods and services that are needed for optimal functioning or to avoid harm.

Why does family violence occur?

Factors that contribute expressly to child abuse include the absence of parenting skills, a lack of understanding of child development, parental emotional immaturity, social isolation, and partner abuse. Risk factors specific to partner abuse include women who believe that it is their duty to keep their families together at all costs, continual exposure to violent behavior in entertainment and the media, and societal attitudes that promote men viewing women as property. Characteristics particular to elder abuse include caregiver resentment and/or exhaustion, impaired caregiver (substance abuse, mental illness, cognitive deficits), and widely held negative attitudes and stereotypes of the elderly.

Characteristics shared by all three types of family violence include low socioeconomic status, substance abuse, and intergenerational history of violence. It is important to remember that violence and its related behaviors are learned. A child who is abused by a parent may become an adult who abuses a partner or child and then, as a caregiver to an elderly family member, may extend the violence further. Presence of risk factors alone does not prove that abuse is occurring.

What are the consequences of family violence?

The damage caused by family violence can be both psychological and physical. Most runaways, teen prostitutes, and juvenile delinquents report that they are child abuse victims. A majority of violent criminals have suffered some form of child abuse. Victims of partner and elder abuse suffer depression, anxiety, and suicide attempts. Physical repercussions include death, broken bones, and sexually transmitted diseases.

▶ EVALUATION

How do I detect that the patient may be a victim of abuse or neglect?

A majority of victims are not going to reveal the abuse or neglect. Abused partners or elders are often overwhelmed, confused, embarrassed, or afraid. The elderly patient may have cognitive impairment that prevents him/her from disclosure. An abused child may have been threatened or coerced by the abuser to keep silent. A high index of suspicion for all types of abuse is important, and it is recommended that all patients be screened, especially those who present with vague somatic complaints and/or behavioral cues.

Although family violence may be difficult to detect, there are some behavioral and physical indicators that will help you make a diagnosis (Table 40–1). These indicators vary depending on the form and victim of abuse.

TABLE 40–1

Behavioral & Physical Indicators of Family Violence

Victim	Form of Abuse	Descriptions
Child	Physical	Lacerations, bruises, welts on face, lips, mouth, torso Abdominal injuries Burns • Cigar or cigarette • Immersion (socklike, glovelike, doughnut-shaped) • Patterned CNS injuries • Subdural hematoma • Subarachnoid hemorrhage • Retinal hemorrhage Fractures of skull, nose, or facial structure; multiple fractures or spiral fractures Extremes in behavior Unusually fearful of adults Contradictory explanations of injury, no explanation Unexplained delay in treatment
	Sexual	Recurrent urinary tract infections Sexually transmitted diseases Bruises on breasts, buttocks, abdomen, or thighs Genital or rectal injuries, irritations, or discharges Difficulty in walking or sitting Sleep disturbances Enuresis/encopresis School failure or truancy Sexual promiscuity Running away
	Neglect	Malnutrition Poor hygiene Inadequate clothing Constant fatigue or listlessness Poor school performance
	Emotional	Discipline problems, aggressive behavior Delays in physical development Failure to thrive

continued

Table 40–1. Behavioral & Physical Indicators of Family Violence *continued*

Victim	Form of Abuse	Descriptions
Partner	Physical	Abdominal injuries (particularly in bathing suit pattern) Lacerations, bruises, welts, human bites Multiple injuries in various stages of healing CNS injuries Spontaneous abortions, miscarriages, preterm labor Fear of retribution
	Sexual	Gynecological problems ● Vaginal and/or urinary tract infections ● Dyspareuria ● Chronic pelvic pain Shame and humiliation Depression, anxiety Somatic complaints ● Chronic headaches, insomnia ● Stomach, pelvic, and back pain ● Atypical chart
	Psychological	Somatic complaints Depression, anxiety Feelings of isolation and self-blame Shame and humiliation Suicidal ideation
Elder	Physical	Lacerations, bruises, welts Bilateral injuries Burns Rope or hand prints Fractures or signs of previous fractures Dehydration or weight loss without a medical explanation Unexplained venereal disease or genital infection Injuries in various stages of healing
	Psychological	Social isolation Chronic pain, psychogenic pain Withdrawal Depression, anxiety Fear of family members Hesitancy to talk openly
	Financial	Coercing the elder to sign a contract, change a will, or purchase goods Lack of necessities despite adequate financial resources
	Neglect	Malnutrition Dehydration Poor hygiene Lack of compliance with medical regimens Decubitus ulcers

What are the components of an evaluation for possible abuse or neglect?

If you suspect that a patient is being abused (or in the very rare instance he/she relates this to you), you must conduct an appropriate interview and physical exam.

How should I conduct the interview?

Phrase your questions in a nonconfrontational way. Do not blame the victim *or* the perpetrator; nor should you confront the perpetrator. The interview should be conducted alone, in a private setting, and you should always explain the limits of confidentiality. Progress from general questioning to more specific questions, allowing the patient adequate time to respond. Be certain that your questions are suitable for the age and educational level of your patient.

If the suspected victim is a child, prepare the child for the interview. Preparation includes clarifying the goal of the interview (i.e., to understand the parents' concern and assess the symptoms and/or injuries) and explaining the necessity of speaking alone to the child. Give the child an age-appropriate explanation of what is going to happen. During the interview, proceed at a relaxed pace and use his/her language when referring to body parts. Remember that questions beginning with "How come?" are more productive than questions beginning with "Why?"

When you are concerned about possible partner abuse, assess the patient with questions similar to the following:

"I am concerned that your symptoms may have been caused by someone hurting you."
"It is pretty common for women to be hurt by their partners. Has anyone been hurting you (by threatening, pushing, hitting, choking, restraining you)?"
"Are you afraid of your partner (have you been threatened by anyone you are in a close relationship with)?"
"Do you feel safe in your current relationship?"
"Has anyone forced you to have sexual activities?"

When you are concerned about possible elder abuse, screen for abuse with questions similar to the following:

"Has anyone at home ever hurt you?"
"Has anyone taken anything that was yours without asking?"
"Has anyone ever scolded or threatened you?"
"Are you afraid of anyone at home?"
"Are you alone a lot?"
"Has anyone ever failed to help you take care of yourself when you needed help?"
"Have you ever signed any document that you didn't understand?"

Describe the physical examination in a patient possibly suffering abuse or neglect.

Whether your patient is a child, adult partner, or elderly person, a thorough physical exam is critical to the diagnosis. Keep in mind the signs and symptoms of family violence as you conduct the exam. More importantly, do not overlook possible injuries that need treatment.

When assessing for child abuse, there are several guidelines to follow. Before the exam, allow time for the child to ask questions. Start the exam with a nonthreatening part of the body and explain each step as you proceed. Conduct the exam with both a nurse and a parent present, because the parent can be a valuable support to the child unless the parent is the abuser. If you suspect physical abuse and your patient is under age 5, order an x-ray survey because clinical fractures often disappear after a week.

A male physician treating a woman abused by a male partner would be well-advised to conduct the physical exam in the presence of a female chaperone.

▶ TREATMENT

Do I have to report the suspected abuse or neglect?

Yes. All states require physicians to report suspected child abuse to the appropriate authorities and most have penalties for failure to report. The laws provide immunity from liability if the report is made in good faith. It is not a breach of confidentiality, because a family's right to privacy does not apply to cases of suspected child abuse. Knowledge about the legal requirements of your state is necessary because there are variations in state statutes. While laws vary in reporting procedures, reporting of elder abuse is also mandatory. As with child and elder abuse, you may be required to report partner abuse to local law enforcement officials. Whenever you suspect family violence, be it child, partner, or elder abuse, always share your suspicions with your preceptor before the patient leaves.

Besides reporting, what is my role in treating family violence?

Your role in the treatment of family violence will differ somewhat, depending on the type of abuse you are treating. When confronted with possible child abuse, support and follow-up are key. This involves providing the family with information about community resources that would be helpful in meeting their specific needs and deficits. Such resources include, but are not limited to, mental health services, financial assistance, and parenting education.

BOX 40–1

Hotline Numbers

National Child Abuse Hotline	1-800-422-4453
National Domestic Violence Hotline	1-800-799-7233
National Organization for Victim Assistance	1-800-879-6682

Other sources can also be of value (Box 40–1). Schedule follow-up visits so that you can make certain that the family is receiving appropriate assistance and provide support. Keep in mind that you may be the only stable contact they have.

If your patient is a victim of partner abuse, remember that she is in a crisis that prevents her from using coping and problem-solving skills. Help her to begin thinking more clearly about her situation and to begin thinking about making changes. Make certain that you refer your patient to appropriate community resources, such as shelters, legal and advocacy services, and mental health agencies. Follow-up visits are imperative to provide the victim opportunities to validate her experience, reassess her options, and begin thinking about making changes. When your patient is ready for change, you can assist her in developing a safety plan. A safety plan consists of a strategy of when to leave and where to go, extra clothing for herself and her children, extra set of keys for the car and home, evidence of abuse (pictures, medical reports), cash, checkbook, and legal documents (such as marriage license, birth certificates, and Social Security cards).

If your elder patient answers affirmatively to any of the questions you posed, you need to determine how the patient feels about his/her situation and how he/she is coping with it. Your goal is to help the patient to begin thinking about the situation more clearly and develop a plan that assures that the abuse stops. As with the other forms of abuse, referrals to pertinent community resources are important. Such resources include legal services, mental health agencies, local offices on aging, and elder social service agencies. If the elderly patient is cognitively impaired, a greater level of intervention is required. You will need to call Adult Protective Services. Make certain that follow-up visits are scheduled so that you can confirm that the patient is receiving needed assistance, assist your patient in dealing with the other systems involved (e.g., social services, legal), and provide support.

What do I need to know about documentation?

Proper documentation is important when providing any medical care, but in suspected family violence cases, it is imperative. Thorough, well-documented medical records provide evidence if there is legal system involvement, and it may be the only evidence of abuse or neglect. Your documentation should include the following:

- Verbatim description of the event
- Location of the abusive event(s)
- Timing and sequence of the events
- Complete medical and relevant social history
- Observed behavior
- Detailed description of injuries, including type, location, number, site and degree of healing, possible causes, and explanations given*
- X-ray and lab findings

Your information should be well organized and legible. The facts should be objective and behaviors should be described and not interpreted. If the police are contacted, the name, badge number, and phone number of the investigating officer and any actions taken should be recorded.

KEY POINTS

- ▶ **The victims of family violence include children, adult partners, and the elderly.**
- ▶ **Violence occurs more frequently in the family than any other place in society.**
- ▶ **Since most victims will not report their abuse or neglect, physicians must maintain a high index of suspicion.**
- ▶ **A nonthreatening and nonjudgmental interview is the basis for assessment and intervention of family violence.**
- ▶ **Physicians are required to report suspect child and elder abuse to appropriate authorities.**

CASE 40–1. **A 3-month-old baby boy is brought to the clinic by his mother. She is concerned about his increased fussiness and redness on his right arm. Upon further questioning, the mother reports that three days earlier, while she was putting clothes into the dryer, the patient rolled off the sofa onto the carpeted floor.**

A. Why does this case make you suspicious of child abuse?
B. What further information should you obtain?

* The use of a body chart to record the location, nature, and size of any injuries is recommended. It is also recommended that healthcare providers take pictures (35 mm or Polaroid-type) of the injuries.

CASE 40–2. **A frail-appearing 80-year-old woman presents to the clinic with a chief complaint of loss of appetite. You note that her clothing is slightly soiled. She is accompanied by her 55-year-old son, who reports that he "takes care" of her. When you begin your questioning, the son immediately responds and interrupts the patient whenever she attempts to answer a question.**

A. What would you include in your physical exam?
B. How would you continue with your assessment?
C. Provided your physical findings and lab are negative, how would you proceed?

USEFUL WEBSITE

National Council on Child Abuse and Family Violence. *http://www.nccafv.org*

41

Asthma/COPD

ASTHMA

► ETIOLOGY

What is asthma?

Asthma is a chronic relapsing inflammatory disorder characterized by hyperreactive airways with smooth muscle hypertrophy. Asthma differs from COPD in that it is an episodic bronchoconstriction resulting from an increased responsiveness to various stimuli and is reversible by bronchodilator therapy. Also, patients with asthma have asymptomatic periods of varying length, based on the severity of the disease.

What triggers asthma symptoms?

There are many different pollutants that trigger a hyperreactive response by the bronchopulmonary tree. Noncontrollable risk factors include allergies, family history of asthma, viral infections, male gender, and low birth weight. Controllable precipitating factors include perinatal smoke exposure, dust mites, animal dander, cockroaches, pollen, pollutants, smoking, secondhand smoke, perfume, drugs (aspirin, NSAIDs, β-blockers, sulfites), exercise, cold air, gastroesophageal reflux disease (GERD), and infections.

What is an asthma attack?

An acute exacerbation of asthma is a sudden worsening of symptoms of varying degrees. Asthma attacks should not be taken lightly for they can result in death. Attack symptoms include difficulty speaking, agitation, diaphoresis, respiration rate of 28 or higher, tachycardia, and pulsus paradoxis of 25 mmHg or higher. Pulsus paradoxis is the difference in blood pressure between inspiration and expiration (inspiration has the lower blood pressure). The intensity of the wheeze is not an indicator of the severity of the attack.

▶ EVALUATION

What should I look for in the office?

Asthma is a disease with a tremendous variability in presentation of symptoms dependant on the severity of the disease. Patients will give a history of wheezing, cough, chest tightness, shortness of breath, and tachypnea. These symptoms seem to be worse at night, early in the morning, or with activity. The symptoms will last for a discrete period of time and then subside. On physical exam, you may hear wheezes (more common expiratory, but can be inspiratory) on lung exam. The patient may have nasal flaring, or be breathing through pursed lips, or using accessory muscles (sternocleidomastoid and intercostals) to assist in breathing.

Which lab tests should I order?

The best way to attempt to document asthma in your clinic is to perform pulmonary function tests in the office. Asthmatics will show an overall decrease in the FEV_1 value and the FEV_1/FVC ratio will be below 0.75. These values indicate an obstructive process. However, after the administration of an albuterol nebulizer treatment, the FEV_1 will increase by more than 12%. This indicates a reversible component of the airway obstruction.

In some types of asthmatics you will see increased immunoglobulin E (IgE) levels, atopic dermatitis, nasal polyps, rhinitis, and aspirin sensitivity. These all indicate an allergic and atopic component to the asthma disease process. Therefore, allergy testing in these individuals would be recommended. This can be done by the skin prick method or by radioallergosorbent testing (RAST). These are IgE hypersensitivity tests to determine allergens to which the patient is hypersensitive.

How do I determine if the patient's asthma is severe?

The severity of disease is determined by the symptoms the patient is experiencing (Table 41–1). Frequency and duration of symptoms, timing of symptoms (during or after exercise, nighttime or daytime), and the response to therapy are all important factors to consider. To determine severity and adequacy of control, ask the patient: How often during the day do you have symptoms? How long do they last? Do they happen at night, during exercise, or in the cold weather? Do they interfere with your daily activities, sleeping habits, or recreational events? How often are you using your rescue inhaler? Does it work?

TABLE 41-1

Determining Severity of Asthma

Asthma Diagnosis	Days with Symptoms	Nights with Symptoms	% of best expiratory flow
Severe, persistent	Continual	Frequent	≤60%
Moderate, persistent	Daily	≥5 per month	60–80%
Mild, persistent	≥2 times/week	3–4 per month	≥80%
Mild, intermittent	≤2 times/week	≤2 per month	≥80%

▶ TREATMENT

How do I treat an asthma attack?

To treat an attack you need to administer oxygen, give racemic epinephrine via a nebulizer, immediately start corticosteroid therapy, and be ready to intubate if the patient becomes fatigued. When reading the blood gases of these asthmatic patients, remember that during an asthma attack they are hyperventilating, so the $PaCO_2$ on blood gas will be low. If the $PaCO_2$ is normal or elevating in a patient that is in some distress, then he or she is beginning to tire and intubation should be strongly considered.

Can asthma be helped without medicines?

Asthma education is a very important part of the treatment of asthma. Education should be focused on the prevention of emergency room visits and acute exacerbations, while aiming for a symptom-free, active lifestyle. Education should focus on the avoidance of triggers, the proper use of inhalers, the importance of daily medicine use, the development of a self-management plan, and an emergency plan in case of an asthma attack.

Environment control measures can also be taken to curtail some triggers that may initiate an asthma attack. The patient should remove carpets, rugs, and stuffed animals, for these harbor dust and other irritants. Pets should be kept outside, and special filters can be placed on furnaces and other air circulation systems. In addition, specially designed mattresses and pillow covers can be used, and bedding should be washed weekly in hot water.

Which drugs help?

There are three methods for quick "rescue" relief of symptoms. First, and most popular, is the short acting β_2-agonist inhalers or nebulizers. Their main use is the treatment of exercise-induced asthma

TABLE 41–2

Long-Term Treatment of Chronic Asthma

Asthma Diagnosis	Chronic Treatment
Severe, persistent	High-dose inhaled corticosteroid with long-acting β_2-agonist. May need oral steroid if severe.
Moderate, persistent	Medium-dose inhaled corticosteroid or low-dose inhaled corticosteroid with a long-acting β_2-agonist
Mild, persistent	Low-dose inhaled corticosteroid or leukotriene agonist
Mild, intermittent	None needed, just rescue therapy. Albuterol for exercise induced.

and trigger-related bronchospasm. Secondly, anticholinergics can be used. These are only used if there is a contraindication or failure of β_2-agonist therapy. Finally, a short course of oral corticosteroids provides anti-inflammatory effects to decrease the swelling of airways.

Describe long-term treatment of chronic asthma.

The long-term treatment of asthma is determined by the severity of the disease. See Table 41–2.

CHRONIC OBSTRUCTIVE PULMONARY DISEASE

▶ ETIOLOGY

What is chronic obstructive pulmonary disease (COPD)?

Chronic obstructive pulmonary disease is a condition of irreversible parenchymal damage to the bronchial tree causing impaired ventilation and gas exchange. COPD is a common term used to describe emphysema and chronic bronchitis. Other systemic illnesses that can cause obstructive airway disease include cystic fibrosis, bronchiectasis, and bronchiolitis obliterans.

▶ EPIDEMIOLOGY

Is COPD a major health problem?

COPD is a very common disease that is increasing in prevalence. Because of the increase in cigarette smoking, environmental pollutants, and other gaseous exposures, COPD now ranks as one of the major causes of activity-restricting diseases. Nearly one fifth of Americans are diagnosed with COPD, and it is currently listed as the fourth leading cause of death in the United States. More than 90% of individuals with COPD have smoked in their lifetimes.

Is emphysema a type of COPD?

Yes. There are two different types of COPD: emphysema and chronic bronchitis. These different types have different physical findings, but ultimately the same outcome. Emphysema, or "pink-puffer," is a condition characterized by abnormal permanent enlargement of the airspaces distal to the terminal bronchiole. There is destruction of the cellular walls but no obvious fibrosis. Therefore, the destruction in emphysema causes overinflation of the airways.

Chronic bronchitis, "blue-bloater," is defined clinically. It is present in any patient (mostly smokers) with a persistent cough for more days than not, with sputum production. The cough lasts for at least three months in at least two consecutive years. The cough is often more prominent in the morning and is known as "smoker's cough." There is an overproduction of mucus that becomes trapped in the airway and cannot escape, making infections more common.

What causes acute worsening of COPD?

Acute exacerbations are a worsening of respiratory status significantly below the baseline where the patient normally functions. Clinic signs of exacerbations are worsening dyspnea and an increase in purulent sputum production. Bacterial infection is the most common cause of acute exacerbations. Etiologic bacteria include *Streptococcus pneumoniae, Haemophilus influenzae, Moraxella catarrhalis, Chlamydia pneumoniae, Mycoplasma pneumoniae,* viruses, and *Pseudomonas* (most severe). Exacerbation can also be initiated by environmental pollutants, congestive heart failure, and pharmacologic noncompliance.

▶ EVALUATION

What would I see on physical exam of emphysema and chronic bronchitis?

Most of the signs and symptoms of emphysema and chronic bronchitis are the same. Similar symptoms include a chronic productive cough, cigarette use, tachypnea, pursed-lip breathing, and accessory muscle use. Symptoms typically are absent during the sleeping hours (except for cough). Physical exam findings include decreased breath sounds, crackles or wheezes, an increase in anterior/posterior chest diameter (barrel chest), and hyperresonance to percussion.

There are a couple of distinguishing characteristics between emphysema and chronic bronchitis. Chronic bronchitis appears earlier than emphysema, usually in patients in their mid-40s. Dyspnea is less common in chronic bronchitis than in emphysema, but the sputum production is more severe. Infections are much more common in chronic bronchitis. On chest x-ray, chronic bronchitis shows prominent vessels and a large heart, while emphysema shows hyperinflation with flattening of the diaphragm and a small heart.

What labs should I order? What will they show?

Chest x-ray will show flattening of diaphragms that are lower than normal, indicating hyperinflation. There will be decrease in vascular markings and a hyperlucency in the lung fields (particularly in the upper lung fields). Pulmonary function tests will show a decrease in the FEV_1 and the FEV_1/FRC ratio below 0.75 (this is the difference from restrictive lung disease, in which the ratio is normal to increased). The decreased ratio indicates air trapping with collapse of the small airways, making it difficult for the patient to exhale the air in the lungs. In addition, there will be an increase in the total lung capacity, residual volume, and functional reserve capacity.

Because of the air trapping and the mucus plugging, there is a mismatch in the ventilation to perfusion ratio. Blood is being perfused, but adequate gas exchange does not occur because of poor ventilation. On arterial blood gas, there will be a build up of CO_2 with a compensatory metabolic alkalosis (increase in bicarbonate). *Note:* A COPD patient needs this increase in $PaCO_2$ to drive the brain's respiratory center. Therefore it is *not* advantageous to correct a high $PaCO_2$ in these patients. If they are talking and appear asymptomatic, then an increase in oxygen is not warranted ("treat the patient, not the numbers"). Patients like these can live with oxygen saturations in the low 90s percentiles.

▶ TREATMENT

How do I treat acute exacerbations of COPD?

There are five steps to treating acute exacerbations of COPD:

1. Give O_2 via nasal cannula or CPAP to keep saturations above 92%. Don't push the O_2 saturation up too high, but attempt to stay around 92%.
2. Encourage bronchodilation with short-acting β_2-agonist every 4 to 6 hours and long-acting β_2-agonist therapy every 12 hours. Inhaled anticholinergics (ipratropium) can be used as adjunctive therapy.

3. Give intravenous fluid resuscitation. Dehydration can make sputum thicker and more difficult to expel.
4. Direct antibiotic therapy toward the most common/likely pathogens.
5. Use systemic steroids to decrease the inflammation. Give IV methylprednisilone (1–2 mg/kg) every 6 to 12 hours for 2 to 3 days. Then switch to oral prednisilone at 60 mg for a total of 2 weeks. Gradually taper the steroid dose for another 2 weeks.

What medications do those with chronic COPD need every day?

There are many treatment options for COPD patients. However, only two have been clinically proven to decrease mortality. The most important part of a treatment program is smoking cessation. The other proven beneficial therapy is the administration of oxygen via nasal cannula or CPAP. A patient must have a PaO_2 of less than or equal to 55 mmHg or an O_2 saturation of less than or equal to 88% for oxygen therapy to be covered by insurance. Adjust the oxygen level administered to maintain the patient's O_2 saturation in the low to mid 90s. Other therapeutic options include inhaled β_2-agonist to help with bronchodilation. Short-acting β_2-agonist can be used for rescue therapy, and long-term β_2-agonist is used for prevention of bronchospasm. Inhaled corticosteroids can also be used to provide an anti-inflammatory effect. There are combination inhalers that provide both a long-acting β_2-agonist and a low-dose inhaled corticosteroid. COPD patients should receive a yearly influenza vaccine and the pneumococcal vaccine every five years.

KEY POINTS

- **A normal or increasing $PaCO_2$ during an asthma attack indicates fatigue in the patient. Be ready to intubate if you feel the patient will tire out.**
- **The difference between COPD and asthma is the reversible nature of asthma in response to bronchodilator therapy.**
- **Do not give β-blockers to somebody with obstructive airway disease. The lungs need the action of the β_2-receptors to stay open.**
- **In obstructive airway disease there is a decrease in the FEV_1/FVC ratio below 0.75. Restrictive airway disease has an increased ratio.**

CASE 41–1. **A 65-year-old man comes into the clinic with increasing shortness of breath. He is a chronic COPD patient with a smoking history of 2 packs per day for 45 years. He has had a horrible sputum-producing cough in the mornings for the last 15 years. His medications are ASA and albuterol. Over the past week he has been battling a runny nose with some dyspnea and wheezing. He is having worsening exertional fatigue when walking one block. His vitals are temperature 37.6°C, respirations 22, pulse 92. His nose is clear with a red oropharynx. He has an increased AP diameter with decreased breath sounds and diffuse wheezing. There is no JVD and heart is RRR without murmur.**

A. What could be causing the acute exacerbation of his COPD?
B. What lab tests should be ordered?
C. How should you treat the acute exacerbation?
D. How would you change his chronic COPD management?

CASE 41–2. **A 15-year-old girl with a history of asthma comes into the emergency room with air hunger and wheezing. It was a windy September afternoon and she had been playing out on her grandfather's farm. She began to wheeze in the field, and had her grandfather bring her to the emergency room. She is currently on albuterol and singulair. During the history, she is only able to answer your questions in three-word sentences. Her vitals are temperature 36.2°C, respirations 14, pulse 120. Her blood pressure is 110/78 on expiration and 82/66 on inspiration. She has allergic shiners and pale and boggy turbinates. Heart is RRR and no JVD. Auscultation of the lungs reveals diffuse wheezes that do not clear with cough. Her capillary refill was less than 3 seconds.**

A. What are the signs of worsening asthma attacks that are cause for concern?
B. What is the immediate treatment for this attack?
C. What lab tests and diagnostic studies do you need?
D. If this patient normally has daily daytime symptoms and twice weekly nighttime symptoms, what chronic treatment should she be on?

REFERENCES

Hunter M, King D: COPD: Management of acute exacerbations and chronic stable disease. Am Fam Physician, 64(4):603–612, 2001.

Kemp JP, Kemp JA: Management of asthma in children. Am Fam Physician, 63(7):1341–1348, 1353–1354, 2001.

USEFUL WEBSITES

American Lung Association. *http://www.lungusa.org*

American Academy of Family Physicians. *http://www.aafp.org*

42

Angina and Coronary Artery Disease

▶ ETIOLOGY

How are coronary artery disease and ischemic heart disease related?

Ischemic heart disease (IHD) is a broad term referring to any situation in which the heart does not receive adequate perfusion to meet its demand. IHD may be caused by atherosclerosis, thrombosis, vasospasm, emboli, or arteritis syndromes such as Takayasu arteritis or Kawasaki syndrome. However, more than 90% of IHD is caused by atherosclerotic lesions and thrombosis secondary to atherosclerotic lesions. Atherosclerotic disease of the coronary arteries is generally referred to as coronary artery disease (CAD).

What is angina?

Angina is cardiogenic pain caused by IHD. It is generally retrosternal and described as heaviness, pressure, or choking more so than as "pain." It may radiate to the arms, neck, or jaw. Patients also may describe back or epigastric pain. Associated symptoms can include nausea, diaphoresis, or dyspnea. The important thing to remember is that angina has a wide variety of presentations, and it must always be strongly considered in anyone with an element of chest pain. (See Chapter 17 for other causes of chest pain.) Angina can be caused by anything that causes IHD, but it is usually caused by CAD. It is very important to note that CAD often is *not* associated with angina; in fact, it may be clinically silent.

What is the pathogenesis of CAD?

A simple synopsis of the currently accepted hypothesis is as follows. Chronic endothelial injury causes endothelial dysfunction, which leads to increased permeability and leukocyte adhesion. Low-density lipoproteins (LDL) and very low–density lipoproteins (VLDL) accumulate in the compromised epithelium, and these particles become oxidized. Macrophages engulf the lipoproteins and become foam cells. Smooth muscle cells proliferate and deposit extracellular matrix, thus forming a mature lesion.

What are the main risk factors for CAD?

Modifiable risk factors include smoking, obesity, physical inactivity, lipid disorders, hypertension, and insulin resistance. Nonmodifiable risk factors include male gender, age, and genetic components.

What are the five main ways that CAD is manifested clinically?

It is useful to divide the clinical manifestations of CAD into five groups: silent ischemia, sudden death, stable angina, acute coronary syndrome, and ischemic heart failure. The underlying cause is atherosclerosis and/or thrombosis in all of them.

What is stable angina?

Stable angina is precipitated by exertion and relieved by rest within five minutes. Other triggers include stress, anger, a heavy meal, or exposure to cold. The keys are: it is not new for the patient, it has a predictable trigger, and it is very short lived.

What causes stable angina?

Stable angina is caused by a *stable* stenosis of 75% or greater of a coronary artery, not by a plaque rupture or by a thrombus.

What is acute coronary syndrome (ACS)?

ACS is a term that encompasses unstable angina, non–ST-elevation myocardial infarction (MI), and ST-elevation MI. It is a useful term to describe a patient, because on initial presentation it is not clear into which subcategory the patient fits. After evaluation, the patient is placed into the appropriate subcategory, rather than the more general ACS group.

■ **Red Flag:** Note that ACS may present without chest pain, especially in the elderly, in diabetics, and in postoperative patients. Symptoms in these individuals may be limited to confusion, dyspnea, or heart failure. These symptoms may be termed "anginal equivalent" in this context.

What causes ACS?

The primary initiating event in ACS is usually disruption of an atherosclerotic plaque. Rupture of the plaque leads to the formation of a thrombus in the coronary artery. If the thrombus does not completely occlude the artery, then the result is unstable angina. If the artery is completely occluded, then an ST-elevation MI occurs because full thickness necrosis occurs. A non–ST-elevation MI is generally partial thickness necrosis caused by transient complete occlusion.

Ironically, the plaques that rupture to cause ACS are usually smaller than those that cause stable angina. Two thirds of the plaques that rupture to form totally occlusive thrombus have stenosis of 50% or less before rupture.

What is unstable angina?

Unstable angina is angina that is new onset, occurs at rest, or is increasing in frequency, duration, or severity. Thus, a patient with well-documented stable angina, who has his usual angina, except that it is now more severe, is classified as having ACS and appropriate evaluation is needed. Angina within two weeks after a myocardial infarction is also considered unstable.

■ **Red Flag:** Unstable angina is considered an MI until proven otherwise.

What is a non–ST-elevation myocardial infarction?

A non–ST-elevation myocardial infarction is unstable angina with elevations in cardiac-specific troponin levels or creatine kinase isoenzyme (CK–MB). Thus, unstable angina cannot be differentiated from non–ST-elevation MI without cardiac enzymes. These patients may or may not have EKG findings such as transient ST elevation or depression, or transient T-wave inversions. These MIs typically do not go on to form Q waves.

What is an ST-elevation MI?

Diagnosis of an ST-elevation MI is made with prolonged angina or "anginal equivalent" and convex ST segment elevation in at least two contiguous leads. The cardiac enzymes will be positive, but these are not needed for the diagnosis. ST-elevation MI's will typically go on to form Q waves.

What is silent ischemia?

Patients with silent ischemia may have transient ischemia (as could be documented on an EKG during the episode), or they may have had an MI without recallable symptoms.

What is Prinzmetal's variant angina?

Prinzmetal's variant angina is a rare form of unstable angina caused by focal spasm of a coronary artery. It often occurs at rest, and patients are often smokers and younger than the typical IHD patient. It is diagnosed by provoking an attack during coronary angiography. It is treated with nitroglycerin and calcium channel blockers.

▶ EVALUATION

See Chapter 17 for the full chest pain differential and work-up.

How should I evaluate someone with stable angina?

First of all, you should be confident that the patient has stable angina as opposed to ACS. If in doubt, proceed to an ACS work-up. Questioning should establish the fact that the symptoms are indeed stable angina. Assess frequency, duration, character, triggers, and associated symptoms such as dyspnea, diaphoresis, and nausea. Assess risk factors such as hypertension, hyperlipidemia, diabetes, age, smoking, obesity, physical inactivity, and family history. Family history is generally considered significant if a first-degree male relative has had IHD under 45 years of age or if a first-degree female relative has had IHD under 55 years of age. Conditions that may exacerbate CAD, such as anemia or thyroid disease, should also be considered. Exercise tolerance and heart failure symptoms should also be assessed in the history.

Physical exam should be thorough, but it is often unremarkable. Especially look for xanthomas, signs of heart failure, murmurs, and bruits. Lab tests that may be useful include urine analysis (you may find diabetes or renal disease, both accelerate atherosclerosis), hematocrit to rule out anemia, lipid panel, glucose, and creatinine. Thyroid should be checked if indicated clinically. Examine chest x-ray for sign of heart failure or cardiac enlargement. A 12-lead EKG may show Q waves from an old infarction or it may be normal. If an EKG is recorded during an anginal episode, it may show ST depression.

Noninvasive testing may be used to establish the diagnosis and guide further treatment. The main types of noninvasive testing are excercise EKG, exercise EKG with perfusion imaging, pharmacologic stress perfusion imaging, and dobutamine stress echocardiography. The gold standard is coronary angiography, which may be indicated by a strongly positive stress test, severely symptomatic patients, or diagnostic dilemmas in which a definite diagnosis is needed.

What type of noninvasive testing should I use for someone with stable angina?

If the patient is able to exercise on a treadmill, then an exercise EKG is usually appropriate. If the person has conditions that will make the EKG difficult to interpret, such as a paced rhythm, conduction abnormalities, or left bundle branch block, then perfusion imaging will be more useful. If the person cannot exercise adequately because of musculoskeletal or other reasons, then pharmacologic stress with perfusion imaging should be undertaken with adenosine or dipyridamole.

How should I evaluate someone with acute coronary syndrome?

ACS patients should be admitted to the hospital. Initial evaluation includes history and physical as in the preceding text. Laboratory evaluations should include urinalysis, basic metabolic panel, complete blood count, coagulation studies, and serial cardiac enzymes. Often CK, CKMB, and troponin I level are taken on admission, 8 hours after admission, and 16 hours after admission. EKG should be obtained within the first five minutes. Chest x-ray should also be done immediately, and the patient should be admitted to a telemetry unit.

How do I interpret cardiac enzymes?

Creatine kinase-MB (CK–MB) rises within 4 to 8 hours of an MI, peaks at 20 to 24 hours, and returns to normal in 48 to 72 hours. However, CKMB is not entirely specific for cardiac tissue. It may also come from skeletal muscle. Typically, if it is not from an MI, it will not return to normal within 48 to 72 hours.

Cardiac-specific troponins are more sensitive and specific than CKMB. They increase within 3 to 10 hours of an MI and peak at 24 to 48 hours. However, they take 7 to 14 days to return to baseline.

When should I suspect silent ischemia and how should I evaluate it?

Suspect it in diabetics, the elderly, and others with multiple risk factors. If in doubt, evaluate with the appropriate noninvasive testing.

▶ TREATMENT

How should I address risk factors?

In addition to the specific treatments discussed in the following text, it is very important to aggressively address all modifiable risk factors including hypertension, lipid disorders, diabetes, obesity, smoking, and physical inactivity. These factors are discussed in other chapters.

How do I treat stable angina?

All patients should be on 81 to 325 mg of aspirin daily (if the patient is allergic to aspirin, use clopidogrel). All patients should also be on a β-blocker unless contraindications exist. Contraindications include asthma (COPD is not a contraindication), atrioventricular nodal block, severe bradycardia, symptomatic heart failure (relative contraindication), and Raynaud's disease. Calcium channel blockers may be used if β-blockers cannot be used. Sublingual nitroglycerin should be prescribed to abort anginal episodes and should also be taken prophylactically when an episode is likely. Long-acting nitrates may be used if necessary. Patients with a strongly positive stress test or symptoms refractory to medical treatment should be evaluated by coronary angiography for possible percutaneous transluminal coronary angioplasty (PTCA) or coronary artery bypass grafting (CABG).

How do I treat ACS?

The first priority in treatment of ACS is a brief initial history and a 12-lead EKG within five minutes of presentation. All ACS patients (without contraindications) should be given aspirin, supplemental oxygen, sublingual nitrates, β-blockers, heparin, IV access, and morphine for pain as needed. Glycoprotein (GP) IIb/IIIa inhibitors may be considered to help stop blood from clotting. If the EKG shows ST elevation over 1 mm in two consecutive leads or new LBBB, then the patient is a candidate for fibrinolytic therapy or PTCA and should be treated as an ST-elevation MI.

How do I treat unstable angina?

Diagnosis of unstable angina is established after cardiac enzymes come back negative. If the patient is asymptomatic for 48 hours then the patient may be evaluated with noninvasive testing or with coronary angiography. If the patient remains symptomatic, evaluation with coronary angiography should be carried out. Based on the results PTCA or CABG may be pursued if indicated.

How do I treat non–ST-elevation MI?

Treatment for non–ST-elevation MI should follow the ACS protocol; however, GP IIb/IIIa inhibitors should be added and evaluation by coronary angiography should be done to evaluate for possible PTCA or CABG.

How should I treat ST-elevation MI?

ST-elevation MI patients should receive the standard ACS treatment as described in the preceding text; however, the main goal is to initiate fibrinolytic therapy within 30 minutes or coronary angiography with PTCA within 1 hour. Absolute contraindications to thrombolytic therapy include stroke or TIA in the last 12 months, hemorrhagic stroke at any time, active internal bleeding, pregnancy, suspected aortic dissection, known CNS tumor or aneurysm, surgery in the last 10 days, or neurosurgery in the last 2 months. Relative contraindications such as systolic blood pressure above 180 mmHg or diastolic below 110 mmHg, CPR, INR greater than 2, and others must also be considered. An ACE inhibitor should be started within 24 hours of the MI. There are many post-MI complications that may occur that are beyond the scope of this chapter.

How should a typical post-MI patient (who has not had complications) be managed?

Post-MI patients should be on a β-blocker, aspirin, ACE inhibitor, and an HMG-CoA reductase inhibitor. A cardiac diet should be instituted, and stool softeners and mild laxatives should be used to avoid constipation. After 12 hours of bed rest, activity should be very gradually resumed. After discharge, enrollment in a cardiac rehabilitation and, if appropriate, a smoking-cessation program is beneficial. Four to six weeks post-MI, an exercise stress test should be carried out with further management based on those results.

KEY POINTS

- **CAD is the leading cause of morbidity and mortality in the United States, and it may be clinically silent.**
- **Aggressive management of risk factors is proven to be very effective in saving lives, and it is one of the most important jobs of primary care physicians.**
- **Unstable angina is a medical emergency, and the patient should be treated as an acute coronary syndrome, including an EKG within five minutes of presentation.**

CASE 42–1. **A 56-year-old woman presents to the emergency room with severe chest pressure of 30 minutes duration, diaphoresis, and nausea.**

A. What is the first thing you should do?
B. What are the main items that need to be addressed in the initial history?
C. What is the initial treatment and work-up if the EKG is negative?

CASE 42–2. **A 62-year-old man presents to your office because he is very concerned about heart disease. His father died of an MI when he was 44 years old, and a brother had a CABG when he was 46 years old. The patient hasn't been to a doctor in about five years. The patient has smoked for 40 years, doesn't exercise but his activity is not limited, denies diabetes, is mildly obese. He denies any significant medical history. He doesn't take any medications and has no allergies. Review of systems is negative. A physical exam is unremarkable. Vitals are temperature 37°C, pulse 88, blood pressure 152/90, and respirations 16.**

A. What diagnostic tests would you order?
B. His tests come back normal. What would you recommend to this patient?
C. He would like to start exercising, but he is worried about "keeling over" when he starts. What do you recommend?

REFERENCES

Lee TH, Boucher CA: Noninvasive tests in patients with stable coronary artery disease. N Engl J Med 344:1840–1845, 2001.
Lee TH, Goldman L: Evaluation of the patient with acute chest pain. N Engl J Med 342:1187–1195, 2000.
Yeghiazarians Y, Braunstein JB, Askari A, Stone PH: Unstable angina pectoris. N Engl J Med 342:101–114, 2000.

USEFUL WEBSITE

American Heart Association site with management guidelines for CAD. *http://www.americanheart.org*

43

Breast Disease

BREAST PAIN/MASTALGIA

▶ ETIOLOGY

What are some common causes of breast pain?

Most types of breast pain can be divided into cyclic or noncyclic. Cyclic pain is most commonly bilateral and associated with physiologic changes. Noncyclical pain is often unilateral and is more likely to occur in postmenopausal women and be associated with a breast or chest wall lesion. Mastitis or plugged lactiferous ducts in nursing women can also present with pain. Other causes include stretching of Cooper's ligaments, fat necrosis from trauma, and chest wall or pectoral muscle pain.

What is fibrocystic breast disease?

Fibrocystic breast disease is a catchall phrase that describes "lumpy, tender breasts." Pain is typically cyclic in nature and peaks in women in their 30s and 40s. It also often resolves with menopause. Pathologically, it is a combination of benign fibrous tissue and cysts that many feel are exaggerated physiologic changes. Fibrocystic changes are not associated with an increased risk of breast cancer.

▶ EVALUATION

Describe a typical history-taking in a woman experiencing breast pain.

History questions should be aimed at the nature of the pain as well as other associated factors. A woman should be asked if the pain is cyclic and if so, does it peak at midcycle or premenstrually. Having the patient keep a calendar or chart of her symptoms can be helpful. She should also be asked about any use of hormonal medications or recent pregnancy. Questions regarding concurrent neck problems, use of the pectoralis muscle group, injury to the chest wall, type of brassiere worn, and other systemic symptoms such as fever or skin changes should also be explored.

What do I look for on physical exam?

The primary goal of physical exam is to look for any signs suggesting a malignancy. A thorough breast exam is paramount, including identifying local areas of tenderness, muscular tenderness, or skin lesions. Placing the woman in the lateral decubitus position allows the examiner to palpate the chest wall apart from the breast to help distinguish the source of tenderness.

List some other studies that should be ordered.

When the physical exam is normal, no further studies are required. Consider an ultrasound exam in women with a focal area of tenderness. Any woman due for screening mammography should have it accomplished. Refer for additional diagnostic testing any woman with a mass on physical exam (as described in the section on breast lumps later in this chapter).

▶ TREATMENT

Do most patients get better?

Mastalgia has a very high spontaneous remission rate of 60% to 80%.

What treatments are appropriate?

Lifestyle changes are the mainstay of treatment for mastalgia. Some lifestyle changes that have been supported by limited randomized controlled trials are: (1) a low-fat (15% of calories) and high–complex carbohydrate diet; (2) avoidance of caffeine; (3) vitamin E supplementation (400 IU twice daily); (4) evening primrose oil (1500–3000 mg daily). Other modifications found helpful are a reduction in the dose of estrogen in hormone replacement therapy or switching oral contraceptives to one with higher progestin activity and the use of topical NSAIDs.

If the mastalgia is severe enough to impact the woman's lifestyle, then consider pharmaceutical treatment. Danazol is the only drug labeled by the Food and Drug Administration for the treatment of mastalgia. It works by inhibiting pituitary gonadatropin secretion and thus estrogen secretion and is prescribed in doses of 100 to 200 mg daily. Danazol has significant side effects including weight gain, acne, hirsuitism, bloating, and amenorrhea. The use of tamoxifen and bromocriptine can also be considered.

NIPPLE DISCHARGE

▶ ETIOLOGY

What is the difference between pathologic and physiologic discharge?

Physiologic nipple discharge is generally bilateral, involves multiple ducts, and is present only with compression. Pathologic discharge is unilateral and often uniductal, spontaneous, and may be bloody or associated with a mass.

What is galactorrhea?

Galactorrhea is milk production unrelated to pregnancy or nursing. It is bilateral and not a symptom of breast cancer or primary breast pathology. It can be caused by nipple stimulation, chest wall trauma, medications, or endocrine abnormalities such as hypothyroidism or pituitary adenomas.

What are the common causes of nipple discharge?

The most common source of a *physiologic* nipple discharge is stimulation (i.e., repeatedly checking for discharge). A *pathologic* nipple discharge is most likely intraductal papilloma followed by ductal ectasia. If a mass is present, the risk for cancer is increased.

▶ EVALUATION

What are pertinent history questions?

It is important to ascertain the color, site, and spontaneity of the discharge. Also, asking about other breast complaints, nipple stimulation or trauma, and medication use is important. Amenorrhea or symptoms of hypothyroidism should also be reviewed.

What do I look for on physical exam?

Perform a complete breast exam. Apply gentle, firm pressure at the base of the areola to try to express any fluid. Pay special attention to whether the discharge comes from one or more ducts. A sample can be tested for the presence of occult blood. In cases of a bloody discharge, cytology can be performed but is often not clinically helpful.

List some other studies I should order.

Women with galactorrhea should have TSH and prolactin levels drawn. Order a mammogram in all women over 35 and younger women if a pathologic discharge is present, although some radiologists prefer ultrasound in women under age 35. Galactography is a mammographic technique that involves injection of contrast into a milk duct and can be used to further evaluate a uniductal discharge. This test is not often performed because of difficulty identifying the duct and a high rate of false negative exams.

▶ TREATMENT

What treatments are appropriate?

Physiologic nipple discharge should be treated with reassurance and advising the patient to avoid checking for the discharge. It often resolves when the nipple is left alone.

Patients with pathologic nipple discharge and otherwise normal evaluation should be referred to a surgical colleague for evaluation and terminal duct excision. A terminal duct excision is both diagnostic and therapeutic if the source of the discharge is benign.

Women with galactorrhea should be treated as appropriate for the primary cause whether that be stopping an inciting medication or treatment of an underlying endocrinological disorder.

BREAST LUMPS

▶ ETIOLOGY

What causes most breast lumps?

The majority of breast lumps are caused by benign disease, although breast lumps are of concern to both the patient and provider because of the risk of a malignancy.

What are the risk factors for breast cancer?

Lifetime risk of developing breast cancer is 1:8 in the United States; thus all women are at risk. Age, age at menarche, family history of first-degree relatives (mother, sister, or daughter), the number of times a woman requires a breast biopsy, a history of atypical hyperplasia, and a personal history of breast cancer are all risk factors (Table 43–1). Protective factors include breastfeeding.

TABLE 43–1

Risk Factors for Breast Cancer

Factors Increasing Risk	Protective Factors
Mother or sister with breast cancer	Breastfeeding > 16 months
Age > 70	Parity > 5
Age at menarche < 12	Exercise
Age at first birth > 30	BMI < 22.9
Age at menopause > 55	Oophorectomy before age 35
Current hormone replacement therapy	
Alcohol use of 2–5 drinks/day	
H/o benign breast biopsy	
H/o atypical hyperplasia on biopsy	
Deleterious BRCA-1/BRCA-2 gene	

H/o = history of, BMI = body mass index

▶ EVALUATION

What are pertinent history questions?

Ask the woman to describe where the lump is and how it was first noticed, how long she has been aware of it, and whether it has changed in size, either gradually increasing or waxing and waning with her menstrual cycle. Benign cysts are often more prominent (and can be tender) premenstrually and recede after the menses. Evaluate risk factors for breast cancer. Examine the woman's fears regarding the lump.

What do I look for on physical exam?

A good clinical breast exam is essential, with careful palpation of the breast tissue, preferably in two positions, determining the characteristics of any masses and the presence of superclavicular or axillary lymphadenopathy. Visual examination of the breast for dimpling and skin changes (peau d'orange) is an often-overlooked portion of the exam.

What does cancer feel like?

The "classic" cancerous lesion is a single, hard lesion that is immobile or adherent to surrounding structures, with irregular borders and a diameter greater than or equal to 2 cm. These features are not diagnostic and all palpable breast masses require further evaluation.

What other studies should I order?

The next step in the evaluation of a breast mass depends primarily on the patient's age and the clinical exam. If a mass is felt to be cystic (smooth, fluctuates with the menstrual cycle, well demarcated, firm, and mobile) options include follow-up exam 3 to 10 days after the onset of her next menstrual cycle with aspiration of the cyst if it persists, immediate aspiration, or ultrasound examination for evaluation of the mass. If the aspirated fluid is not bloody and the mass totally resolves after aspiration, no further evaluation is required. If it does not resolve, further evaluation such as ultrasound should be performed. If the mass is solid on ultrasound examination, then the patient must have a tissue biopsy for definitive diagnosis.

In *women under 35* years of age, the breast tissue is denser and mammography is difficult to interpret, so ultrasound evaluation is preferred. In *women over 35* years of age, a mammogram is performed to evaluate the lesion in question as well as to search for any other clinically occult lesions. Mammographic features that suggest malignancy are increased density, irregular margins, spiculation, and accompanying clustered irregular microcalcifications. *A palpable breast mass with a normal mammogram requires further evaluation* including a biopsy.

KEY POINTS

- **Mastalgia is a benign symptom with a very high spontaneous remission rate.**
- **Fibrocystic changes are related to physiologic changes rather than true "disease."**
- **Women with fibrocystic disease are not at increased risk for breast cancer.**
- **Characteristics associated with malignancy are unilateral, uniductal bloody discharge and association with a breast mass.**
- **Although some characteristics and risk factors impact the chance that a lesion is malignant, all breast masses deserve a complete evaluation and adequate follow-up.**

CASE 43–1. **A 55-year-old woman presents for her well-woman exam with a complaint of noting a mass during her breast self-exam. You note a 1.5-cm, firm, irregularly shaped mass in her left breast.**

A. What further historical information would you like?
B. What clues does your clinical exam give you?
C. What do you do if the remainder of her evaluation is normal?

CASE 43–2. **A 40-year-old woman presents with a complaint of breast discharge.**

A. What other historical information would you like?
B. How will your evaluation change based on your physical exam?

CASE 43–3. **A 28-year-old woman presents with breast pain. It is cyclic in nature and often associated with a "lumpy" feeling to her breasts and tenderness. It peaks just before her menses. She is on oral contraceptives.**

A. What is the likely cause of her mastalgia?
B. What treatment recommendations can you make?
C. What are your further options for treatment if her pain is restricting her lifestyle?

REFERENCES

Fletcher SW, Barton MB: Evaluation of breast lumps. Up To Date 11(2), 2003.
Morrow M: The evaluation of common breast problems. Am Fam Physician 61:2371–2378, 2385, 2000.
Pena KS, Rosenfeld JA: Evaluation and treatment of galactorrhea. Am Fam Physician 63:1763–1770, 2001.
Shirley R: Breast pain. Up To Date 11(3), 2003.
Shirley R: Nipple discharge. Up To Date 11(2), 2003.

44

Cancer Prevention and Screening

What does cancer prevention and screening involve?

The primary goal of cancer screening is to prevent morbidity and mortality from cancer. This is done through primary prevention (preventing the cancer from starting) and secondary prevention or screening ("catching" the cancer once it has started). A secondary goal is to avoid harm in the process. You should be proactive not only for the patient's benefit, but for personal reasons as well; failure to do so is one of the most common reasons for a malpractice claim against a family practitioner.

How do I know what to do or if it is cost-effective to do anything at all?

Several organizations and specialties make recommendations concerning screenings for specific cancers. The American Cancer Society website concentrates on information for patients, but physicians will also find useful information there. Health insurance programs generally refuse to cover newer screens that have not yet proven sensitivity and specificity or cost-effectiveness.

Most evidence-based recommendations come from the United States Preventive Service Task Force (USPSTF). The USPSTF is an independent panel of experts in primary care and prevention that systematically reviews the evidence of effectiveness. Their recommendations are graded as: A (Definitely Do), B (Do), C (Unsure), D (Don't Do), and I (Insufficient Data). Furthermore, the Task Force periodically updates the existing recommendations and adds new reviews. Because recommendations can become dated quickly, the USPSTF website provides physicians with easy access to the most current recommendations for cancer screening and prevention.

A key in deciding what or how much to do is to consider the likelihood of getting the patient to actually perform the intervention. Knowing that eating fruits and vegetables prevents cancer is one thing; getting patients to change eating habits is another. Hence, some USPSTF critiques focus specifically on the effectiveness of counseling.

What is a key first step?

Make a risk assessment, initially and ongoing, then counsel accordingly (Table 44–1). Physicians need to be aware of which diagnoses are associated with cancers, such as ulcerative colitis and cirrhosis. Tobacco is linked not only to lung cancer but also to cancer of the bladder, cancer of the gastrointestinal (GI) tract from mouth to rectum, and cancer of the cervix, as well as leukemia. Thirty percent of all cancer deaths are from smoking. Alcohol is linked to mouth, larynx, liver, colon, and breast cancer. Some estimates indicate that another 30% of all cancer deaths per year result from poor diet and insufficient exercise. Diets high in fat and low in fruits and vegetables are linked to several cancers including GI, lung, bladder, and breast. Obesity is associated with a number of cancers, so achieving and maintaining a non-overweight BMI with a low-calorie diet and exercise is "anti-cancer."

TABLE 44–1

Guidelines for Cancer Prevention and Screening: Risk Assessment and Counseling*

Items to Cover	Comments	USPSTF Rating (year applied)
Family History	Especially: breast, colon, prostate & melanoma	None
Tobacco Use	Frequent history with liberal cessation education	A (2003)
Alcohol Excess	Frequent history and education	None
Sun Excess	Hx: easy or severe burns, unprotected sun exposure. Counseling proportionate to risk.	I (2003)
Diet	Advise 5 servings daily of fruit and vegetables and low fat; and low calorie if overweight	I (2003)
Vitamins and Supplements	Advise against hi dose β-carotene, vit A and D. Condone other vitamins; caution about costly, unproven items.	I (2003)
Exercise	Regular exercise for all	I (2002)
Breast Self-exam	Teach and advise to do monthly.	I (2002)
Testicular Self-exam	Advise young men to seek care for discovered scrotal abnormality.	I (1996)
Environment & Occupational Exposure	Be alert for exposures to radon, asbestos, lead and Agent Orange.	None

USPSTF = United States Preventive Service Task Force, Ratings = A (Definitely Do), B (Do), C (Unsure), D (Don't Do), and I (Insufficient Data)
*Do all items initially at age 20 then periodically thereafter.

Describe other steps to take when considering a patient's cancer profile.

- Document risks on the patient chart problem list.
- Use system prompts (e.g., chart forms and computer triggers) as reminders and quick references to outstanding and completed interventions.
- Include all over-the-counter supplements in your medication history.
- Determine each patient's perspective about prevention. Many prefer indifference or neglect, while others have developed an excessive, even phobic approach. The former may need encouragement to be more serious about prevention; the latter often need advice about harm including wasting money.
- Think "cancer" when you encounter cancer-prone clinical situations (e.g., painless hematuria, iron deficiency anemia in adults, nonhealing skin lesions, unexplained symptoms such as pain, weight loss, and anorexia, and change in bowel or urine habits).
- Use written patient educational materials. It takes a fair amount of time to discuss some of the recommendations or why some screens are not recommended. This time is often not paid for by the insurance. Furthermore, it is prudent to add prevention information when the patient comes for other reasons; unfortunately these encounters may not allow enough time for these interactions.

What about vitamins and related supplements?

Use caution when making strong recommendations, because there is not good supportive evidence for many recommendations and practices. Vitamins and minerals obtained from food are generally more effective than those from supplements. Other variables such as dose, duration, and product further confuse patients. The USPSTF recommendations are Don't Do (D) for β-carotene (may cause lung cancer) and Insufficient Data (I) for all others. However, the USPSTF states there is little reason to discourage people from taking most supplements with the caveat that high doses of vitamins D and A may be harmful. As there may be other benefits and no harm, advising or condoning a daily multivitamin with 0.4 mg of folate is reasonable. There is limited support for adding extra C (500–1000 mg), E (400 units), and selenium (200 μg). Patients may appreciate a brief mention of the unproven effectiveness and unnecessary expense of many other over-the-counter supplements that claim to prevent cancer.

What are the next steps and recommendations about specific cancers?

See Table 44–2 for an action-oriented summary.

Breast Cancer. Despite some studies to the contrary, the USPSTF concluded that mammography reduces mortality and recommends screening every one to two years for women aged 40 and older (B rating). Evidence is strongest for ages 50 to 69; benefit beyond age 75 is assumed not proven. A clinical breast exam is given an "I" rating because no trial has examined the benefits compared to no screen. Routine self-breast exam is likewise rated "I" because supportive evidence is poor, and false positives are problematic. Other groups, however, recommend these exams, and they have become standard procedures for most practices. Patients taking or considering hormone replacement therapy (HRT) should be advised about the slight associated increase risk of breast (and endometrial) cancer. For most women there is no or negligible net benefit and possible harm may result from long-term HRT. The USPSTF (2002) rates it "D" for the prevention of chronic disorders, with an "I" for postmenopausal women who have had a hysterectomy.

Cervical Cancer. Cervical cancer is the tenth leading cause of cancer death. Human papillomavirus (HPV) infection is the most important risk and is a necessary precursor. Tobacco use increases the risk twofold to fourfold. The precancerous and early cancer lesions can be detected by cervical cytology, which reduces the incidence and mortality. The conventional method is a smear of cervical scrapings fixed on a glass slide (Pap smear). Newer technologies include "rinsing" the smear into a liquid. This technique may be more sensitive but perhaps not as cost-effective. One well-accepted recommendation starts cervical cytology exams within three years of sexual activity onset. Although most guidelines include starting at age 21 even if the woman is not sexually active, it is probably safe (and sometimes best) to waive this screen for women with a reliable history of being always abstinent, especially if the exam would be traumatic. The rest of the pelvic exam has not been shown to be an effective cancer screen. Women at high risk of HPV should have a Pap smear every year, others every two to three years. For benign reasons, cervical cytology exams are not recommended for women who have had a hysterectomy or for those over 65 with previous negatives. HPV testing is available but not recommended as a cancer screen (USPSTF rating "I").

Skin Cancer. Of most concern is malignant melanoma. Squamous and basal cell carcinoma are also common in the elderly and may require extensive surgery. However, according to the USPSTF the evidence is insufficient to recommend a total body skin exam or to advise preventive measures to everyone. Nonetheless, it seems prudent to do a periodic history risk assessment on all patients, then

TABLE 44–2

Guidelines for Cancer Prevention and Screening: Clinician Exams and Testing

Action	Age 20–39	40–49	50–74	75+	Comments	USPSF rating (year applied)	Medicare Coverage
Weight & height	+	+	+	+	Screen for obesity; use BMI	B (1996)	
Breast exam (F)	+	+	+	?	Every 1–2 yrs; use the time also to obtain risk hx and discuss mammogram	I (2002)	Yes
Skin exam	+ *	+ *	+ *	+ *	+ Do "spot" checks when examining for other reasons; * Do full exam q 1–2 yrs if fair skin, freckles, nevi, family history	I (2001)	No
Rectal exam (M)			?	?	Value low; ? Only if high-risk prostate ?	I (2002)	Yes
Mouth exam		*	*	*	* Tobacco, excess alcohol q 2–3 yrs	None	No
Testes exam (M)	*				* Cryptorchism	I (1996)	No
Cervical cytology (F)	+	+	+ to 65		Every 2–3 yrs if low risk (3 prior neg, low STD risk); otherwise yearly	A (2003)	Yes
Mammogram (F)		+	+	+	Every 1–2 yrs; annual if high risk	B (2002)	Yes
Fecal blood &/or sigmoid or colonoscopy		*	+	+	Blood annual; Sig q 5 yr; Colon q 10 yr * Family history	A (2002)	Yes
PSA or discuss (M)		*	+	?	* Family history	I (2002)	Yes

\+ Indicated in all
* High risk only
USPSTF = United States Preventive Service Task Force, Ratings = A (Definitely Do), B (Do), C (Unsure), D (Don't Do) and I (Insufficient Data)
Note: Frequency intervals are suggestions unless A or B rating.

examine and counsel those at high risk. History items include family history and excess unprotected sun exposure, especially severe sunburns. Also, when performing exams for other reasons, pay attention to other risks such as skin type, freckles, and the presence of multiple nevi especially atypical nevi (which resemble melanoma in some ways). The strength of the counseling should be proportionate to the risk. Advise those at very high risk to stay out of the sun if possible or use sunscreen and protective clothing whenever in the sun for more than a few minutes.

Prostate Cancer. This is the most common cancer in men, with a lifetime risk of 17% for diagnosis and 3% for death. Although more diagnoses are being made and the survival time is longer, the USPSTF (2002) finds insufficient evidence to give credit to early screening. Risk factors include: African-American, family history (increases risk twofold), and diets high in fat, red meat, and dairy. Protective factors may include a diet high in soy, tomatoes, selenium, or vitamin E. Although a screening digital rectal exam has historically been advised, this exam has not been shown to reduce mortality. Because this exam is extremely onerous to most men, a physician may not find it unreasonable to forego a digital rectal exam. PSA blood testing is the main screening test, but the value of this test is unclear, with estimates that up to 50% of prostate cancers detected this way will never cause symptoms. Most experts agree that physicians should at least discuss the pros and cons of prostate cancer screening with the patient. A recent trend to reduce unnecessary interventions is to follow up mildly increased PSA levels with a total and free PSA, because the percent-free PSA is inversely proportionate to the cancer risk. Obtaining serum levels may also be helpful.

Colon Cancer. The etiology of colon cancer is complex and multifactorial. Proposed risk factors include sedentary lifestyle, obesity, tobacco, alcohol, and diet (e.g., high fat, low folate and fiber). The screening choices are colonoscopy, fecal occult blood testing (FOBT), sigmoidoscopy, or sigmoidoscopy and FOBT combined. The USPSTF rates each of these as A, not favoring any one. Colonoscopy emerges as the preferred screen, because it may be more sensitive. Except for a bothersome bowel prep, it is relatively painless with sedation, and Medicare and some other insurances will cover the cost of the exam. Most doctors generally refer patients to a gastroenterologist for this screen. Sigmoidoscopy is often done in the family practitioner's office. FOBT should be done on three (not just one) separate stools after a few days of minor diet modifications and avoidance of aspirin, NSAIDs, and vitamin C supplements. Specimen cards with instructions and applicators are usually dispensed from the office. Virtual colonoscopy (CT of the colon after introduction of some air per rectum) is a promising substitute for actual colonoscopy.

Testicular Cancer. Most testicular tumors are first noted by the patient (usually white American) and treatment is often curative. However, neither regular clinical exams nor advising all young men to do regular self-exams are of proven value. The USPSTF recommends that physicians should advise all adolescents and young men to seek care if they discover any scrotal abnormality. Although most testicular cancers occur in men without a risk, regular self and clinical exams may be worthwhile for those at high risk (e.g., cancer of the other testis, multiple atypical nevi, and cryptorchism). At risk is not only the undescended testis that has spontaneously descended or been surgically placed but also the other normal testis.

Other Cancers. There are no recommended screens for any other cancers in asymptomatic average risk patients. In fact, the USPSTF rates the following "D" (all in 1996): pancreas (physical exam or ultrasound), thyroid (physical exam), bladder (urinalysis), lung (chest x-ray), ovary (physical exam, ultrasound, tumor marker). A physical exam screen for mouth cancer was rated "I". For women considering contraceptive options, it may be worthwhile to discuss cancer relative to oral contraceptive use. Evidence suggests that ovarian and endometrial cancers are decreased but that breast and cervix cancers are increased. The net increased risk is negligible and the overall effect may be favorable (USPSTF).

What about screening for exposure to and advising against environmental carcinogens?

Spending office time on this is likely low yield, at least as a routine, universal action. It is reasonable to defer responsibility to governmental agencies. In general, unproven or negligible risks are pesticides, toxic wastes, nuclear power plants, microwaves, cell phones and towers, power lines, video terminals, and aspartame. Some proven or highly suspicious risks are radon, asbestos, lead, and Agent Orange. Some advice to give on an as-needed basis might include:

- Check the home for radon.
- Avoid "do-it-yourself" remodeling if you risk possible asbestos exposure.
- Take lead-avoidance precautions.
- Contact the U.S. Department of Veterans Affairs with questions about Agent Orange.

Can a patient be too old for these screens?

Yes, although it may be difficult to ascertain what age is too old. The screens in question are primarily those for breast, colon, and prostate cancer. Most of the studies on efficacy have not included many of the very old. It is generally safe to forego these screens if the patient's estimated life expectancy is less than five years. It is not unreasonable to conclude that a PSA is contraindicated in the very old, even for someone with a longer life expectancy than five years.

If I encounter a patient with diagnosed cancer, what are some key first-step questions I should be asking myself or my preceptor before I interact with the patient?

Ask about the facts of the cancer in this patient. What stage? What is the "TNM" status (tumor size, nodal involvement, metastic disease present)? What is the prognosis? Realize, even with oncology input, that precision will be lacking and that clinicians generally overestimate the time until death. What treatments or surgery have been donc or are ongoing? Is an oncologist involved?

If the patient with cancer is likely to die in the next few years, what are some keys for end-of-life care?

Key Error. Insufficient discussion by the clinician. Consider taking some time first with the patient, then with your preceptor, to discuss the items in the following list. This should benefit not only you but also the patient and preceptor.

Key Discussion Topics (remember to cover all)

- News (bad and good): Education about diagnosis, extent and what to expect. Add realistic "hope" if present.
- Mapping (the care plan): Deciding about treatment or palliation, symptom relief, place of care, advanced directives, etc.
- Making the most of life remaining: encouragement and counseling

Key Actions

- Initiate the discussion (patients and physicians frequently avoid opening this door very wide).
- Discuss early (don't wait until the patient is "falling apart").
- Do not abdicate all responsibility to the oncologist.
- Understand the patient (see following section).
- Determine the patient's capacity to make decisions.
- Talk to the Health Care Proxy and significant others.
- Sit down (taking the extra time to listen and discuss).
- Schedule frequent office visits.

Key Topics to Explore for Understanding the Patient

- The patient's current understanding of the illness (i.e., what, where, how bad, what is expected). Studies have shown wide disparities between patient, family, and physician perceptions about illness information and the extent to which topics have been discussed.

- How much information about diagnosis and treatment is desired?
- Which psychological stage is the patient in (shock, denial, anger, bargaining, depression, acceptance)?
- Unanswered questions
- Sense of humor: is any left?
- Spiritual history
- What would make life more satisfying?

Keys for Symptom Relief

- Do not ignore symptoms, and ask about them frequently.
- Pay particular attention to pain (liberal use of narcotics is often indicated), depression, anxiety, insomnia, nausea, anorexia, diarrhea, dyspnea, itching.
- A good web reference to end-of-life care with over 100 "fast facts" about specific symptoms and clinical scenarios is the End of Life/Palliative Education Resource Center (see Useful Websites at the end of this chapter). A free registration is required.

KEY POINTS

- ▶ **Cancer screening and prevention are critical must-do roles for the family physician.**
- ▶ **Only a few office interventions are proven effective.**
- ▶ **Valid reasons exist for the judicious inclusion of several unproven interventions.**
- ▶ **Risk assessments determine indications for individual patients.**
- ▶ **A proactive, anticipatory approach is important in caring for the patient with cancer.**

CASE 44–1. A 55-year-old woman is being seen in the office for a diabetes checkup. No cancer diagnosis is noted. She does not bring up prevention nor volunteer any worrisome symptoms. Other patients are waiting to be seen, but you can spend one or two minutes on "other things."

A. What reference might you make to cancer during this time?
   Mammogram order
   Age-specific educational handout
   Follow-up appointment for routine health maintenance
   If flu season and in a high-risk category, do nothing about cancer but give a flu shot instead
   Any of the above

B. How can the medical record and office resources assist you in addressing cancer?
   Routine health maintenance flowsheets
   Patient education materials
   Progress note reminder of items to cover next visit
   Problem list notation of risks
   All of the above

CASE 44–2. A 60-year-old man is being seen in the office for a refill of his blood pressure medication. Six months ago he was diagnosed with small-cell lung cancer with mediastinal involvement. He had radiation treatment and now feels fairly good; he's taking walks every day and eating well. He has an appointment with the oncologist in two months. Five minutes are available to "do something" relative to cancer.

A. What is the best use of this five minutes?
   Education about exercise including longer walks and lifting weights
   Review of alternative medicine options for cancer treatment
   Review of cancer prevention, e.g., colon cancer screening, diet, PSA
   Depression screen
   Talk about how his favorite baseball team is doing

B. Which of the following is *not* important to easily find in the medical record for this patient?
   Problem list notation of the cancer type, extent, and treatment
   Advances directives information
   Family history pertinent to cancer
   Name of consultants
   Cancer-related symptoms if problematic

USEFUL WEBSITES

American Cancer Society. *http://www.cancer.org*
United States Preventive Services Task Force. *http://www.ahcpr.gov/clinic/prevenix.htm*
End of Life/Palliative Care Education Resource Center. *http://www.eperc.mcw.edu*

45

Heart Failure

▶ ETIOLOGY

What is heart failure?

Heart failure (HF) is a clinical syndrome, which is the final common pathway for various diseases of the heart. It is defined as an abnormality of cardiac function that is responsible for failure of the heart to adequately pump blood to the tissues (systolic heart failure) or to do so only by utilizing abnormally elevated diastolic volumes (diastolic heart failure). HF is classified as left ventricular, right ventricular, systolic, or diastolic. Systolic HF is characterized by a failure of adequate contraction of the left ventricle (LV) and, therefore, low ejection fraction (EF) (<50%). Diastolic HF refers to abnormal filling of the LV and elevated filling pressures. Because diastolic HF has a normal EF, it is sometimes referred to as "high output" HF. This chapter will focus on left ventricular failure because it is the most common type of the four.

How is the severity of HF classified?

There are two main systems for classification of HF (Box 45–1). The New York Heart Association (NYHA) classification system is a measure of severity of symptoms related to everyday activity. A second more recent classification system defined by the American College of Cardiology (ACC) and the American Heart Association (AHA) focuses on the evolution and progression of HF. This system is an important advancement because the new classification system emphasizes the ability to prevent HF, halt its progression, and identify patients at risk for more severe disease.

What are common causes of LV failure?

When determining why a patient has gone into HF you must determine both the underlying causes of HF as well as the precipitating event. Prompt treatment of the precipitating factor can save a patient's life. For example, a patient with long-standing hypertension and structural heart disease becomes acutely anemic and goes into heart failure. Hypertension is the underlying cause of HF, but the anemia added stress to the heart and caused it to fail. Long-standing hypertension is the most common cause of HF. Other

BOX 45–1

Main Systems for Classification of Heart Failure

NYHA Classification:

Class I (Mild)—Ordinary physical activity is not hindered by symptoms of HF.
Class II (Mild)—No symptoms at rest. Ordinary activity may result in exacerbation of symptoms. Slight limitation of physical activity.
Class III (Moderate)—Remains comfortable at rest. Mild activity results in exacerbation of dyspnea and fatigue.
Class IV (Severe)—Symptoms at rest. Unable to perform any physical activity without discomfort.

ACC/AHA Classification:

Stage A—Patients at high risk for development of HF, but without evidence of structural disease.
Stage B—Structural abnormality of the heart, but have never had symptoms.
Stage C—Structural abnormality of the heart, and current or previous symptoms.
Stage D—End-stage symptoms of HF and are refractory to treatment.

underlying causes are coronary artery disease, congenital heart disease, cardiomyopathies, viral myocarditis, and valvular lesions (especially aortic stenosis). Acute stressors that precipitate HF include anemia; infection; thyrotoxicosis; pregnancy; arrhythmias; myocarditis (viral or rheumatic); infective endocarditis; physical, dietary, fluid, environmental and emotional excesses; acute hypertension; myocardial infarction; and pulmonary embolism.

▶ EVALUATION

What are the criteria for the diagnosis of HF?

The Framingham criteria are well established and useful for the diagnosis of congestive heart failure (Box 45–2). The patient must meet one major and two minor criteria for the diagnosis of HF.

Describe the important historical findings.

Dyspnea on exertion or rest is the most common symptom of LV failure and most likely results from a combination of pulmonary venous congestion and decreased forward cardiac output.

BOX 45–2

Framingham Criteria for CHF

Major Criteria:

PND
Neck vein distension
Rales
Cardiomegaly
Acute pulmonary edema
S3 gallop
Increased venous pressure > 16 cm H_2O
Hepatojugular reflux

Minor Criteria:

Extremity edema
Night cough
Dyspnea on exertion
Hepatomegaly
Pleural effusion
Vital capacity reduced by 1/3 from normal
Tachycardia > 120 bpm

Major/Minor:

Weight loss > 4.5 kg over 5 days of treatment

Pulmonary edema increases resistance in the airways and stimulates J receptors in the lung that mediate rapid shallow breathing. Shallow breathing leads to respiratory muscle fatigue and accumulation of lactic acid, which further worsens the feeling of shortness of breath. Ask the patient if her exercise tolerance has changed and how far she can walk before becoming short of breath.

Dulled mental status can result from decreased cerebral perfusion.

Change in urination can occur as a result of decreased renal perfusion throughout the day and increased renal perfusion at night when blood flow is redistributed while lying supine. Ask the patient how many times he gets up at night to use the restroom.

Paroxsysmal nocturnal dyspnea (PND), orthopnea, or nocturnal cough result when fluid accumulates in the dependent areas and then redistributes to the lungs when the patient is supine. Ask the patient how many pillows he uses to sleep, or if he finds it necessary to sleep in a recliner. For PND ask the patient if he ever awakes from sleep with severe breathlessness.

Always inquire about precipitating factors of HF, such as chest pain, anemia, thyroid problems, recent illness, and emotional stresses.

What are important physical findings?

Signs and symptoms of heart failure lie on a continuum from the acute attack to long-standing disease (Box 45–3). The acute patient may show signs of severe distress with difficulty breathing, extreme exercise intolerance, and refusal to lie flat. Hypotension may be present in acute heart failure along with cyanosis and jugular venous distension (JVD).

How do I differentiate between diastolic and systolic HF?

Diastolic HF patients often have the same signs and symptoms as systolic HF patients, except that on echocardiography they have a normal ejection fraction (Table 45–1).

What labs and tests should I order?

In heart failure it is important to discover the underlying cause of dysfunction, looking for treatable causes of the disease. A thorough

BOX 45–3

Signs & Symptoms of Heart Failure

S3 and/or S4: Although not specific to heart failure, these extra heart sounds are often present.

Displacement of apex: Can occur in the presence of cardiomegaly. If so, you can palpate the apex of the heart more laterally than in healthy patients.

Rales: Moist rales are often heard throughout the lung fields in patients with pulmonary edema. Rales may be absent in patients with long-standing heart failure.

JVD: Distension of the jugular veins is typical of right-sided heart failure. As central venous pressure increases, the height of distension will also increase. In the case of hepatic venous congestion, pressing on the liver and observing the rise in jugular venous distension may elicit the hepatojugular reflux.

Edema: Edema of heart failure is considered dependent in nature, often happening in the legs bilaterally and symmetrically. This is a pitting type of edema and is often worse in the evenings.

Hepatomegaly: Hepatomegaly with increasing central venous pressures leading to increase in liver congestion. Ascites and jaundice can result from the increased venous pressures and hepatic injury, respectively.

TABLE 45–1

Differentiating Diastolic and Systolic Heart Failure

Characteristic	Diastolic HF	Systolic HF
Age	Elderly	All ages, typically 50–70
Sex	Female	Male
LV ejection fraction	>40%	<40%
LV cavity size	Normal/concentric LV hypertrophy	Dilated
LV hypertrophy on EKG	Present	Sometimes present
CXR	Congestion with or w/o cardiomegaly	Congestion with cardiomegaly
Gallop rhythm	S4	S3
HTN	+++	++
Diabetes mellitus	+++	++
Previous MI	+	+++
Obesity	+++	+
Chronic lung disease	++	0
Sleep apnea	++	++
Long-term dialysis	++	0
Atrial fibrillation	+	+

+ = occasionally associated with, ++ = often associated with, +++ = usually associated with, 0 = not associated with

Data from Jessup M, Brozena S: Heart failure. N Engl J Med 348:2007–2018, 2003.

work-up would include an echocardiogram, CBC, BUN, creatinine, thyroid studies, and a chest x-ray. A chest x-ray may reveal cardiomegaly with increased vascular marking from pulmonary vein distension. Virtually every new patient with heart failure will get an echocardiogram to determine ejection fraction to use as a measure of cardiac function. Follow-up echocardiograms are often used to track the progress of disease. Brain natriuretic peptide is a useful test for HF when clinical evidence is ambiguous.

What is the differential diagnosis of HF?

Dyspnea on exertion can be present in normal, unfit people, those with chronic lung diseases, anemia, and obesity. Orthopnea can also be seen in chronic lung disease. Edema can be seen in patients with renal disease, liver failure, malnutrition, arthritis, trauma, varicose veins, or thyroid dysfunction. Many of the other signs and symptoms of heart failure are somewhat specific to this disease, making it a fairly straightforward clinical diagnosis.

BOX 45–4

Pharmacotherapy for Congestive Heart Failure

Diuretics: Fluid overload is often treated with diuretics to relieve edema and lower central venous pressures. Loop diuretics as well as spironolactone, a potassium-sparing diuretic, are used most commonly to treat heart failure. Successful treatment of fluid overload requires careful monitoring of daily I/O and weight measurements. Spironolactone was shown in the RALES trial to lower mortality in class III and IV left-sided heart failure when used with other standard therapies. This is thought to be related to its aldosterone antagonist effects of helping to down-regulate the RAAS system.

ACE inhibitors: These drugs have proven effective in patients with left ventricular systolic failure as well as in patients with left ventricular dysfunction without failure. Contraindications to ACE inhibitor use include hyperkalemia ($K^+ > 5.5$ mmol/L), pregnancy, renal failure, and hypotension. ACE inhibitors have proven to decrease mortality in patients with CHF.

β-blockers: Because of their negative inotropic properties, it may seem counterintuitive to use β-blockers in HF. The rationale behind their use is to down-regulate the β-adrenergic receptors in heart tissue, resulting in increased cardiac functioning. Patients may complain of increase in symptoms early in their treatment with β-blockers, but you should instruct patients to continue the drugs to allow for receptor down-regulation to occur. You should withhold administration until you have treated the acute instability. Contraindications to use of these drugs include lung disease caused by bronchospasm, symptomatic bradycardia, or heart block.

Digoxin: This positive inotrope is useful in patients with left ventricular systolic dysfunction to improve cardiac output. It does not affect mortality.

Vasodilators: In patients unable to take ACE inhibitors, vasodilators can achieve some benefit. Hydralazine and isosorbide dinitrate have been used, but do not have as profound an effect as the ACE inhibitors.

The cornerstone of the medical treatment of heart failure caused by systolic dysfunction is the use of ACE inhibitors and β-blockers. Calcium channel blockers have no place in the treatment of systolic dysfunction and in fact will cause a decline in cardiac output.

▶ TREATMENT

How do we treat HF?

As with any chronic disease, treatment begins with risk factor modification. Cessation of smoking, continuation of physical activity and exercise, and dietary modification including sodium restriction to less than 3 grams a day are crucial to the prevention of further progression of disease. Patients should limit exercise in heart failure to dynamic activities such as walking or jogging. Patients should avoid isometric exercise (weightlifting). If you know the etiology of the patient's heart failure, you should work to treat the underlying condition. In the case of coronary artery disease, catheterization with angioplasty will help improve myocardial function. More severe cases may require bypass surgery. In patients with severe left ventricular failure, surgical placement of a ventricular assist device may be necessary.

Pharmacotherapy is appropriate during acute exacerbation of heart failure, as well as for long-term treatment of the disease (Box 45–4).

KEY POINTS

- **Always identify the underlying pathology as well as the acute stressor that has caused an exacerbation or first presentation of CHF. Identifying and treating an acute stressor can be lifesaving.**
- **Use the NYHA and ACC/AHA classification systems to grade the severity and prognosis of CHF.**
- **Use the Framingham criteria to help diagnosis of CHF.**
- **All patients with CHF should be placed on an ACE inhibitor (unless there are contraindications); this has been proven to prolong life.**
- **Consider use of spironolactone and β-blockers as well.**
- **Digoxin can decrease morbidity, but does not decrease mortality in CHF.**

CASE 45–1. **A 65-year-old man presents at the emergency department with a two-day history of "feeling run down." Further history reveals he has a 40-year history of smoking one pack per day, has had problems with his cholesterol for "as long as I can remember," and has high blood pressure. Review of systems uncovers that he has gotten short of breath with even the slightest exercise, and is sleeping on two to three pillows a night.**

A. What is your differential diagnosis?
B. What are the signs and symptoms of heart failure?

CASE 45–2. **A 53-year-old woman comes into your office complaining of "coughing up blood" for the last two days. Additional questioning reveals an episode of chest pain lasting "only a few minutes" that occurred one week ago. Past medical history is significant for type II diabetes. Vital signs are within normal limits. Exam reveals rales throughout the lung fields and an S3 on cardiac exam.**

A. What lab test or imaging studies will you order?
B. What is the most common etiology of heart failure?

REFERENCES

Braunwald E, Fauci AS, Isselbacher KJ, et al.: Harrision's Principles of Internal Medicine. New York: McGraw-Hill, 2001.
Jessup M, Brozena S: Heart failure. N Engl J Med 348:2007–2018, 2003.

USEFUL WEBSITES

eMedicine. *http://www.emedicine.com/EMERG/topic108.htm*
National Heart, Lung and Blood Institute. *http://www.nhlbi.nih.gov/health/public/heart/other/hrtfail.htm*

46

Dementia

What is dementia?

Dementia is a state of *progressive* mental decline that can affect assorted cognitive functions but by definition must affect the patient's *memory* (although there are exceptions to this, such as frontotemporal dementias). The typical demented patient loses cognitive function gradually. Dementia causes loss of higher-level cortical skills inversely to how they were learned. For example, as a child we learn walking, talking, toilet training, concrete thinking, simple mathematics, abstract thinking, complex mathematics/problem solving—generally in that order. The demented patient usually loses aspects of his/her memory first, then complex problem solving, abstract thinking, etc. on down the list. Use the criteria found in the DSM-IV to definitively diagnose dementia.

▶ ETIOLOGY

What causes dementia?

It is important to stress that dementia tends to be a progressive disease. In fact, 95% of all dementias are categorized as irreversible. Alzheimer's disease (AD) causes 60% to 70% of dementias (if this is the case, it is called *dementia of the Alzheimer type*). Vascular disease causes about 20% of dementia cases, making it the second most common cause. A mixed vascular/Alzheimer picture is also fairly common. Alcoholism, Huntington's disease, Pick's disease, and Parkinson's disease make up the majority of the irreversible dementias.

Unfortunately, only 5% of dementias are reversible. However, the reversible causes are extremely important because when properly diagnosed, significant function can be restored to the patient. They make up the bulk of the disorders we are trying to rule out with lab tests (see Evaluation section of this chapter).

What are the reversible causes of dementia?

Reversible causes of dementia include pharmaceuticals, depression (pseudodementia), thyroid disorders, parathyroid disorders, vitamin B_{12} deficiency, electrolyte disturbances, trauma (subdural/epidural hematomas), and normal pressure hydrocephalus.

▶ EVALUATION

Of what should I be aware before beginning the history?

The dementia history is remarkably complicated by the fact that, by definition, the patient has cognitive decline. You must rely on a second source of information, ideally a family member or another party with whom the patient has daily contact. The demented patient usually knows he is losing his memory and wants to demonstrate to the physician that his thinking is unhindered. The thought of cognitive impairment is abhorrent to almost everyone—most people say that they would rather die than "lose their mind." Patients will often rationalize their deficits: for example, when testing long-term memory by asking about past presidents, a demented individual might minimize her deficits by saying that she was "never really interested in politics."

What questions should I ask during the history?

Be sure to ask about the risk factors for the two most common causes of dementia: Alzheimer's disease and vascular dementia. For dementia of the Alzheimer type, risk factors include older age, family history, Down's syndrome, and female gender. For vascular dementia, think of the risk factors for stroke: hypertension, diabetes, hyperlipidemia, tobacco use, and male gender. A thorough review of systems may help tease out some of the reversible causes. Ask the patient and family members about specific instances where the patient's memory has failed. Ask about activities of daily living. Sometimes patients suffer from agnosia (failure to recognize familiar objects), aphasia (difficulty with language), and apraxia (impairment in voluntary movement). Sometimes personality changes can be associated with dementia. Because dementia is a progressive disease, it is important to ask if the symptoms have worsened over time. It is also helpful to know in what time frame the symptoms have arisen. If the symptoms have a sudden onset, it is likely that there is another process at play instead of, or confounding, the dementia.

Describe the physical exam.

You should perform a thorough neurological examination to determine any comorbid conditions that you should treat. A thorough mental status evaluation (MSE) is also indicated. Depression and psychosis are common sequelae of dementia. Other physical exam maneuvers should be directed toward the reversible causes of dementia.

What labs or other tests should I order?

A good general set of labs for the work-up for dementia includes CBC, electrolytes, creatinine, calcium, TSH, vitamin B_{12} levels, and blood urea nitrogen (BUN). Remember, it will be rare (in only 5% of patients) to find a clinically significant disturbance in any of these tests pertaining to the dementia. These results are still absolutely necessary to obtain, but you should remember that the last word comes from your clinical diagnosis and not the lab tests.

The mini mental status exam (MMSE) is a common instrument used to quantify cognitive function and decline. A perfect MMSE is 30; a score of 23 or less suggests dementia. When you interview a patient and have any doubt about his cognitive function, administer the MMSE to obtain a baseline. More important than the actual number on the MMSE is the change (or lack of change) in the number from previous visits. The MMSE is a good instrument to track the progression of the disease, so compare previous MMSEs to the current one.

Medical literature provides moderate evidence that either a head CT or MRI is an appropriate test. However, some physicians believe that unless the patient exhibits focal neurologic signs or symptoms, has an acute onset, or has seizures, a head CT or MRI is not indicated. The current standard of care is to obtain a CT or MRI to rule out normal pressure hydrocephalus, unsuspected cerebrovascular disease, and subdural hematoma.

Neuropsychological testing is another cognitive testing method. This consists of a long battery of tests that are usually interpreted by a trained neuropsychologist. They can be beneficial to further quantify the patient's level of functioning. The expense and access issues are the downsides to neuropsychological testing.

What is the differential diagnosis for dementia?

Not many syndromes can be confused with dementia. Psychoses and other psychiatric disorders can sometimes masquerade as dementia, so look for psychotic symptoms. Many demented patients develop psychoses of various forms, but these often present later in the disease. Once again, obtaining a good history and continuity of care for the patient are essential when diagnosing dementia.

What is the connection between depression and dementia?

Depression can express itself so that it looks like dementia. This occurrence is called *pseudodementia*. Compared to dementia, pseudodementia tends to: (1) have a more rapid onset, (2) cause the patient to be apathetic to your questions (instead of trying and missing the question, the patient won't even try and typically says "I don't know" frequently during cognitive testing), (3) cause the patient to exaggerate his symptoms instead of trying to hide them. The "good" thing about pseudodementia is that the dementia symptoms resolve with antidepressant treatment.

How does delirium differ from dementia?

It is important to distinguish delirium from dementia because the treatments differ. Compared with dementia, delirium typically has a rapid onset; is more associated with "sundowning," which means that symptoms worsen in the evening; is associated with waxing and waning of consciousness; has an underlying medical cause; and has a shorter course.

▶ TREATMENT

What is the best pharmacologic treatment for dementia?

If the clinical picture is suggestive or even suspicious for AD, then an acetylcholinesterase inhibitor is indicated. In general, dementia is frequently underdiagnosed. Furthermore, even patients that have been correctly diagnosed are not receiving adequate pharmacotherapy with the acetylcholinesterase inhibitors. Four cholinesterase inhibitors are currently available: tacrine, galantamine, donepezil, and rivastigmine. These medications provide only a modest improvement in the cognitive functioning of patients. Their main function is to slow the rate of progression of the disease. Vitamin E in large doses (1000 IU twice a day) has also shown some success in decreasing the rate of progression of AD. Vitamin E is not recommended in patients who are taking anticoagulation medication.

What are some common comorbid conditions/behaviors? How are they treated?

Depression: As previously mentioned, depression is common among demented patients. The low side effect profile of the selective serotonin re-uptake inhibitors (SSRIs) make them an appropriate management option for depression.

Psychotic symptoms: Psychotic symptoms are treated best with the new atypical antipsychotics.

Wandering: This is a disturbing and dangerous behavior for the patient and caregiver. Appropriate use of locked rooms, doors, and gates can be beneficial. Sometimes this behavior is the straw that breaks the camel's back for the caregiver, leading to the caregiver placing the patient in an assisted living facility. Psychotropic medications are generally not helpful to reduce wandering.

Medical complications: Demented patients tend to be a more aged population; thus they have their share of physical diseases (particularly cardiovascular issues). Any medical problems should be dealt with in the same manner as for the nondemented population.

Agitation: This nebulous term describes patients with dementia who are upset, frightened, or angry. At worst, patients can get physically violent and inconsolable. Appropriate cholinesterase therapy is the first line in prevention of this state. Benzodiazepines have somewhat fallen out of favor but can be an important mediator in acute problems with agitation. The new atypical antipsychotic agents are also commonly used for agitation.

What is the family physician's role in patients with advanced disease?

Dementia is a chronic, unrelenting disease that causes significant financial and psychological stress on the caregivers. Overburdened caregivers suffer higher rates of depression and suffer emotional distress as they watch their loved one deteriorate. The family physician should offer reassurance and keep an open dialogue with the caregivers about if, when, and how the patient needs to be transferred to some type of assisted living facility. It is important to know what types of facilities are available in your community. Finally, elder abuse is a reportable offense in most states. If you suspect abuse, it is your duty to report it to the proper authorities.

KEY POINTS

- **Alzheimer's disease is the most common dementia.**
- **Reversible causes of dementia, while not very common, must be ruled out as the cause for the dementia.**
- **All patients with Alzheimer's disease should be treated with anticholinesterase inhibitors.**
- **"Caregiver burden" is a well-documented phenomenon of dementia and should be addressed with families.**

CASE 46–1. **A 76-year-old man is brought to your office by his adult daughter. She tells you that he has had difficulty keeping track of his finances recently. She thinks this is odd because he is a retired accountant and has had no trouble with this before. She states that he is able to feed and clothe himself. Physical exam is normal. MMSE is 23. A CBC, CMP, TSH, and vitamin B_{12} are all within normal limits. A CT of the head is also normal.**

A. What is the most likely etiology of this condition?
B. What are some good questions to ask for the history?

CASE 46–2. **A 76-year-old man with a history of tobacco abuse, hypertension, and diabetes mellitus type II is brought into your clinic by his wife, who states that he would "forget his head if it wasn't attached." This problem apparently has been around for a few years but took a turn for the worse several months ago. The problem has stayed relatively the same since that time. The physical exam is normal except for a blood pressure of 146/90. A CBC, CMP, TSH, and vitamin B_{12} are normal. His blood glucose is 192.**

A. What is the most likely etiology of this condition?
B. What is the next step in diagnosis/management?

USEFUL WEBSITE

Alzheimer's Association. *http://www.alz.org*

47

Depression and Anxiety

▶ ETIOLOGY

What biological, psychological, and social factors help explain the cause of mood disorders?

Biological. Ample information suggests that genetics plays a role in the development of mood disorders. Twin studies have shown that the rate of mood disorders in identical twins is 67% to 76%, but only 19% in fraternal twins. Individuals with a family history of mood disorders are at a higher risk of developing a disorder themselves. Many medical conditions are also related to mood disorders (e.g., cardiovascular disease, multiple sclerosis, cancer, thyroid disorders, AIDS, endocrine changes).

Psychological. Individuals who are continually under a great deal of stress, have a negative outlook on life, or have a passive temperament are more likely to suffer from a mood disorder. These individuals often have cognitive distortions including unrealistic expectations, overgeneralization of adverse events, personalization of negative or difficult events, and overreaction to stressors. Behaviorally, individuals who are continually under stress believe that any action on their part would be futile and therefore they continue to do nothing (learned helplessness).

Social. Among the many implicated social issues are difficult marriages, divorce, problems with children, and economic difficulties. Many individuals do not have the social resources (e.g., friendships, family) or buffers that aid in coping (e.g., spirituality).

When evaluating for anxiety and depression, what comorbid conditions should I look for?

Alcohol and Drug Abuse. Many individuals attempt to cope with their anxiety/depression through the use of substances, and many people who abuse drugs and alcohol become depressed and/or agitated.

Suicidal Thoughts and Plans. Suicide rates are high for depressed and anxious individuals. While assessing the patient's suicide risk, determine whether the patient: (1) has thoughts of dying or suicide, (2) has a plan, (3) has the means to carry out the plan, and (4) is able to sign a safety contract. If the patient has a plan and is unable to sign a contract, he/she must be placed somewhere for treatment.

Homicidal Thoughts and Plans. It is not uncommon for individuals with anxiety and depression to have difficulties with anger control and/or psychosis. For example, new mothers who suffer from postpartum depression may harm themselves and/or their children because of depression-induced psychosis. If the patient has a plan and means to carry it out, consider a safety contract and contacting appropriate authorities.

Abuse. Many individuals who are abused will admit to being depressed and/or anxious but, unless asked specifically, they will often not divulge that they are victims of abuse. It is also common for adults who were victims as a child to have difficulties with anxiety and/or depression.

What are the most common anxiety disorders?

Panic disorder, with or without agoraphobia, is diagnosed when the patient has recurrent panic attacks (shortness of breath, fear of imminent death or a feeling of impending doom, pounding heart, sweating, chest pain, paresthesias, trembling, nausea, and fear of losing control). *Agoraphobia* is the fear of having another panic attack, which then limits the patient's ability to leave the house or go places where immediate escape might be difficult.

Acute stress disorder (ASD) and *post-traumatic stress disorder* (PTSD) are characterized by the re-experiencing of an extremely traumatic experience (e.g., rape, murder, motor-vehicle accident), followed by hyperarousal and subsequent attempts to avoid these re-experiences. The main distinction between ASD and PTSD is the duration of symptoms. With PTSD, the symptoms last longer than one month. It is important to assess and treat for ASD because treatment results are much better with early intervention.

Specific phobia is excessive anxiety that is provoked by exposure to a specific feared object or situation. Common phobias include fear of animals or insects, natural environment (e.g., heights, storms, water), blood-injection injury (often characterized by a strong vasovagal response), or situations (e.g., public transportation, tunnels, bridges, elevators, flying, driving). *Social phobia* is an excessive anxiety provoked by exposure to social or performance situations.

Obsessive-compulsive disorder (OCD) is characterized by obsessions (which cause anxiety, e.g., germs on the hands) and compulsions (behaviors aimed at reducing the anxiety, e.g., hand washing). *Generalized anxiety disorder* (GAD) is a condition of excessive worry and anxiety for more days than not over a period of at least six months.

How do I evaluate patients for depressive disorders?

A mnemonic that helps in remembering all of the possible symptoms of a major depressive episode is ***SIGECAPS***. A patient must have five or more of these symptoms, including depressed mood and/or anhedonia:

Sleep disturbance—early morning awakenings or restless sleep
Interest—little interest in activities they used to enjoy (anhedonia)
Guilt—feeling guilty or worthless
Energy—feeling tired or fatigued
Concentration—impaired concentration and/or indecisiveness
Appetite—weight change and/or changes in their normal eating patterns
Psychomotor disturbance—any psychomotor agitation or retardation
Suicidal thoughts—recurrent thoughts of death, suicidal ideation, and suicide attempt

What are the common types of depressive disorders?

Major depressive disorder is present when the individual has had two or more major depressive episodes. *Dysthymic disorder* is characterized by at least two years of low-grade depression (i.e., does not meet the criteria for a major depressive episode). *Cyclothymic disorder* is characterized by at least two years of numerous periods of low-grade depression and hypomania. *Seasonal affective disorder, grief reaction,* and *adjustment disorder with depressed mood* are other disorders caused by the time of the year, response to loss, and response to a significant change (e.g., divorce), respectively.

Bipolar I disorder is characterized by one or more manic episodes and is usually accompanied by major depressive episodes. Manic episodes must include at least three of the following symptoms:

- Inflated self-esteem or grandiosity
- Decreased need for sleep
- More talkative than usual or pressure to keep talking
- Flight of ideas or subjective experience of racing thoughts
- Distractibility
- Increase in goal-directed activity (socially, at work, or sexually) or psychomotor agitation
- Excessive involvement in pleasurable activities that have a high potential for painful consequences (e.g., spending, gambling, sexual indiscretions)

Bipolar II disorder is characterized by one or more major depressive episodes and at least one hypomanic episode. Hypomanic episodes use the same criteria as manic episodes, only hypomania does not cause marked impairment in social or occupational functioning or require hospitalization. See Figure 47–1.

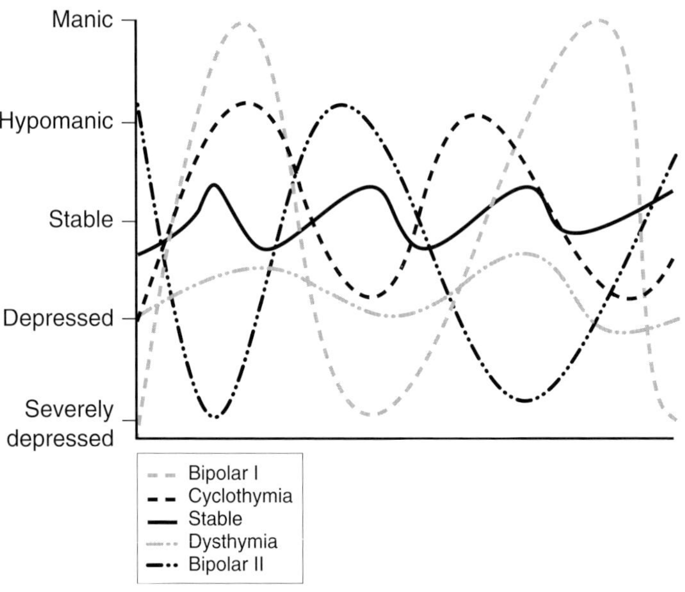

Figure 47–1. How the common types of depressive disorders fluctuate as compared to a stable (nondepressive) psychological status.

▶ TREATMENT

What pharmacological treatments are best for major depressive disorders?

The selection of antidepressant should be made with respect to safety, tolerability, efficacy, ease of use, and cost. Selective serotonin re-uptake inhibitors (SSRIs) have become accepted as the most commonly used first-line antidepressant class (Table 47–1). These agents are well tolerated with minimal sedative, anticholinergic, or cardiovascular side effects. They are especially safe and useful in elderly and medically ill patients. They can be dosed once daily with minimal dosage titration. SSRIs also target other psychiatric disorders, such as anxiety, which often coexist with depression.

Discuss timing related to the use of antidepressants.

Once an appropriate antidepressant is initiated it is crucial to educate the patient with respect to onset of effects and adverse effects. This education will help reduce the high noncompliance rate with antidepressants. Although studies have shown nonstatistical

TABLE 47–1

Overview of Common Antidepressants

Drugs	Advantages	Disadvantages	Comments
SSRIs			
Citalopram (Celexa) Escitalopram (Lexapro) Fluoxetine (Prozac) Paroxetine (Paxil) Sertraline (Zoloft)	• Relatively safe in overdose • Generally well tolerated • Effective in both MDE and AD • Effective in PMDD • Safe in medically ill, elderly and post MI or CHD • Safe in pregnancy • Safe in breastfeeding: Zoloft and Paxil	• GI intolerance • CNS activation • Sexual dysfunction • Serotonin withdrawal syndrome: Paxil (consider slow taper) • Serotonin syndrome • Drug interactions: Prozac and Paxil • Cost (except fluoxetine)	• Prozac: most stimulating. Paxil: most sedating. • First-line for MDE and AD • To minimize the GI intolerance and CNS activation that occur in the beginning of therapy, start at a lower dose to minimize GI intolerance and CNS activation • Start at ½ of depression dose in AD patients
Bupropion (Wellbutrin)	• Weight neutral or loss • No to minimal sexual dysfunction • Useful in SSRI-induced sexual dysfunction • Useful in smoking cessation	• Risk of seizure in overdose • CNS activation: anxiety, insomnia, tremor, nausea, headache • Cost	• Avoid in seizure disorders, head injury, or bulimia nervosa • Avoid in agitated, insomniac patients
Mirtazapine (Remeron)	• Relatively safe in overdose • Minimal anxiety, insomnia, nausea, or sexual dysfunction • High sedation; useful in insomnia • Increase appetite; useful in elderly • Generic available	• High sedative effects • Weight gain • Lipid elevation • Rare cases of agranulocytosis	• Useful in elderly • Useful in anxious, agitated, insomniac patients
Nafazodone (Serzone)	• Relatively safe in overdose • No significant sexual dysfunction • Very useful in reducing symptoms of anxiety	• BID dosing requiring dose titration • Drug Interactions • FDA black box warning: hepatotoxicity • Cost	• Second or third-line agent • Useful in anxiety, agitation, sleep disturbance, insomnia, sexual dysfunction

continued

Table 47–1. Overview of Common Antidepressants *continued*

Drugs	Advantages	Disadvantages	Comments
Venlafaxine (Effexor)	• Relatively safe in overdose • "Dual mechanism" agent: low dose acts as selective serotonin reuptake inhibitor (SSRI), higher dose norepinephrine kicks in. • May be more effective than single action antidepressants • Effective in generalized anxiety disorder	• BP elevation at higher dose • GI intolerance • CNS activation • Sexual dysfunction • Cost	• Useful in severe depression • Useful in SSRI failure or refractory to other antidepressants • Monitor BP especially at higher dose • Useful in treatment of menopause symptoms
TCAs	• Well-established efficacy • Sedative effects useful for insomnia • Effective for chronic pain syndrome and neuropathy • Effective in migraine prophylaxis	• Often fatal in overdose • High rates of treatment discontinuation • Sedation, orthostasis, anticholinergic effects, and weight gain • Substantial dosage titration • Need plasma drug level monitoring • High rates of noncompliance	• NOT first-line treatment • Mostly used for pain and migraine management • Useful in treatment of insomnia with low dose • AVOID in medically ill, post MI, elderly
Buspirone (Buspar)	• Effective in generalized anxiety disorder • No sedation issues • No cognitive and psychomotor impairment • No abuse or dependence issues	• Delayed onset of effects • NOT effective for other types of anxiety disorder	
Benzodiazepines:			
Alprazolam (Xanax) Clonazepam (Klonopin) Lorazepam (Ativan)	• Provide rapid relief in anxiety disorder	• Sedation • Dependence and abuse issues • Cognitive and psychomotor impairment	• Recommend PRN and short-term usage

AD = anxiety disorder, CHD = coronary heart disease, MDE = major depressive episode, MI = myocardial infarction, PMDD = premenstrual dysphoric disorder early response rates to antidepressants as early as one week, the full antidepressant effect is not evident for four to six weeks of therapy. Thus, the patient often must wait before improvement is experienced.

Treatment duration should allow adequate time for both resolution of depressive symptoms (remission, 6–8 weeks) and prevention of relapse (6–12 months); therefore, a depressed patient should be treated for 6–12 months and then reassessed for the need for further management. Long-term maintenance treatment (2 years to lifelong) is indicated for a patient with three or more major depressive episodes.

Are some depressions treatment-resistant?

Most cases of apparent treatment-resistant depression are a result of inadequate treatment. Common underlying factors include underdosing, not allowing enough time for response, and poor compliance. Intolerance to antidepressants has been implicated as one of the major causes for antidepressant discontinuation. Most of the adverse effects are transient, or can be minimized by dosage reduction or counteracted with another agent. Strategies to improve response include (1) increasing doses, (2) switching to another SSRI, a different class, or a dual-mechanism agent, or (3) adding another agent to augment antidepressant response.

Can antidepressants be used during pregnancy or lactation?

Studies have indicated that exposure to SSRIs during pregnancy is not associated with increased risks of major malformation, miscarriage, stillbirth, or prematurity compared to controls. However, it is still prudent to hold off drug therapy during the first trimester if possible, otherwise, SSRIs are preferred in this setting. In regard to breastfeeding, SSRIs (sertraline, paroxetine) and tricyclic antidepressants (TCAs; amitriptyline, nortriptyline, desipramine, clomipramine) have not been shown to have adverse effects on nursing infants.

Which pharmacological treatments are best for anxiety disorders (AD)?

It is well established that AD is a chronic disease that requires long-term maintenance treatment. Antidepressants with serotonin or norepinephrine properties such as SSRIs, venlafaxine, mirtazapine, nefazodone, and TCAs also have anxiolytic effects. Again, SSRIs, with the exception of fluoxetine (Prozac), are considered the first-line treatment for different types of AD. Sertraline (Zoloft) and paroxetine (Paxil) are the most studied. Fluoxetine, the most stimulating/activating SSRI, and bupropion (Wellbutrin), an agent with mainly dopamine activity, are not ideal for AD. Buspirone (Buspar), an antianxiety agent with different mechanisms of action than the above agents, is useful only in GAD.

Because of potential problems with physical dependence and addiction, long-term use of benzodiazepines for AD should be discouraged. They can be used as short-term or on an as-needed basis at the beginning of a maintenance antianxiety agent (e.g., with SSRIs) when antianxiety effects have not yet fully developed or when flare-ups occur.

What pharmacological treatments are best for bipolar disorder?

Pharmacological treatment of bipolar disorder includes mood stabilizers and adjunctive agents. Both lithium and valproate are considered first-line treatment for bipolar disorder. Lithium is most useful in patients with pure mania, a previous response to lithium, non-rapid-cycling types, and without neurological impairment, psychotic symptoms, or a history of substance abuse. In contrast, valproate is considered the best first-line treatment in patients with mixed or rapid cycling episodes, and in patients with neurological impairment, a history of substance abuse, or the bipolar type of schizoaffective disorder. Valproate is also an appropriate alternative to lithium in pure mania. Other anticonvulsants such as carbamazepine (Tegretol), lamotrigine (Lamictal), gabapentin (Neurontin), and topiramate (Topamax) have shown efficacy in bipolar disorder.

Adjunctive agents are mainly used in the treatment of acute mania. Atypical antipsychotics (e.g., olanzapine) are commonly used because of their fast action. They may also have some mood stabilizing properties. They are especially useful for those manic patients who are also psychotic or aggressive. Benzodiazepines (e.g., lorazepam) are also helpful initially for agitation and to reduce the patient's symptoms until the mood stabilizer is up to therapeutic dosages.

What psychosocial interventions are best for depressed and anxious patients?

Cognitive, behavioral, and interpersonal therapies are effective in mood and anxiety disorders. Recent research has also provided strong evidence regarding the effectiveness of marital and family therapy. Marital therapy is especially helpful if marital discord is implicated in, or precedes the onset of, the condition. Family therapy is indicated in the case of a symptomatic child or adolescent. In the case of adjustment disorders and some other conditions (e.g., simple phobia), psychotherapeutic approaches are often sufficient or the only thing that is effective.

Both research and treatment guidelines encourage the use of psychotherapy alone or in combination with medication. The

Agency for Health Care Policy and Research (AHCPR), Veterans Health Administration–Department of Defense (VHA-DOD), and the American Psychiatric Association recommend combination treatment for moderate to severe depression and psychotherapy for mild depression. You should review the patient's condition and any treatment results by eight weeks and modify the treatment if the patient has not improved. Other interventions include encouraging the patient and family members to increase psychosocial support, normalize sleep patterns, begin an exercise program, decrease or eliminate stimulants (e.g., caffeine) and alcohol/drugs, and develop effective problem-solving, coping, and relaxation strategies.

KEY POINTS

- **Depression is a prevalent illness, requiring global screening in the primary care setting.**
- **Depression and anxiety are often comorbid conditions, frequently compounded by a number of other psychosocial issues (e.g., substance abuse).**
- **The current recommendation for treatment of anxiety and depression is a combination of psychotherapy and pharmacotherapy.**
- **Close follow-up until remission is achieved is recommended.**

CASE 47–1. A 27 year-old woman comes to your clinic worried that she has a sexually transmitted disease (STD). When you ask about her sexual behavior she reports that she is "God's gift to man" and that she had intercourse with four different men the night before. She is chewing gum, blowing bubbles, and smiling as she talks to you. You ask if she is always in this good of a mood and she replies, "Oh no! I usually feel like this for a while and then I have no energy and feel really guilty and can hardly get out of bed."

A. What additional information do you need to determine what disorder this woman may have? How do you distinguish between bipolar I and bipolar II disorders? What questions could you ask to elicit this information?
B. What comorbid conditions do you need to be concerned about?
C. Assume that the woman answers all questions so that she does indeed fit the criteria for bipolar I disorder. What is your recommended treatment plan?

CASE 47–2. **A 47-year-old man complains of difficulty sleeping, having horrific nightmares, and "reexperiencing" the car accident he was in six weeks ago. The patient denies suicidal thoughts. He states that he wants you to "give him something to help with his nerves."**

A. What is the most appropriate diagnosis for this patient?
B. What is the difference between acute stress disorder and post-traumatic stress disorder?
C. What is the most appropriate treatment?

REFERENCES

Keller MB, McCullough JP, Klein DN, et al.: A comparison of nefazodone, the cognitive behavioral-analysis system of psychotherapy, and their combination for the treatment of chronic depression. N Engl J Med 342(20):1462–1470, 2000.

Papolos D, Papolos J: Overcoming Depression: The Definitive Resource for Patients and Families Who Live with Depression and Manic-Depression. New York: Harper Collins, 1997.

USEFUL WEBSITES

Anxiety Disorders Association of America. *http://www.adaa.org*
Depression and Bipolar Alliance. *http://www.dbsalliance.org*

48

Diabetes Mellitus

What is diabetes mellitus?

Diabetes mellitus is a disease of abnormal glucose metabolism resulting in hyperglycemia. It is caused by a deficiency in insulin secretion or a combination of insulin resistance and inadequate insulin secretion. More than 13 million Americans report a diagnosis of diabetes mellitus; however, this number does not include the additional 30% or more of diabetics who are undiagnosed and untreated. The dangers of diabetes come from the vascular changes associated with the disease. These vascular changes are a major cause of retinopathy and blindness, end-stage renal disease, peripheral and autonomic neuropathies, and lower extremity amputations. They are also major contributors to stroke and cardiovascular disease.

How is diabetes classified?

Previously, diabetes classification was based on age of onset; if the patient was in his/her teens or younger, then it was most likely juvenile onset (now type 1); if he/she was older then it was most likely adult onset (now type 2). However, with the increasing prevalence of obesity, teenagers commonly develop type 2 diabetes. Similarly, an elderly patient may also present with new-onset type 1 diabetes and diabetic ketoacidosis (DKA).

▶ ETIOLOGY

What is type 1 diabetes?

Type 1 diabetes is a result of pancreatic islet B cell destruction and, ultimately, absolute insulin deficiency. Pancreatic islet B cells are responsible for insulin secretion. The cause for this cell destruction is autoimmune in 90% of the cases. In type 1 diabetes, since the pancreas is no longer able to secrete insulin, all insulin must come from exogenous sources. Type 1 diabetics require daily insulin to prevent severe hyperglycemia and ketoacidosis. They are considered insulin dependent.

What is type 2 diabetes?

In type 2 diabetes, peripheral tissue is insensitive to insulin and pancreatic B cells fail to produce adequate amounts of insulin in the presence of elevated glucose levels. Because most type 2 diabetics retain the ability to secrete some endogenous insulin, those who use exogenous insulin will not likely develop ketoacidosis from not taking their insulin. They are therefore considered "insulin requiring" and not "insulin dependent." Type 2 diabetes accounts for 90% of all diabetics. Gestational diabetes mellitus (GDM) is defined as hyperglycemia during pregnancy that usually resolves after delivery. Other types of diabetes that are much less common are those caused by genetic defects in B cell destruction, genetic defects in insulin action, and diseases of the exocrine pancreas that are either drug or chemical induced.

▶ EVALUATION

How is diabetes diagnosed?

The Expert Committee on the Diagnosis and Classification of Diabetes Mellitus has established criteria for the diagnosis of diabetes (Table 48–1). The fasting plasma glucose (FPG) is the preferred screening and diagnostic test because it is inexpensive and easy to use. The 75-g oral glucose tolerance test (OGTT) tested at two hours is more sensitive and more specific than the FPG, but it is poorly reproducible and more expensive than the FPG. The OGTT is not recommended for routine use, but may be used to further evaluate a patient with an impaired fasting glucose (IFG) or in a patient with a normal FPG where diabetes is still suspected. An IFG describes the range of FPG levels between "normal" and that diagnostic for diabetes. Finally, an elevated random (any time of day) plasma glucose of 200 mg/dL, in the presence of the classic symptoms of polyuria, polydipsia, and unexplained weight loss, is diagnostic of diabetes. A HbA_{1C} should *not* be used to diagnose diabetes.

What history and physical exam findings are important in the diagnosis of diabetes?

When you suspect type 2 diabetes, the history should focus on questions about general well-being including unexplained weight loss, fatigue, or increased thirst; recurrent or persistent infections including vaginal candidiasis or intertrigo; slow-healing skin injuries or infections; recent visual changes or blurred vision; polyuria; and tingling, burning, or numbness in the hands and feet. Many type 2 diabetics are overweight with increased fat distribution about the

TABLE 48–1

Criteria for the Diagnosis of Diabetes and Impaired Glucose Tolerance

Test	Classification			
	Normal	Impaired Fasting Glucose	Impaired Glucose Tolerance*	Diabetes†
Fasting plasma glucose	<100 mg/dL	100–125 mg/dL	———	≥ 126 mg/dL
2-hr plasma glucose OGTT (75 g)	<140 mg/dL	———	140–199 mg/dL	≥ 200 mg/dL
Random PG + symptoms of DM‡				≥ 200 mg/dL

PG = plasma glucose, OGTT = oral glucose tolerance test
*As determined by the 2-hr plasma glucose on the 75-g OGTT
†In the absence of symptoms of DM, these criteria should be confirmed by repeat testing on a different day.
‡Symptoms of DM = polyuria, polydipsia, and unexplained weight loss

chest, abdomen, face, and neck; although not all type 2 diabetics are overweight. Your examination should include a search for evidence of neurologic or cardiovascular complications that result from long-standing occult type 2 diabetes. If patients with type 2 diabetes present acutely, particularly if they are elderly, they may demonstrate confusion, dehydration, and hypotension.

The patient with type 1 diabetes typically presents more acutely than the type 2 diabetic. Symptoms usually occur more rapidly and include weight loss, weakness or fatigue, polyuria, polydipsia (frequent drinking because of thirst), polyphagia (frequent eating), blurred vision, paresthesias, and nocturnal enuresis. Examination usually reveals a loss of subcutaneous fat with muscle wasting, secondary to the diversion of amino acids to form glucose and ketone bodies. Postural hypotension and signs of dehydration may also be present. The above signs and symptoms develop more acutely when absolute insulin deficiency is more rapid in onset. If ketoacidosis is present, anorexia, nausea, and vomiting usually occur. Depending on the degree of hyperosmolality, the patient's level of consciousness may vary from alertness to coma. A fruity breath odor of acetone may also be present.

On whom should I perform routine screening?

Many times, the type 2 diabetic is asymptomatic at the time of initial presentation and therefore may not be diagnosed until complications appear. Current evidence does not support the routine screening of asymptomatic individuals, but use clinical judgment to screen those individuals who are considered at high risk of having or developing diabetes. Nonpregnant adults who should be screened, using an FPG, include those with a body mass index (BMI) greater than 25 kg/m^2 along with additional risk factors of: age over 45; physical inactivity; first-degree relatives with diabetes; members of high-risk ethnic groups such as Native Americans, Latinos, African Americans, Asian Americans, and Pacific Islanders; history of delivering a baby weighing more than 9 lb; hypertension; an HDL cholesterol less than than 35 mg/dL and a triglyceride level greater than 250 mg/dL; polycystic ovary syndrome (PCOS); a previous impaired glucose tolerance or IFG test; or a history of vascular disease.

The American Diabetic Association (ADA) recommends screening high-risk women (marked obesity, personal history of gestational diabetes mellitus [GDM], glycosuria, or a strong family history of diabetes) at the first prenatal visit. An FPG greater than or equal to 126 mg/dL or a random plasma glucose greater than or equal to 200 mg/dL confirmed on separate days, unless accompanied by polyuria, polydipsia, and unexplained weight loss, are considered diagnostic of diabetes. Average-risk women and those who are considered high-risk, but who were not found to have GDM at the first screening, should be tested between 24 and 28 weeks of gestation. Testing can be done by a 100-g OGTT or by using a 50-g glucose challenge test to screen for women with a one-hour result of greater than or equal to 140 mg/dL, and then performing a 100-g OGTT on those that exceed this threshold. The diagnostic criteria for the 100-g OGTT are as follows: greater than or equal to 95 mg/dL fasting, greater than or equal to 180 mg/dL at one hour, greater than or equal to 155 mg/dL at two hours, and greater than or equal to 140 mg/dL at three hours. Two or more of these values must be present to confirm the diagnosis of GDM. Low-risk women—age below 25 years, normal prepregnancy weight, no known first-degree relatives with diabetes, no history of abnormal glucose tolerance, member of a non–high-risk ethnic group, and history of normal obstetric outcomes—do not require screening.

Children with the following risk factors should be screened using the FPG, starting at age 10 and continuing every two years as long as the risks persist.

- BMI above the 85th percentile for age and sex
- Weight for height above the 85th percentile, or weight greater than 120% of ideal for height

plus any two of the following risk factors:

- Family history of type 2 diabetes in a first-degree or second-degree relative

- High-risk ethnic group as mentioned earlier in this section
- Signs or conditions associated with insulin resistance (hypertension, dyslipidemia, PCOS, acanthosis nigricans)

Once diabetes is diagnosed, what should the initial evaluation include?

During the initial evaluation, classify the disease as either type 1 or type 2 diabetes and question and examine the patient for the presence or absence of diabetic complications.

- Present history: Symptoms of diabetes; results of diagnostic testing
- Past history: History of hypertension, dyslipidemia; medications that may affect blood glucose levels
- Social history: History of exercise; eating patterns; presence of any factors that might interfere with management—lifestyle, economic, cultural, education; use of tobacco, alcohol, or controlled substances
- Family history: History of diabetes, atherosclerosis
- Review of systems: Prior or current infections of skin, foot, dental, and genitourinary system; symptoms of end-organ disease associated with diabetes including eye, cardiovascular, nerve, kidney, genitourinary, cerebrovascular, and foot complications; reproductive and sexual history

What do I look for on physical examination after diagnosis?

The physical examination should focus on height and weight; blood pressure, including orthostatic measurements; the eye (for cataracts and retinopathy); mouth; thyroid; heart; abdomen (for hepatomegaly); peripheral pulses; feet (for ulceration, infection, or sensory loss, as measured with a monofilament); skin; and neurologic system (dulling of vibration, pain, temperature, and possible loss of ankle jerks). Also seek signs of diseases that can cause secondary diabetes (e.g., hemochromatosis, Cushing's, and pancreatic disease).

What subsequent labs and studies should I order?

Initial testing should include an HbA_{1C}; fasting lipid profile (total cholesterol, HDL cholesterol, LDL cholesterol, and triglycerides); urine screen for microalbuminuria (in those who have had type 1 diabetes for more than five years and in all type 2 diabetics); serum BUN and creatinine; TSH in all type 1 diabetics and in type 2 patients as clinically indicated; EKG, if clinically indicated; and a urinalysis for ketones, protein, sediment, or signs of infection.

▶ TREATMENT

What are the goals of treatment?

The results of several clinical trials, including the Diabetes Control and Complications Trial and the United Kingdom Prospective Diabetes Study, have shown that glycemic control can delay the onset and slow the progression of microvascular and neuropathic complications of diabetes. Glycemic control can be monitored through blood glucose self-monitoring, at a frequency that is determined by the overall stability of the disease, by the patient's motivation, and by the HbA_{1C}. The goals for the management of diabetes and its comorbid diseases are preprandial plasma glucose of 90 to 130 mg/dL, postprandial plasma glucose less than 180 mg/dL, HbA_{1C} less than 7%, total cholesterol less than 200 mg/dL, LDL cholesterol less than 100 mg/dL, HDL cholesterol less than 40 mg/dL, triglycerides less than 150 mg/dL, blood pressure below 130/80 or below 120/75 if renal insufficiency is present, smoking cessation, and prevention of retinopathy, proteinuria, and damage to the structures and skin of the foot.

What treatment steps are appropriate for managing diabetes?

Diabetes management should include a team that consists of the patient, the patient's family, the physician, and other healthcare professionals including a diabetic educator, ophthalmologist, and podiatrist. The team should instruct the patient in the self-management of his disease and the potential complications of noncontrol. The overweight adult diabetic should focus initially on restricting calories and increasing exercise. The nonobese adult diabetic may need to reduce the percentage of carbohydrates in her diet, but she may not have to change her overall calorie consumption. Exercise is important for the nonobese adult diabetic, as well. If diet and exercise do not result in a significant drop in the HbA_{1C}, the patient should begin medication therapy.

What types of medication are available?

The oral medications for treating type 2 diabetes fall into three main categories: those that affect glucose absorption (acarbose), those that stimulate insulin secretion (the sulfonylureas), and those that alter insulin action (metformin and thiazolidinediones).

Acarbose reduces postprandial hyperglycemia by interfering with carbohydrate digestion. Undigested carbohydrates that reach the lower bowel can cause significant flatulence. Although this side effect should discourage the diabetic from consuming excess carbohydrates, a significant number end up discontinuing the medication. Hypoglycemia is a common side effect, and is of concern in the elderly and those with cardiac disease.

Metformin can be used for the obese type 2 patient or for those not responding to maximum dosages of sulfonylureas. It improves fasting and postprandial hyperglycemia and hypertryglyceridemia, but is not associated with the weight gain or hypoglycemia seen with other diabetic medications. It is contraindicated in patients with renal, hepatic, or cardiorespiratory insufficiency, or alcoholism. The *thiazolidinediones* sensitize peripheral tissues to insulin. They are effective as monotherapy, but are often prescribed in combination with metformin or insulin. Weight gain and edema are common side effects and patients need to be monitored for changes in liver function.

Insulin therapy is used in all type 1 diabetics; in type 2 diabetics who have failed treatment with diet, exercise, and oral hypoglycemic medications (HbA_{1C} remains ≥8); and in gestational diabetics who have failed diet management. Diabetics on insulin should monitor their blood sugars daily. The different types of insulin are prescribed based on their onset of action, their time to peak effect, and their duration of action. For type 2 diabetics, the longer-acting insulins such as NPH insulin (0.1–0.2 U/kg) and insulin glargine (10 U) are most often started as a single evening or pre-bedtime dose. If the initial nighttime dose does not bring the blood sugars within the expected range, the longer-acting insulin dose may be increased or the shorter-acting insulins, regular or insulin lispro, may be administered along with meals. Some insulins come as a combination of a short-acting and a longer-acting insulin, for example 70% NPH and 30% regular. While these combinations may make insulin administration easier, individually titrating each component becomes more difficult. Blood glucose measurements obtained by self-monitoring are used to adjust the insulin dosage and to help prevent hypoglycemia. Type 2 diabetics are often continued on one or two of their oral hypoglycemic medications after insulin is started. (More specific information on insulin management for type 1 and type 2 diabetes can be obtained from the DeWitt reference cited at the end of this chapter.)

What should I do when I see a diabetic for a follow-up visit?

When a patient who has been diagnosed with diabetes comes in for follow-up visits, assess the following: the patient's understanding of his/her diabetes; control of blood sugars through diet, exercise and/or medication; the presence or control of risk factors such as hypertension and dyslipidemia; compliance with medications and any problems that the patient may be experiencing with the medications; and any physical signs of end-organ damage. Examine the patient's feet at each visit. The frequency of monitoring laboratory tests is usually determined by the overall control of the diabetes, the existence of comorbid conditions, and the need to screen for medication side effects. HbA_{1C} reflects the state of glycemia over the preceding 8–12 weeks; you should monitor at least every 3–4 months for those with HbA_{1C} greater than 2% above the upper limits of normal, and every 6 months for those with greater control. Measure lipids every 3–4 months until the patient meets her goal, and then annually. Screen urine for microalbumin annually and then, once positive, at each visit. Perform dilated eye exams annually. Provide pneumococcal vaccine as recommended and influenza vaccine annually. Consider aspirin therapy on an individual basis.

When should I admit the patient to the hospital?

Two main causes for hospitalization are diabetic ketoacidosis (DKA) and hyperosmolar coma. In addition to the classic symptoms described earlier in the chapter, the diagnostic parameters for DKA are hyperglycemia greater than 250 mg/dL, acidosis with blood pH less than 7.3, serum bicarbonate less than 15 mEq/L, and serum positive for ketones. Hyperglycemic hyperosmolar state occurs in type 2 diabetics and is less common than DKA. It is characterized by hyperglycemia without ketosis. Other diagnostic parameters include hyperglycemia greater than 600 mg/dL, serum osmolality greater than 310 mOsm/kg, no acidosis, with a blood pH greater than 7.3, serum bicarbonate greater than 15 mEq/L, and a normal anion gap (<14 mEq/L).

KEY POINTS

- **Diabetes classification can no longer be assigned simply by using the patient's age.**
- **An HbA_{1C} is great for monitoring glycemic control, but should not be used as a screening test for diabetes.**
- **The management of diabetes requires ongoing medical care and education of the patient and his/her family in order to prevent acute complications and to reduce the long-term complications.**
- **Insulin should not be considered the treatment of last resort.**

CASE 48–1. **A 54-year-old obese African-American woman presents with a history of recurrent vaginal candidiasis. Her genitourinary review of systems is unremarkable, including a history of polyuria. In addition, she has not experienced the classic symptoms of polydipsia or unexplained weight loss. You suspect that she may have diabetes.**

A. What testing would confirm a diagnosis of type 2 diabetes?
B. What further history should be obtained once the diagnosis of diabetes is obtained?
C. Which specific areas should the physical exam focus on once the diagnosis of diabetes is made?
D. Which baseline labs should be ordered in a newly diagnosed type 2 diabetic?
E. What would be the first steps in the management of her diabetes?

CASE 48–2. **A 68-year-old type 2 diabetic comes in for a follow-up visit. He is currently on the highest recommended doses of metformin and rosiglitazone and has been for the last four months. He states that he has had difficulty following his diabetic diet since the death of his wife, six months ago. He also has been unmotivated to walk or exercise. His blood pressure is 140/88 and was 135/82 on his previous visit. His physical exam is otherwise unremarkable.**

A. What nonmedication interventions could be used to help this patient regain control of his diabetes?
B. Which blood tests should be ordered on this patient for routine follow-up of his diabetes?
C. What medications could be used to treat his hypertension? How might this change if microalbuminuria were found on examination?
D. If the decision were made to start him on insulin therapy, how might this be done?

REFERENCES

American Diabetes Association: Standard of medical care in diabetes. Diabetes Care 27 Suppl 1:S15–S35, 2004.

DeWitt DE: Outpatient insulin therapy in type 1 and type 2 diabetes mellitus. JAMA 289:2254–2264, 2003.

Masharani U, Karam J: Diabetes mellitus and hypoglycemia. In Tierney L (ed): Current Medical Diagnosis and Treatment, 42nd ed. New York: McGraw Hill, 2003, pp 1152–1192.

USEFUL WEBSITES

American Diabetes Association (Clinical Practice Guidelines). *http://www.diabetes.org*

U.S. Department of Health and Human Services, Agency for Healthcare Research and Quality. *http://www.preventiveservices.ahrq.gov*

49

Family Discord/ Dysfunction

What is meant by the term "dysfunctional family"?

A family that is dysfunctional has difficulty fulfilling its necessary obligations to: (1) satisfy the needs of family members for affection and intimacy, (2) satisfy the sexual needs of the parents, (3) produce, protect, raise, and socialize children, (4) provide for the material maintenance (shelter, food, clothing) of the members by forming an economic unit, (5) promote a sense of autonomy so that each member can become independent, and (6) encourage each member to develop a sense of right and wrong and a values system that society approves.

What causes families to become dysfunctional?

Dysfunction may result from impaired learning and/or poor modeling within the families in which the parents were raised. It can also result from stressful life events that overwhelm the family's ability to cope. Stress may arise from the family's normal life cycle development tasks and/or from unexpected external crises. Some family systems can face crises better than others because their resources and their system dynamics help them to adapt better.

What is a family system?

A system is a set of interrelated units that exist in such a way so that the state of each unit depends on the state of the other units. Furthermore, a system must be understood as a whole that is both greater than and different than the sum of its parts. For example, the cardiopulmonary system consists of separate units that are interdependent and where disease in one part of the system affects the rest of the system. Likewise, treatment directed toward individual units can either positively or negatively affect the other parts.

In similar fashion, the family system contains separate, interdependent units (family members with their unique personal attributes) that have specific roles, obligations, and interrelationships. The character of the family is greater than, and different than, the sum of the characteristics of the individual members. Furthermore, the actions of any one member ripple out to affect the others.

How do family systems work?

Doherty and Baird suggest five functional axioms that apply to family systems.

Axiom 1. *The family as a whole is more than a collection of individuals* (discussed earlier).

Axiom 2. *Families have repeating interaction patterns (sometimes called rules) that regulate members' behavior and that often become rituals.* These govern the family's everyday life, establishing regularity and stability. Some rules may be troublesome, like "it's okay to interrupt one another's conversation at any time," "the spouse of an alcoholic is expected to make excuses for his/her lapses in responsibility," or "the only way to get attention in the family is to become ill."

Axiom 3. *A family member's symptoms may serve a function within the family, becoming incorporated into family interaction patterns as essential ingredients to maintain harmony and regularity.* For example, a brittle diabetic child's precarious health may hold an unstable marriage together, or the marital union between partners may be based on the patient and caretaker roles of the spouses. Recurring psychosomatic or psychosocial problems and poor treatment compliance may indicate that the patient's symptoms serve a hidden family purpose.

Axiom 4. *The ability to change is a hallmark of healthy family functioning.* Change is a constant challenge for the family as it progresses through its life cycle and as it confronts inevitable family crises. Healthy families can change their rules, roles, and relationships to help them adapt to changing circumstances.

Axiom 5. *Families share joint responsibility for their problems.* Family members are simultaneously actors and reactors, especially in maintaining chronic problems. To help a family, the physician who thinks and acts from a systems perspective must assume that everyone bears responsibility for family problems.

How will I recognize a family that functions well when I see one?

Families that function best demonstrate a number of common characteristics. They are intimate, affectionate, and loyal, balancing closeness with separateness between members. Members also balance the amount of time they spend together with time away from the family, and they have both personal and family friends. These families respect each other's viewpoints, choices, and perceptions and permit both individual and joint decision making, often taking the children's feelings and ideas into account. They are capable negotiators and excellent problem-solvers who manage problems by changing roles and rules. When conflict occurs, they resolve it quickly.

The parents, who share equally in making decisions, are definite family leaders. Internal boundaries are clear and provide each member with personal time and space. Family roles and household responsibilities are stable, but often shared. Family rules are accepted by all and are predictable, fair, and stable, but can be flexible when needed. Likewise, discipline is more democratic with predictable or negotiated consequences, and some degree of leniency.

Healthy families are also open to the external environment. They focus on the family at the same time that they engage the outside world—school, church, community organizations, governmental organizations, charities, etc.

Over time the level of closeness within healthy families evolves as children mature, become more like peers, and then often assume roles as caretakers for their parents.

Communication in healthy families is empathic. Members listen attentively to others and speak for themselves. They feel free to discuss themselves and their own feelings and relationships. No topic is "out-of-bounds." Verbal messages are clear and accompanied by congruent nonverbal messages. Members track each other's conversation with few, if any, irrelevant, distracting side comments or negative nonverbal messages.

What characteristics and behaviors describe a family that is "at risk" for dysfunction?

Dysfunction occurs more often as the family moves toward extremes of cohesion (emotional bonding) and flexibility (adaptability to change), although the key variable appears to be whether all family members are satisfied with the system as it exists. If they are, the family will function adequately until someone expresses dissatisfaction. Then families at the extreme are more threatened with disruption. Balanced families can meet the functional needs of family members much more effectively.

Cohesion. The family that is *disengaged* demonstrates extreme emotional separateness and evidences little of the following characteristics: family loyalty, involvement between family members, sharing of feelings, parent–child closeness, or time spent together. Members prefer to go their own ways and to make independent decisions.

At the other extreme, the family that is *enmeshed* demonstrates extreme emotional closeness. Their energy is mainly focused inside the family, family loyalty is demanded, and decisions are made by the whole group. Members are very dependent on one another, permit little private space, blur generational boundaries, and have few individual friends.

Flexibility. The family that is *chaotic* demonstrates erratic leadership, often with unsuccessful parental control and ineffective discipline. Decisions are subject to endless negotiation and are often made impulsively. Roles are unclear and are subject to frequent, unpredictable reversals. Rules, likewise, frequently change for no logical reason.

At the *rigid* extreme of adaptability, the family is governed by authoritarian, highly controlling parents. Rules don't change and discipline is enforced with strict consequences. Decisions are imposed by the parents after limited negotiation. Roles are strictly defined and generally follow traditional male–female stereotypes.

How can the family physician focus on family systems and family assessment?

Most family physicians do not provide family therapy. You can, however, practice family systems medicine. Because often you will care for family members over time, you have an opportunity to collect and record much information about the family, such as the following:

Family context information. Collect and record all the data defined by the *CHERESH* acronym (see Chapter 5).

Family genogram. The family tree or genogram allows you to create a visual record of family structure, developmental issues, relationship patterns, genetic and medical disorders, and stressful life events.

Family relationships. Note fractures in relationships like divorce and separation. Identify conflict between family members and relationships that are overly close, especially those that cross subsystem boundaries (such as a mother–daughter relationship that is closer than the wife–husband relationship).

Family life cycle stage. Make note of the family's life cycle stage. The family progresses through developmental stages that require it to accomplish specific tasks new to each stage (Table 49–1). If the family fails to accomplish these tasks it may have difficulty with further family development. Since transitions from one stage to another require change and adaptability they create stress that may make the family more vulnerable to other crises.

Hold family conferences. Family conferences are a very effective setting in which to gather information about the family and its dynamics and to communicate vital information. Leading a conference can be daunting for the uninitiated. This reluctance can be assuaged by proper preparation and by following an organized format, such as the one outlined in Box 49–1.

Text continued on p. 315

TABLE 49–1

The Family Life Cycle Stages and Developmental Tasks

Life Cycle Stage	Developmental Tasks
Young adult	*Establish self-identity.* Separate from their family of origin without cutting themselves off entirely or fleeing to a substitute emotional refuge. *Develop a support system.* Establish a network of intimate peer relationships. *Establish self in work.* Develop a "job identity."
The new couple	*Balance intimacy with autonomy.* Decide what they will share in terms of ideas, feelings, bodies, friends, etc., and what they will reserve for their own privacy. *Balance freedom with commitment.* Decide what is open to negotiation and what is not in terms of time, money, friendships, dedication to work, school, etc. *Identify shared values.* Decide on role responsibilities (e.g., who will cook, shop, clean house, earn income, maintain the car, pay bills, etc.); on the importance of religion; on the place of work in the family; and on the role children will play. They must also relinquish the "fantasy partner." *Define new relationships with families of origin.* Give priority to the spouse relationship over extended family relationships.
Childbearing/preschool family	*Allow and enjoy the neonate's dependence.* *Share the spouse's attention* with the new infant and overcome feelings of abandonment and neglect. *Reexamine the couple relationship.* This begins during pregnancy and involves reexamining expressions of intimacy and sexuality, and includes integrating new positions and roles (e.g., "father" and "mother" must integrate with "husband," "wife," and "lover.") *Rework relationships with families of origin.* A child reconnects the couple with the lineage family and "readmits" the couple's parents to the family. They often want a greater part in the life of the growing family, visiting more often and giving more advice (often about settling down, child rearing practices, etc.). *Deal with the increasing autonomy of the growing child.* The child tests his/her ability to influence the parents' behavior with struggles for autonomy that reinforce the separateness of child from the parents.
School-age family	*Deal with boundary issues between the family and society.* School represents the larger society, and as such it imposes expectations on the family, introduces new stimuli, and is often the first contact for the child with people different from his/her family.

continued

Table 49–1. The Family Life Cycle Stages and Developmental Tasks *continued*

Life Cycle Stage	Developmental Tasks
	Maintain the couple relationship and ongoing role commitments. It is easy to become child-centered and forget the pair bond since the children's presence decreases the ease and opportunities for privacy and for nurturing marital intimacy. Parents must find a way to support and nurture each other as well as the children.
	Focus on "styles of mastery." Much time, energy, and money is spent on lessons, sports, and other learning activities. The achievement, competence, conformity, and creativity of the parents are mirrored in the growing child's development.
Family with teens	*Face problems with identity.* The individual developmental tasks of the child and the adults are curiously similar during this period. The adolescent is trying to establish a self not previously integrated and the adult is evaluating beliefs and decisions in light of several decades of personal, familial, and social change. The similarity in developmental issues often explains the frequent intensity and bitterness of parent–adolescent interchanges. If parents are more secure in their own self-identity, they are less threatened as children deal with identity crises and are more capable of supporting children going through difficult adjustments.
	Face problems with sexuality. Teens are overwhelmed by great physical and emotional changes, seek a means to express new aspects of self, and are often embarrassed and burdened by the seemingly overwhelming consequences of success and failure. Adults face changes in desire and question their continuing attractiveness and sexual performance.
	Face problems with independence. Teens increasingly assume responsibility for their own actions and become aware of the effects of their actions on others in and out of the family. Adults need to give up control and responsibility for their child's behavior.
	Face problems with dependence of the older generation. When teens and parents are struggling with their identity, sexuality, and independence, the grandparents are often "fighting for their lives." Parents are often expected to support the grandparents while at the same time losing the support given to them by the older generation. Parents often find themselves in a double squeeze from the teens on one side and the grandparents on the other. This double squeeze can lead to the parents becoming isolated from the generations on either side of them.
Launching family	*Shift from dependence to interdependence.* Young adults increasingly gain skills in handling responsibilities and can begin to teach the parents. At this time, young adults resolve their searches for identity and the parents resolve their midlife transitions.

continued

Table 49–1. The Family Life Cycle Stages and Developmental Tasks *continued*

Life Cycle Stage	Developmental Tasks
	Realign family subsystems and reassign role responsibilities. The family learns to do without the daily presence of one of its eldest junior members. Changes in personal space in the home and others taking over the jobs formerly done by that person affect all routines of daily living. Parenting responsibilities decrease and parents must develop or extend other meaningful interests and activities to take the place of all the time and energy they expended on the children's development. *Responsibilities of parents to their own parents are often decreasing.*
Empty nest family	*Return to being a couple alone.* This is often the time of highest marital satisfaction, but if the marital bond is weak, the increasing prominence given to the couple relationship may strain the bond more than it can manage. Each spouse must recommit to the marriage. *Face the challenges of aging.* This occurs with decreasing physical and psychological resources and the need to reorganize living situations and actively prepare for the reality and consequences of aging. *Assume the role of grandparents.* *Deal with the death of their aging parents.*
Aging family	*Maintain ego integrity in the face of potential despair.* The aging couple gives meaning to life through relationships with each other. Sexual relationships and relationships with children and grandchildren continue, and the couple is active in outside interests, but with declining participation. *Adjust to losses with greatly decreased reserves.* They suffer losses in health, work, mobility, support systems, and often their spouse. *Make major adjustments in living arrangements and financial security.* *Continue activity and comfortably disengage.*

BOX 49–1

A Suggested Plan for Preparing and Leading a Family Conference

Preliminary work

- Background preparation
  - Identify your family contact person.
  - Establish a reason for the conference.
  - Decide who will attend.
  - Schedule the appointment with date, time, place.
- Review the family structure
  - Prepare the genogram—get to know the players and how they are connected.
  - Make note of the family's life cycle stage to anticipate normative crises.
- Develop conference goals
  - Define a limited number of goals for the conference.
  - Develop tentative assumptions about the family and their concerns.
  - Establish an agenda for leading the conference.

A suggested agenda for leading a family conference

- Break the ice
  - Greet the family and familiarize everyone with the room including seating and location of rest rooms, if needed.
  - Make a personal connection with each family member by way of a personal word, a handshake, a smile, and good eye contact.
- Define the goals
  - Ask each person who wishes to speak to articulate their goals for the session.
  - Restate each goal so that it is clear, concise, and realistic.
  - Add any other necessary goals from your own list.
  - Consider writing the goals on a white board or newsprint pad so that they remain in full view of everyone, don't get forgotten, and can be saved.
  - Prioritize the goals, selecting the most important ones for this session.
- Discuss the concern(s)/ issue(s)
  - Ask each person for his or her point-of-view.
  - Encourage each family member to ask questions.
  - Ask the family how they may have managed similar problems in the past.

continued

BOX 49–1. A Suggested Plan for Preparing and Leading a Family Conference *continued*

- Identify resources that can help manage the family's concern(s)/issue(s)
  - List family strengths.
  - Note medical resources.
  - Record economic resources.
  - List other community resources—e.g., support groups, financial help, housing, food, governmental and private agencies, private philanthropy, faith-based organizations, etc.
- Develop a management plan
  - Ask the family if they have thought about a plan.
  - Contract with the family to assist them in creating a plan to manage their concerns, including referral or reappointment, if that is needed.
  - Ask for any remaining questions about the plan to assure that steps for implementation are clear and understood.

What role can the family physician play in helping families to manage stress and dysfunction?

Most medical students begin their clinical rotations with a biomedical focus, in which families are relegated to the background, and communicating with them is not considered integral to the physician's role. By graduation, however, you should realize that patients belong to families and that family members influence each other in a whole host of areas, including infectious diseases; health behaviors; psychosocial stresses and strains that affect health; social support for prevention and recovery from illness; defining the nature and seriousness of symptoms; and deciding on where and when to obtain healthcare. You also should recognize that the family is the social group most immediately affected by illness and medical treatment and that it is a valuable source of information for diagnosis and treatment. Be willing to engage families and communicate medical findings and treatment options, ask for relevant diagnostic and treatment information, listen to questions and concerns, advise families about medical and rehabilitation needs, and channel communication through key members.

More advanced students and family practice residents will be able to manage the family's stress and emotional reactions. You will be able to discuss medical data and the family's feelings and concerns; elicit family expressions of concern and feelings about a family member's condition and its effect on the family; empathize with family concerns and normalize them when appropriate;

form hypotheses about the family's level of functioning around a member's problem; encourage family coping efforts; tailor medical advice to the family's unique needs, concerns, and feelings; and identify family dysfunction and make a referral when appropriate.

What are some key first steps in helping a family that is experiencing problems?

Engage a family that is suffering stress or that exhibits dysfunction by forming a covenant with them during a family conference that specifies both the physician's and the family's roles and responsibilities. During that discussion, consider the following management options.

Referral to another health professional. Most family physicians refer families with serious problems like alcoholism and chemical dependency, domestic violence, and chronic family discord. Once they decide to refer, the physicians will help select an appropriate therapist/consultant, connect the family with the consultant, provide any useful information that helps the therapist/consultant work with the family, support and monitor the family's treatment progress, and continue following the family when therapy is completed.

Further family assessment and treatment. After an initial family conference, the physician may decide that he or she needs to learn more about the family before making a decision about referral or further counseling. This may include gathering information about how the family functions as a unit, the impact of the family on a family member's problem, or the impact of the member's problem on the family. Gathering this information usually requires one or more additional family conferences.

Following an adequate assessment some family physicians will determine that they can help the family with primary family-oriented counseling, which is a level of care that emphasizes support, education, and prevention. This type of counseling is most useful for families who generally function well, but who face a crisis that requires major change in their roles and relationships and that challenges their adaptive resources. This counseling does not emphasize specialized therapy's powerful interventions that create fundamental change in the family's structure or interaction patterns.

Individual assessment and treatment. In addition to family assessment and treatment, individual family members may benefit from personal psychological evaluation and treatment. Individual management for problems such as depression and anxiety will improve the member's ability to contribute more effectively to the success of family therapy. In some cases family problems are discovered during the course of managing a family member who came to the physician for a personal concern. In this case the physician will continue to assess and treat the index patient, and subsequently engage the other family members.

What are some clinical presentations that are "red flags" for family assessment?

Family assessment is particularly important in those clinical situations where the family system may cause a patient's problem(s) or where the patient's problem(s) may significantly impact the family. Some of those settings are described in this section.

When family members must become *caregivers* for another family member, family study can help the physician to anticipate compliance, since motivation to care for family members is influenced by the family system. It can also help to anticipate problems in the caregivers, since the stress of caring for the ill person may precipitate health problems in those providing the care.

Family assessment is mandatory when the history reveals *overt symptoms* of family distress. Overt symptoms include such problems as impending divorce or separation; an environment of excessive arguing, fighting, and baiting; noncommunication between family members; incest, child abuse, and other forms of domestic violence; juvenile delinquency and runaways; and major school failure or behavior problems.

Family study is also useful in settings where *covert symptoms* predominate. Covert symptoms include overutilization of healthcare facilities, doctor shopping, excessive somatization, and the "positive review of systems" where the patient responds affirmatively to nearly all queries.

Chronic family stress may also be a root cause for *chronic depression* that is unresponsive to treatment. The usual patient in this setting has suffered decades of depression with poor results from management. Not infrequently prior physicians have become incorporated into the dysfunctional family pattern and may have perpetuated the problem by prescribing medications, such as tranquilizing drugs, that can make the depression worse.

Family study is also useful for people with *chronic anxiety* who present multiple times for multiple complaints where no organic disease is discovered. Many such patients have a history of long-term anxiolytic use, and in almost all situations family functioning has deteriorated and family interaction patterns are distortedly organized around the anxiety symptoms.

Chronic fatigue is a symptom that requires thorough medical and psychological evaluation, but early in that process the physician needs to assess personal and family life stresses. If the medical evaluation is negative, then the physician can concentrate more fully on family-centered evaluation and treatment.

Suspect family dysfunction when parents continue bringing their normal children to the office with *recurring pediatric complaints,* and many attempts to educate the parents have been ineffective.

Certain settings for *insomnia* may relate to family issues. For example, a middle-aged man who complains of insomnia may have an underlying depression related to a midlife crisis, a divorce, and alcohol abuse as an aid to sleep.

In settings of *serious, especially terminal, illness* the family always experiences the impact of managing the problem and then coping with the loss.

Some cases of *sexual dysfunction* result from misinformation and basic misunderstanding about normal anatomy, physiology, and the sexual response. Other cases result from specific organic problems. However, a large number are still caused by significant relationship issues between the couple and within the family.

A final caveat: any *consistent problem that defies medical explanation* after repeated, thorough evaluation, including specialty consultation, may be a clue to family dysfunction as a root cause.

KEY POINTS

- **Family dysfunction can affect the health of individuals within the family.**
- **Family dysfunction can be detected by family physicians.**
- **Family dysfunction can be treated by family physicians in their practice or via referral to an appropriate therapist.**

CASE 49–1. **A 47-year-old man presents to your office complaining of fatigue of three-month duration. His symptoms correspond to the time that his wife assumed the caregiver role for her 82-year-old mother, in the couple's home. His mother-in-law requires round-the-clock care, and his wife has done the bulk of the care herself. They have a son who is graduating from college in the near future as well. The patient previously had been in good health, and the family had heretofore had no major problems.**

A. What is the likely cause of this patient's fatigue?
B. What treatments or interventions would you recommend for this patient?

CASE 49–2. **A 25-year-old woman who works as a teacher in your community, and who you have cared for since childhood, presents for evaluation after missing her last menstrual period. A home pregnancy test was positive. You confirm her pregnancy and date it at six-weeks gestational age. She returns in two weeks with her husband for her first prenatal visit. Both are excited, since they have been married for two years, and now expect their first child. You have also cared for the husband since he was a child, and you know their families, also patients of yours. You are aware that the husband is an only child with a distant, alcoholic father and a mother who has doted on and protected her son. Mother and son remain very close. The wife's parents are divorced and she remains close to her father, a prominent local businessman, but is estranged from her mother. She is the oldest of four siblings and remains close to her two brothers, but does not get along well with her sister, the youngest in the family, who remains very close to their mother.**

A. Which family life cycle stages are represented in this case, and what are the developmental tasks for each stage?
B. What are the family system concerns, if any, that need investigating in this family?

CASE 49–3. **Several days ago you admitted a 75-year-old man to the hospital because he had become increasingly confused, begun wandering outside the home, kept leaving the stove on when he went to make tea, and was increasingly belligerent with his youngest daughter, with whom he lives. Following an appropriate medical and neuropsychiatric evaluation he was diagnosed with moderately severe Alzheimer's dementia. When you discuss this with the daughter she breaks down in tears. She is becoming "worn out" in her attempt to care for her demented father, feels guilty about her inadequacy, and also notes that the stresses of caregiving are starting to negatively affect her relationship with her husband. Her older siblings (a brother and two sisters) have made it clear that they do not want their father**

continued

CASE 49–3 *continued*

admitted to a long-term care facility. Since she is not employed outside the home, she is the one most able to provide care for her father. After all, she says, "It is the least she could do for all her father has done for her." You suggest a family conference to help the family reach some resolution.

A. Who should be invited to this conference?
B. How will you prepare for this meeting?
C. What questions do you want to answer about this family's functioning?
D. How will you run this conference?

REFERENCES

Doherty WJ, Baird MA: Family Therapy and Family Medicine. New York: Guilford Press, 1983.

McGoldrick M, Gerson R, Shellenberger S: Genograms: Assement and Intervention, 2nd ed. New York: Norton, 1999.

Mengel MB, Holleman WL, Fields SA (eds): Fundamentals of Clinical Practice, 2nd ed. New York: Kluwer Academic/Plenum Publishers, 2002.

The Working with Families Institute. Working with Families: case-based modules on common problems in family medicine. Toronto: University of Toronto Press, 2003.

50

Frailty

Discuss the demographics of frailty.

The latest census projections estimate that the elderly population will increase to 54 million persons by 2020, double the growth rate of the total population during the same time period. By 2020 one in six Americans will be elderly, by 2050 one in five. More importantly, according to the same projections, the number of persons over 85 (the oldest old) will increase to 18 million, or about 5% of the total population. Because of this anticipated increase in the elderly population and its increasing ethnic diversity, the coming years will produce an unprecedented need for services and goods required by individuals in their seventh through tenth decades, those most likely to be frail.

What is the definition of frailty?

There is no agreed-upon definition of frailty. However, most clinicians agree that frailty is a physiologic vulnerability resulting from reduced reserve and capacity to withstand stress. These declines in reserve appear to involve the neuromuscular system, the neuroendocrine system, and the immune system.

Frailty in its later stages is also known as *failure to thrive* in the elderly. Frailty has been associated with anorexia, unplanned weight loss (10% or more over six months), weakness, poor energy, or low activity. The result of these signs can include chronic undernutrition, sarcopenia (decreased muscle mass), osteopenia, balance and gait abnormalities, deconditioning, and slow gait speed. Any one of these signs can lead to a wide range of adverse outcomes that include functional decline, institutionalization, and death.

Frailty is associated with older age, being female, being African-American, having less education and lower income, and having higher rates of comorbid chronic diseases.

▶ ETIOLOGY

What causes frailty?

Medicine does not completely understand the etiology of frailty, but strongly associates it with aging and not with specific diseases. Aging affects the musculoskeletal system via weight loss, sarcopenia, and a decline in skeletal muscle mass. Diminished taste, poor dentition, dementia, delirium, chronic wasting illness, or social isolation may precipitate chronic undernutrition, leading to this progressive weight loss and decline. The most profound effect occurs in the oldest age groups, resulting in decreased strength and endurance, weakness, and fatigue. Additionally, the loss of skeletal muscle may result in a reduction in strength, decreased bone density, and the slowing of resting metabolic rate, thereby disrupting thermoregulation and resulting in the heat and cold intolerance seen in the very old. Because fat replaces lean muscle mass, there may be an association with the glucose intolerance and insulin resistance seen in middle and older age groups.

The immune system changes with age, including a decline in the overall number of T cells and a decreased effectiveness of T-memory cells. These changes may influence the body's response to newer antigens. The oldest and most frail individuals also display lower CD_4 counts. This decline may explain the shorter duration of effectiveness of immunizations in older individuals. Furthermore, the production of antibodies declines with age. These changes result in the frail older individual's increased vulnerability to infection and mortality, perhaps caused by protein/calorie undernutrition or chronic exposure to high levels of stress hormones.

The neuroendocrine system maintains homeostasis by regulating hormonal and neuronal responses to stressors. Many of these functions change with age; the most obvious is the loss of estrogen at menopause. Other components of this system suffer with age by slowing responses to normal stimuli and sluggish negative feedback loops. You can appreciate the complexity of this system by considering the role of the sympathetic nervous system and its part in response to physical and emotional stress. Long-standing exposure to high levels of stress hormones including cortisol, epinephrine, and norepinephrine can contribute to suppressed immune function, increased insulin resistance, and loss of lean muscle mass. Other important hormones that decline in old age include growth hormone, testosterone, and dehydroepiandrosterone (DHEA), which has been associated with reductions in lean body mass.

Interrelated changes in these three systems likely increase the vulnerability to stressors and reduce the ability to adapt to changes in the environment. When age and other nonalterable contributors combine with secondary organism stressors including dementia, depression, cancer, chronic infection, and CHF, they contribute to neuroendocrine dysregulation, sarcopenia, and immune dysfunction and the clinical syndrome of frailty.

Are disability and frailty the same thing?

Do not confuse frailty with disability. Frailty may be the cause of disability in many cases, and disability the cause of frailty in others, but the two are not synonymous.

▶ EVALUATION

How is frailty diagnosed?

Frequently the patient presents complaining of "weakness" or "wooziness" with resultant functional decline and/or inability to complete usual tasks such as preparing and cleaning up after a meal, making the bed, or doing laundry. Clues in the medical history may include a past history of inflammatory bowel disease, connective tissue disease, cancer, ischemic heart disease, congestive heart failure, cirrhosis, chronic obstructive pulmonary disease, tuberculosis, stroke, Parkinson's disease, recurrent urinary tract infection, large bone fracture, depression, delirium, or dementia.

Medication classes that cause particular trouble with the elderly include diuretics, β-blockers, narcotics, benzodiazepines, neuroleptics, anticholinergics, glucocorticoids, or any combination of medications that add up to six or more (polypharmacy).

The social history may reveal that the patient lives alone, is poor, and has limited family or community contact. She may have long-standing alcohol use and/or a history of tobacco use. The recent loss of spouse or other losses including a change in residence that resulted in the loss of a familiar living situation can increase vulnerability to frailty. A history of blood transfusion between 1980 and 1995 should be noted. Family history may not be particularly helpful.

A review of systems may be positive for fatigue, fever, or weight loss. Dry mouth, poor dentition, or swallowing difficulties can make it more difficult to eat. Shortness of breath can limit mobility and slow eating; joint pain or muscle weakness can impair mobility and increase functional dependence; skin rashes or ulcers can contribute to generalized discomfort and make skin susceptible to infection; focal neurologic deficits or cognitive impairment can result in memory, judgment, and safety issues.

What should the physical examination cover?

Survey vital signs including weight and height. Assess affect, the ability to transfer, and any evidence of abuse or neglect. Assess skin and mucous membranes for signs of dehydration. Evidence of heart failure can be found upon exam of the heart and or peripheral vasculature. Lungs exam positive for rales, wheezes, or diminished breath sound may indicate acute infection, failure, or restrictive lung disease. Abdominal exam is noteworthy for pain, masses, ascites, or organomegaly. Examine joints for inflammation, deformity, or decreased range of motion. A neurological exam might show signs of dementia, depression or focal deficit including motor, sensory, language, or memory impairment.

Specialized exams such as the "get up and go" test, timed walks, or a Folstein mini mental status examination can help to quantify functional impairment.

▶ TREATMENT

How is frailty treated?

Treatment of frailty is directed at the cause if a cause is found and/or at the prevention of adverse outcomes associated with (especially) hospitalized frail elders. Adverse outcomes include confusion, delirium, falls, disability, and dependency. Preventive approaches include minimizing stressors that worsen frailty including deconditioning, dehydration, isolation, medication side effects (including those of anesthesia), and stress associated with unfamiliar environments. The only generally agreed-upon treatments target sarcopenia and include regular exercise with or without dietary modifications that emphasize adequate amounts of calories and protein. The patient is encouraged to eat whatever nutritionally dense foods he/she enjoys including meats, carbohydrates, fruits and vegetables, and nutritionally dense deserts such as custards, ice cream, puddings, and fortified milk shakes. Nutritional supplements are sometimes recommended but physicians should take care that the supplement does not diminish appetite nor replace meals. Encourage the patient to consider multivitamins.

Regular exercise is possible and is helpful even in the very old, deconditioned nursing home patient. Weight (resistance) training coupled with nutritional supplementation over 10 weeks in nursing home patients aged 85 and older improved muscle strength by more than 125% compared to less than 3% in the control group. Increased muscle strength and mass improves walking speed and bone density. Regular aerobic exercise reduces insulin resistance and improves aerobic conditioning. Flexibility training improves coordination and joint range of motion. Balance training including tai chi, dancing, and specialized physical therapy can prevent falls.

An interdisciplinary team including midlevel providers and rehabilitation and nutritional specialists can achieve the best treatment together. Many frail elders live in a community where visiting nurses and other support such as meals on wheels can be helpful.

What if frailty does not improve?

Often, there is no acute illness identified in the frail elderly and even after medications are adjusted and social circumstances are improved, a failure to thrive may continue. Frailty associated with multiple chronic diseases and perhaps exacerbated by an acute event (e.g., a hip fracture) can result in an inability to participate in rehabilitation, poor intake, undernutrition, weakness, weight loss, and death. Patients, families, and healthcare providers are encouraged to plan for this end-stage with well-considered advance directives and a thoughtful palliative care plan.

KEY POINTS

- **Ongoing frailty seems to be a physiologic syndrome of aging associated with high levels of disability, dependency, and death.**
- **This syndrome results in decreased reserves and worsening ability to cope with both physiological and psychological stress.**
- **Frailty, in its preclinical stage, is preventable with regular exercise and diet adequate in protein and calories. Treatment can forestall disability.**

CASE 50–1. **An 82-year-old man, recently widowed, had been living alone in a new home closer to his daughter. Medical history includes congestive heart failure and osteoarthritis of the knees. The patient was recently hospitalized for total knee replacement. Unfortunately, he fell while walking to the bathroom with a portable IV. He suggests that his pain medication caused confusion. Bed rest led to weakness, incontinence, poor appetite, and weight loss. The patient was discharged to a nursing home for rehabilitation.**

A. What were the prehospitalization signs of frailty?
B. What were precipitants of acute frailty?

CASE 50–2. **An 89-year-old woman, widowed, lives alone in a retirement community. She complains of weakness and frequent falls over the past several months. Past medical history is positive for colon cancer, chronic obstructive pulmonary disease, and recent weight loss. The patient is slightly confused and normotensive, with marked kyphoscoliosis. "Get up and go" was difficult, requiring more than 20 seconds and much help to arise from a chair. There was obvious muscle wasting. Mini mental status exam score was 21 (cognitively impaired), weight 115 lb, height 5 ft 6 inches. A colonoscopy performed three months earlier was negative; labs including TSH were normal. Physical therapy and occupational therapy were initiated, but the patient was inconsistent in her attendance at therapy sessions. Dietary supplements were "forgotten" in the refrigerator. After several months and many falls, she moved into an assisted living facility where her weight, diet, and exercise can be monitored.**

A. What physical exam findings indicate that this patient is frail?
B. Can you predict any adverse outcomes related to this patient's frailty?

REFERENCES

Fiatarone MA, et al.: Exercise training and nutritional supplementation for physical frailty in very elderly people. N Engl J Med 330:1769–1775, 1994.

Fried L, Darer J, Walston J: Frailty. In Cassell C (ed): Geriatric Medicine, An Evidence-Based Approach, 4th ed. New York: Springer, 2003, pp 1067–1075.

Goldstein A, Damon B: We the Elderly. US Department of Commerce, Bureau of Census. Accessed Dec. 12, 2003, at http://www.census.gov.

Heuser M, Adler W: Immunological aspects of aging and malnutrition. In Verdery R (ed): Clinics in Geriatric Medicine. Vol. 13, Num. 4, Saunders, 1997, pp 697–715.

Verdery R: Clinical evaluation of failure to thrive in older people. In Verdery R (ed): Clinics in Geriatric Medicine. Vol. 13, Num. 4, Saunders, 1997, pp 769–778.

Young, H: Challenges and solutions for care of frail older adults. Online Journal of Issues in Nursing 8(2). Accessed Dec 12, 2003, at http://www.nursingworld.org/ojim/topic21/tpc21_4.htm.

51

Healthcare Maintenance

What is the general approach to a healthcare maintenance visit?

Primary care physicians often see patients who present for a health maintenance visit. These patients may use other, less specific terms such as "checkup" or "a physical." Students are generally well versed in addressing patient needs for specific complaints. It is often more challenging to approach a patient without such complaints. A systematic approach to these patients will allow for a structured, thorough, and focused visit that meets the current and future needs of your patients.

Each of these visits will begin with a modified history. This history may be relatively comprehensive if the patient is new or may represent a review of important developments in the interval from the prior healthcare maintenance visit to this visit. Information gathered from the history will help direct the physical examination, limited screening tests directed toward prevalent, asymptomatic disease conditions, and patient counseling/education.

HEALTHCARE MAINTENANCE FOR CHILDREN

What is the general approach to a healthcare visit for a child?

The pediatric well visit provides the physician with an opportunity to address five fundamental tasks:

- Identification of congenital medical conditions (especially in younger children)
- Assessment of key growth and developmental markers
- Screening for common or significant asymptomatic disease
- Provision of childhood vaccinations as scheduled
- Counseling, education, and anticipatory guidance

These five tasks are the foundation of pediatric well care.

What are the differences between a pediatric and adult visit?

One significant difference between a pediatric visit and an adult visit is the presence of the parent(s), who will often provide a considerable portion of the pertinent information. You should recognize this role and allow parents an opportunity to share medical information concerning their child as well as to express their concerns. It is equally important to remember that most pediatric patients can participate in sharing their histories and you should actively engage them throughout the visit. Balancing these activities is often challenging.

Most pediatric patients will have only limited experience with visits to the doctor's office. The pediatric patient may also be uncertain about why she is there and what will happen. This is a second significant difference between pediatric and adult visits. A successful pediatric visit begins with making the child as comfortable as possible with the manner in which the history and examination will occur. The physician can facilitate this by explaining exactly what will happen in terms that the child can understand. In addition, a few simple guidelines will facilitate the encounter:

- Allow sleeping children to remain asleep for as much of the examination as possible.
- For children who are uncomfortable in the exam room, perform the history and as much of the physical examination as possible with the child comfortably on the parent's lap.
- Tailor your examination to progress from least to most invasive. In general, observation is less invasive than touching (e.g., watching an infant grasp objects in the parent's hand is less invasive than listening to the patient's heart or lungs). Touching is less invasive than manipulation (e.g., feeling for femoral pulses is less invasive than checking for hip dysplasia). Portions of the examination that can be completed in the parent's lap are less invasive than those that require separation from the parents.

What is the schedule for well-child visits?

The American Academy of Pediatrics (AAP) currently recommends 24 well-care visits between birth and 18 years of age. The majority of these visits fall in the preschool years (birth through 4 to 6 years old). An overview of the content of these visits is provided in Table 51–1.

What are the recommended childhood vaccines?

The recommendations for childhood vaccinations are reviewed and revised regularly. The Centers for Disease Control and Prevention (CDC) publishes the most recent harmonized schedule with details

TABLE 51–1

Well-Care Visits, Preschool Years

	Birth	2–4 wks	2 months	4 months	6 months	9 months	12 months	15 months	18 months	2 years	3 years	4 years	5 years
Intake Hx	X	X[a]											
Phys Exam	X	X	X	X	X	X	X	X	X	X	X	X	X
Growth		X	X	X	X	X	X	X	X	X	X	X	X
Developmental Screen	X	X	X	X	X	X	X	X	X	X	X	X	X
Vaccination[b]	X	X	X	X	X		X	X	X			X	X
Screening													
Hearing	X[c]										X[d]	X	X
Vision											X[e]	X	X
Lead							X[f]						
TB							X[g]						

[a]Should be done at the first visit regardless of age.
[b]See Useful Websites section at the end of this chapter for specific vaccination schedule.
[c]Newborn hearing screen often done in newborn nursery.
[d]Infant should be screened for signs of decreased hearing at every visit; formal hearing screen should be performed by age 5.
[e]Infant should be screened for signs of decreased vision at every visit; formal vision testing should be performed by age 5.
[f]Infants should be screened by history for risk factors; high-risk patients should have serum lead levels tested. Testing thereafter should be based on prior results and risk status.
[g]Infants should be screened by history for risk factors; high-risk patients should have PPD placed. Testing thereafter should be based on prior results and risk factors.
This table is based on the protocol used in the author's practice, which is recommended by the AAP and referenced through the NIH (http://www.nlm.nih.gov/medlineplus/ency/article/001928.htm).

about the vaccines on its website (see Useful Websites section at the end of this chapter).

How soon should the newborn examination occur?

The initial newborn examination occurs shortly after birth. In the outpatient setting the first examination is usually within the first month of life. Both the history and the physical examination will be more comprehensive than on most subsequent visits because you will not need to repeat much of the information you gather and record.

What should be included in a newborn history?

Birth History. The history should include a brief review of the prenatal course including maternal prenatal care history, maternal medical conditions, and complications, if any, of the prenatal period. Also include a review of the delivery including gestational age at delivery, method of delivery (vaginal, assisted vaginal, caesarian) and any complications of the labor or delivery process. Make note of any resuscitative measures performed at the time of delivery.

Newborn Nursery Course. Briefly review the infant's history while still in the hospital, including any abnormalities noted, any testing completed, hepatitis B vaccination if given, and how many days the newborn remained in the hospital. Also note birth weight and discharge weight. Many hospitals have standardized discharge forms that summarize this information. When it is available, you should carefully review this information as a part of the first outpatient visit.

Interval History. The first month with a new child is an exciting and challenging experience. This is especially true if the parents are new to parenthood and the child is their first. Place special emphasis on normal infant activities including eating (what, how much, and how often), sleeping (especially sleep patterns through the night), urination (often measured as the number of diapers used each day), defecation (again, often measured as the number of diapers with stool each day), and crying (how much, how often, and parents' ability to console the infant). In addition to gathering information about each of these areas, the physician will have an opportunity to educate parents concerning normal parameters for each.

What should be included in a newborn physical examination?

As the first evaluation in the office, the initial examination serves as a baseline and is therefore comprehensive.

Vital Signs. These include temperature, pulse, respiratory rate, length, weight, and head circumference.

- You can check temperature in a variety of locations. Note the specific location along with the reading.
- Pulse and respiratory rate are both measured most accurately with the infant resting quietly, preferably in a parent's arms or lap.
- Length is often most easily measured by marking the disposable paper on the exam table. A mark can be made at the crown of the head. The infant's legs can be fully extended and a mark made at the heel. The infant is then removed and the distance between the two marks is recorded.
- The additional weight of clothing and diapers can be significant for infants, so weight should be measured with the infant fully disrobed.
- Head circumference is measured as the circumference from brow (above the eyebrows) to temple (above the ears) and around the occiput (roughly equivalent to the position of a hat band).

General Observation. Is the child healthy appearing, comfortable, and normal appearing?

Head and Neck. Observe the face for rashes. Check the ear canals for patency and the ears for position. Also note the preauricular pits when present. Check the mouth and soft palate for defects and make note of the mucosal lining for both moisture and oral thrush, if present. Both anterior and posterior fontanelles should be open. Palpate the neck for adenopathy. Note the head lag when the child is gently raised from the table.

Eyes. Check for red reflex and for normal eye movement in all directions. Note the reaction of pupils to light.

Cardiovascular. Although it is often difficult for students to distinguish heart sounds in a rapid infant cardiac cycle, you should make note of S1 and S2 and murmurs in all infants, if present. Congenital heart defects may not be apparent at birth and may be picked up for the first time in the physician's office. Palpate peripheral pulses with particular note made of femoral pulses (both quality and symmetry).

Pulmonary/Thoracic. Note normal breath sounds and adventitial (rales, rhonchi, wheezes) sounds if present. Make note of the chest wall contour especially at the sternum; palpate the clavicle for uneven contour, which may indicate a fracture. Examine the breasts and palpate for breast tissue.

Abdomen. Make particular note of the umbilical stump if present. The stump generally detaches by 2 to 4 weeks of age. Examine the umbilical region for umbilical hernia noted as either a palpable defect below the umbilicus or as a visible bulging of the area below the umbilical stump.

Genital Examination. Examine males for the presence of both testicles. Inspect the site of circumcision when applicable. In uncircumcised males the foreskin should be retracted to examine the glans. In females, note patency of the vagina. Examine the inguinal region for the presence of congenital hernias.

Anus. Check the anus for patency and note any rashes that might represent either diaper contact dermatitis or candidiasis.

Spine. Examine the entire course of the spine for evidence of spina bifida. Pay particular attention to the uppermost and lowermost portions of the spine.

Skin. Make note of the tone of the skin as well as the presence of any congenital/birthmarks. Make particular note of face, scalp, posterior neck, and the sacral spine.

Extremities. Examine all extremities for symmetry and shape. Make note of muscle tone and symmetry of movement and normal posture. Examine hips for evidence of hip dysplasia via the Barlow and Ortolani tests. The Barlow test is performed with the hips flexed to 90 degrees and adducted. Downward pressure is applied to the knees. In infants with unstable hips an audible and/or palpable click is noted. The Ortolani test is performed with the hips flexed to 90 degrees. The hips are then gently adducted and then abducted. Again, note is made of an audible and/or palpable click.

What are the routine newborn screening tests?

Most newborns will have undergone a number of screening tests while in the newborn nursery. Confirm that the tests were completed and document the results at the first visit. Most infants will have been tested for congenital hearing defects. In addition, a blood sample was drawn to screen for variety of congenital conditions most frequently including thyroid disease, phenylalanine level, and hemoglobinopathy. Each state requires different tests. You should be familiar with the newborn screening protocol in your state as well as the mechanism for obtaining the results.

What vaccines are given to newborns?

Most children will have received the first hepatitis B vaccine prior to discharge from the newborn nursery. You should confirm that this occurred. As noted in the vaccination schedule, the infant will receive the second hepatitis B vaccine at this first visit if it falls on or after the fourth week of life.

What are the markers of normal development?

Developmental milestones may be measured on standardized instruments such as the Denver II, or the physician may develop his or her own protocol for assessing the developmental status of the pediatric patient. See Table 51–2 for a brief summary of age-appropriate milestones.

What is the content of anticipatory counseling?

The first visit establishes the pattern of counseling that you will follow at all subsequent visits. Review age appropriate developmental, safety, and healthcare issues. Solicit and address parental concerns.

In addition, you must make a note of the timing of the next scheduled visit and be sure to address developmental, safety, and health issues that will arise prior to the next visit (anticipatory guidance). Pay particular attention to issues of injury prevention, violence prevention, sleep positioning, and nutrition.

What should be included in follow-up visits?

Subsequent visits will follow the pattern developed in the first visit but will focus most closely on changes and developments that occurred in the interval between the prior well visit and this visit.

History. Primary focus should be placed on interval history. There is no need to repeat the prenatal or birth history unless a question has arisen that requires clarification. Open-ended questions concerning interval illnesses, injuries, or developments will allow parents to report such information. The history will also focus on parental reports of developmental tasks. It is often useful to review age-appropriate milestones prior to entering the exam room. This will serve to direct and focus the history.

Physical Examination. Growth parameters (height, weight, and head circumference in infants) remain critical and should be recorded on a standardized growth chart to document the adequacy of growth. In addition to the elements of the examination described above, several other elements will arise as the child grows. The United States Preventive Services Task Force (USPSTF) recommends particular attention to blood pressure monitoring (starting at age 3) and vision screening (starting at ages 3 to 4). Additionally, children should be screened for strabismus beginning at approximately 3 months of age. Use of the cover–uncover test may be helpful. The child fixates with both eyes on a distant object (eye chart, picture, or toy). As one eye is covered the other eye should move to fixate on the object. Repeat on the opposite side. Beginning at the age of 8 to 10 years, children should be screened for signs of pubertal development and may also be screened for scoliosis.

TABLE 51–2

Key Developmental Milestones by Visit, Birth to 2 Years

	Motor	Language	Social
Birth–1 month	Symmetric movement	Vocalizes	Looks at faces
2 months	Lifts head	Laughs	Smiles
4 months	Head is steady; grasps toys or objects, develops raking grasp	Squeals	Begins to watch others' movements
6 months	No head lag when pulled to sitting; sits alone; passes objects from one had to the other	Turns to voices; early single-syllable sounds	Begins self-feeding
9 months	Pulls self to standing; stands with assist; pincer grasp (thumb and finger)	Combines syllables; begins to use specific speech such as baba	Waves, points, and plays games with hands
12 months	Stands alone; begins to walk	Specific use of speech; early word development	Begins to drink from a cup
18 months	Walks well; begins to run; goes up steps; stacks objects	Multiple words; may begin to combine words	Uses utensils, drinks well from a cup, imitates parental activity
2 years	Walks and runs with facility; jumps in place	Begins to combine words and point to pictures when prompted	Dresses self with assistance, can do grooming with assistance

Screening. The USPSTF recommends no additional screening laboratory tests in the general population between birth and 10 years old. For populations with specific risks additional screening tests may include hemoglobin/hematocrit, PPD, blood lead level, and HIV testing. For a detailed description of the populations at risk refer to the USPSTF website listed at the end of this chapter. In addition, the American Academy of Pediatrics recommends routine urinalysis beginning at 1 year of age.

Vaccinations. Review vaccination history at every visit to ensure that children are on schedule and that those who are not are appropriately scheduled for catch-up vaccinations. A review of the protocol for catch-up vaccinations can be found at the USPSTF website listed at the end of this chapter.

Counseling. The USPSTF recommends counseling for injury prevention; car safety (car seats for children under 5; seat belt and shoulder harness use for children over 5); bicycle helmet use; smoke detector use; flame retardant sleepwear; water temperature (maximum 120–130°F); window/stair guards; pool fences (when applicable); storage of potentially toxic or dangerous items such as chemicals, weapons, and matches; poison control phone number; dietary recommendations; regular physical activity; dental care; and passive/active tobacco counseling.

HEALTHCARE MAINTENANCE FOR ADOLESCENTS

What is adolescence?

Adolescent patients are a unique population combining many of the challenges of both pediatric and adult patients with the addition of many unique challenges of their own. While the terms adolescent and teenager are often used interchangeably, many of the developmental changes associated with adolescence begin prior to the "teen" years. Pubertal development, for example, is not considered abnormal ("precocious") unless it occurs before the age of 8 in young women. For this reason, adolescence is best understood as the developmental transition period between childhood and adulthood rather than a specific age-delimited event. The USPSTF defines this group as 11 to 24 years old for the purpose of their recommendations.

What are the health risks of adolescence?

Adolescence challenges patients, parents, and physicians as a period of physical, cognitive, and psychosocial transition from childhood to adulthood. Most adolescents are healthy when they leave childhood and remain so as they enter adulthood. The major causes of adolescent mortality—accidents, suicide, and homicide—are not medical in the strict sense of the term, but are behavioral. Much morbidity in this period is, likewise, behavioral. Sexually transmitted disease and pregnancy, drug use and accidents, dysmorphic body image, and eating disorders all represent facets of adolescent behavior with high medical and social costs.

What is the purpose of the adolescent well visit?

The well-adolescent visit allows the physician to assess the status of development while simultaneously identifying behaviors that may have both immediate and significant long-term consequences for the patient. The adolescent well visit presents several unique challenges to the physician. Many adolescents will not present for a well visit, making it necessary to address these issues as a part of a visit for other acute issues. While parents of adolescents continue to play a critical role in the well-being of their children, the adolescent patient may be unwilling to provide all the necessary information with the parent in the room. You must tailor discussion of healthcare issues with adolescents to the appropriate level of cognitive and psychosocial development.

How can the adolescent visit be facilitated?

A few key guidelines will facilitate the adolescent visit:

- All adolescent visits must include at least some time alone with the physician to ensure that accurate and complete information is obtained.
- All adolescents should be assured that, to the extent possible, information they share will remain confidential.
- Both parents and adolescents should be given an opportunity at each visit to identify important issues they would like to have addressed.
- Parents should be made aware of both the "time alone" and confidentiality components of the visit and the important role these play in providing comprehensive care for each adolescent. Parents should also be made aware that this is standard and does not reflect a particular concern or judgment about their child.

What are the transitions of adolescence?

Adolescence is the transitional phase from childhood to adulthood and can best be understood as the period of development when this transition occurs. As such, adolescence is defined less by a specific age range or an identifiable set of problems than by the time period and developmental tasks necessary to enter adulthood. Broadly understood, these developmental tasks fall into three major categories: (1) physical development, (2) psychosocial development, and (3) cognitive development. While clearly interrelated, these three major categories each represent a significant challenge to both adolescents and their caregivers.

What are the physical developmental changes of adolescence?

Physical development includes growth in stature, increased muscle mass, and development of secondary sex characteristics. For women it includes development of adult stature (usually at or shortly after first menstruation), breast development (thelarche, average age 11 in North America), initiation of menstruation (menarche, average age 12.5 in North America), and onset of fertility. For men this includes adult stature (common age 16 but variable), secondary sexual characteristics (axillary, facial, and pubic hair development), increased muscle mass, and development of adult male vocalization. While a full discussion of these changes is beyond the scope of this review, the most apparent adolescent change is physical development. An understanding of the basic changes, normal milestones, and Tanner staging (Table 51–3) of these changes is important for any complete evaluation of an adolescent patient.

What are the psychosocial changes of adolescence?

Psychosocial development for adolescents centers on three key interrelated developmental tasks: (1) development of an independent sense of identity, (2) separation from family, and (3) integration into peer group(s). While the exact path taken by each adolescent varies, and many of the behaviors associated with these changes are culturally dependent, the fundamental tasks are shared by all adolescents. Development of an independent sense of identity gives rise to many of the risk behaviors stereotypically associated with adolescents. No longer willing to accept at face value the prescribed (or proscribed) activities of family, adolescents begin to independently explore and experiment. For some adolescents, this exploration will take the form of undesirable behaviors such as drug use or sexual activity; for others, the experimentation may be more constructive such as involvement in sports, new academic endeavors, or new religious or social activities. Experimentation in itself is not undesirable or destructive. It is, instead, the beginning of behavior, with which we associate adults seeking out and discovering new knowledge.

Younger children have much of their lives and environments determined by their families. Adolescents begin for the first time to define peer groups, activities, and environment not by the requirements of their families but by their own independent judgments. This activity is generally informed by the values and expectations of their families but is implemented by the adolescents rather than by the

TABLE 51–3

Tanner Staging

	Tanner Stage I	Tanner Stage II	Tanner Stage III	Tanner Stage IV	Tanner Stage V
Pubic Hair	Prepubertal	Light straight thin hair	Darker, curlier, and thicker	Adult pubic hair but limited distribution	Adult distribution including medial thighs and lower abdomen
Breast	Prepubertal	Breast bud development	Enlarged breast and areola	Areola forms a secondary contour	Adult contour with nipple enlargement and elevation
Penis	Prepubertal	Enlargment	Increased length	Glans enlargement and increased circumference	Adult size and contour
Testes	Prepubertal	Scrotal enlargement with pink textured skin	Increased scrotal volume	Continued increased volume and darker pigmentation	Adult contour

family. The control has begun to transition from family to adolescent. As might be expected this transition is conflictual although variable in the degree of conflict. While the conflict need not be uncontrolled or even overt, there is an inherent conflict in the process of separation from one's family. Questions designed to elicit information concerning such experimentation serve the dual purpose of identifying potential risk-taking behaviors *and* providing a gross measure of adolescent development in this domain. Adolescents who exhibit no such behavior are developmentally less advanced than their peers who are actively engaged in such behavior.

With the role of family in adolescent social behavior attenuated, the role of self-selected peers takes on increased importance. Generally this follows a predictable pattern of group, same-gender interactions followed by group, mixed-gender interactions leading to sequential pairs ("dating") and culminating in long-term pairing. Again, questions designed to elicit information concerning this behavior provides both "risk" information (for example, early onset sexual activity) and also normative developmental information.

What are the cognitive developmental changes of adolescence?

Cognitive development is complex. For purposes of routine adolescent care, pay attention to two specific cognitive developmental tasks that mark significant transitions from childhood to adulthood. Cognitive understanding in childhood is largely concrete—the world is seen in black and white. People are good or they are bad. I like you or I dislike you. Very little childhood understanding involves intermediate or "shades of gray" interpretation. Adult understanding, or formal operational thinking, involves interpretation and judgment that encompasses much subtler distinctions (e.g., "He's a good guy but I can't stand it when he . . .").

A second defining characteristic of childhood cognitive understanding is the limited ability to project future consequences from current actions. The ability to fully understand the future implications of current actions develops significantly after adolescents' ability to engage in a variety of potentially risky behavior.

What is the general approach to obtaining a history from an adolescent patient?

Adolescent patients are generally a very healthy population. They do not usually have numerous or complex medical problems. The most critical component of the visit is therefore the history and particularly an expanded version of the social history. An organized approach to the history will allow the physician to obtain important medical, developmental, and social information; explore potentially sensitive issues in a nonthreatening manner; and introduce the adolescent to a broad outline of topics that would be appropriate for the adolescent to raise in the future should she/he decide to do so. Below is an outline of one such approach. This is not the only possible approach, but it covers the major areas of concern, is brief enough to fit in a regular office visit, is flexible enough to allow for follow-up if necessary, and reflects the developmental model discussed above. It can be remembered with the mnemonic ***FACE TIME***, a reflection that the key to caring for adolescents is the ability to talk with and listen to these patients when they present to your office.

A note on questions: The following key questions are by no means exhaustive nor are they intended to be the only possible phrasing. In obtaining an adolescent history, the practitioner must be attuned to cues from the adolescent that would require further questioning. It may also be necessary to ask the same question more than once, in more than one way, to ensure that the adolescent and the practitioner understand the question in the same way.

Family. Although adolescents are beginning to make the transition toward an independent self-identity, family retains a central role in their lives. Assessment of all adolescents requires an understanding of both the structure and function of the family as well as the adolescent's role in and attitudes toward her family. *Key questions include:*

With whom do you live?
How do you get along with your parents? Siblings?
Where in your home is "your" space"?
How much time do you send at home?
Do you fight with your parents? How do you handle disagreements?

Academics. School, for those still in school, represents the largest single commitment of time for most adolescents. Assessment of adolescents' academic attendance, performance, involvement, and plans allows for identification of those adolescents at risk for school failure as well as providing a unique window on adolescent psychosocial and cognitive development. *Key questions include:*

Are you in school?
What grade?
How are you doing?
What do you like/dislike?
Do you feel safe at school?
What do you want to do when you're done?

Community. Although family remains central to adolescents' sense of identity, many begin for the first time during this time period to independently choose their peer groups, activities, and sources of social interaction. This area of questioning includes both peer interactions that are potentially risky (for example, gang involvement) as well as those which have been shown to be protective (for example, involvement in athletics or religious organizations). Keep in mind that the single biggest predictor of risk behaviors for adolescents is the participation of their peers in that behavior. *Key questions include:*

What do you do when you're not in school?
Who do you like to spend time with?
What do you and your friends do when you're together?
Do you play any sports?
Tell me about any school activities you are involved with.

Experimentation. Adolescence is marked by a strong tendency toward experimentation. New peers, increasing independence, and decreasing direct supervision mark this period as one of increased opportunity for participation in a variety of new (and potentially dangerous) activities. While experimentation is a normal and desirable trait in young adults, the combination of experimentation with limited cognitive understanding of potential long-term consequences makes for a dangerous combination. An important key to risk behavior identification lies with peer behavior. All questions should include questions about peer activity (see the next section about toxic habits). *Key questions include:*

Are you sexually active? Are your peers?
Have you ever run away from home?
Do you ride a bike? With a helmet?
Do you drive? With a seat belt?
Have you ever been stopped while driving? Been ticketed?
Have you ever been in a fight?

Toxic Habits. Adult behavior regarding substance use and abuse is almost entirely predictable based on behavior established during adolescence. Because many of these behaviors are first tried while adolescents are unable to fully appreciate the short or long-term consequences of such behavior it is critical that physicians screen for such behavior. Again it is important to note that adolescent behavior is often predicted by the behavior of their peers. For this reason, questions should include peer substance use as well. (From a practical standpoint it is preferable to begin by asking about peer behavior. It is always easier to report your friends' behavior than to admit to such behavior yourself.) *Key questions include:*

Have any of your friends tried tobacco? Do any use regularly?
Have any of your friends tried alcohol? Do any of them drink regularly?
Have any of your friends tried any other drugs? Do any of them use other drugs regularly?
Have you tried tobacco?
Have you tried alcohol?
Have you tried any other drugs?

Image. Self-image is of paramount importance in adolescence. The reasons for this are multiple but the uncertainty associated with separating from family while simultaneously attempting to form new peer relationships places particular pressure on adolescents to compare themselves with others. While this is normal in adolescence it can manifest in psychologically and physically threatening manners such as anorexia nervosa or bulimia. *Key questions include:*

Have you ever tried to lose weight?
Have you ever been on a diet?
Have you ever made yourself vomit after eating? Used a laxative when not constipated?
If you could change one thing about yourself what would that be? Why?

Medical/Mental Health. While most adolescents are healthy, a review of the patient's past medical history is important. For those adolescents with preexisting medical conditions, increasing independence means increasing personal responsibility for their own medical care. Many previously well-controlled conditions (e.g., asthma) become less well controlled in adolescence as parents play a lesser role in management. Some medical conditions may appear for the first time in adolescence (e.g., dysmenorrhea or STDs). Pay particular attention to routine healthcare maintenance needs of adolescents. Review and update vaccination records as needed (hepatitis B, MMR, and tetanus are often needed). Review risk factors for such long-term health risks as cardiovascular disease (cholesterol screening may be indicated in this age group). Sexual health screening is necessary for this age group. For young women who have begun having sex annual pap smears and STD screening are indicated. Because suicide is the second or third leading cause of death among adolescents (depending on the population studied), screening for symptoms of depression may be important in this age group. *Key questions include:*

Can you tell me about any medical problems you have had?
Do you ever experience sleep disturbance, loss of interest in normal activities, feeling of guilt or anxiety, decreased energy, difficulty with concentration, anhedonia and appetite changes, psychomotor agitation, or depression and suicidal ideation?

Environment. No understanding of adolescent well-being is complete without an understanding of where they live. By this we mean home environment including safety, community and resources, school and adequacy, peer interactions and abuse, and risks to safety such as guns and other weapons or lack of smoke detectors in the home. Key questions will require the practitioner to be aware of the environmental risks prevalent in their community. This is a cornerstone of family medicine and in keeping with the understanding that all health care must be understood in the context of a biopsychosocial model of the patient, the family, and the community in which he or she lives. For all patients, ask about a few environmental risks. *Key questions begin with:*

Are there weapons in your home?
Do you or your friends carry weapons?
Do you feel safe in your home?
Do you feel safe with your peers? With your significant other?
Are there smoke detectors in the house?

What are the components of the physical examination for well adolescents?

The adolescent physical examination often reveals less than the history but can be an important addition to a comprehensive history. The USPSTF–recommended components for general populations include height, weight, and blood pressure. In a broader physical examination several key areas of the exam should be noted with particular care.

- Vital signs: Note height, weight, and blood pressure, and examine hearing and vision.
- Skin: Acne is a very common condition in adolescence. Although generally of limited medical concern, it can cause considerable concern to the adolescent. In addition, note should be made of secondary sexual characteristics of axillary and facial hair.
- Thoracic: Breast development will begin in this age group and should be noted. Among adolescent males unilateral or bilateral gynecomastia is common and should also be noted. It is generally a nonpathologic sign.
- Spine: Examination of the spine for scoliosis often begins in this age group.
- Genitourinary: Examine for physical signs of pubertal development.

What are the recommended screening tests for well adolescents?

For the general population the USPSTF recommends no additional screening tests. For sexually active females the USPSTF recommends Pap smear and chlamydia screening. The American College of Obstetricians and Gynecologists currently recommends that Pap smears begin within three years of first sexual activity or 21 years old, whichever comes first. For sexually active adolescents the USPSTF also recommends screening for syphilis, HIV, and gonorrhea. Screening for hepatitis B may be indicated in unvaccinated patients. For high-risk populations the USPSTF recommends PPD screening.

What vaccines should be reviewed with well adolescents?

Most children will have completed their vaccinations prior to adolescence. An additional Td is recommended at 10 to 12 years old. Note the status of all vaccinations at least once with a particular emphasis on varicella, Td, MMR, and hepatitis B. For high-risk populations the USPSTF also recommends pneumococcal, influenza, and hepatitis A vaccination. (See Useful Websites at the end of this chapter for details concerning high-risk definitions.)

What counseling should occur during a well-adolescent visit?

Adolescents should receive counseling concerning issues uncovered during the history. Be sure to note these issues for future reference. In addition, for the general population the USPSTF recommends counseling concerning seat belt use, bicycle/motorcycle helmet use, smoke detectors, gun storage, regular physical activity, dental care, and dietary issues including fat, cholesterol, caloric balance, and calcium and folate intake (in pregnant patients or those with childbearing capability).

HEALTHCARE MAINTENANCE FOR ADULTS

What are the general health issues of adults?

Adults represent a much more diverse population than either children or adolescents. If childhood is the age of congenital disease and adolescence is the age of behavior-related morbidity, then adulthood represents the age of acquired illness. Environment, genetic predisposition, activity (and inactivity), as well as age itself contribute to a population that will increasingly have significant medical conditions.

What are the subpopulations of adults?

Because such a uniform approach to this group of patients is not entirely possible, the USPSTF has divided this population into two age groups, 25 to 64, and 65 and older. Although these groupings are helpful, you may find it useful to consider two additional subgroups, adults up to 40 and those over 80. The first group represents a generally healthy group of patients with relatively low risk for the most common causes of morbidity and mortality among adults (cardiac disease, cancer, renal disease, infectious disease such as pneumonia and influenza among others). This group will have considerably fewer screening tests. As the population ages, it seems apparent that those over the age of 65 are not a homogenous group either. Recognize that the "young elderly" do not always fit the stereotypical profile of a geriatric patient and that the "older elderly" may have additional concerns that do not always apply to their younger peers.

You can view care of adult patients as a continuum rather than a series of distinct groups. Those age groups are useful for organizational purposes but you must always interpret them in the context of an individual patient and her medical story. In addition, the specific medical issues of each age group are influenced by the medical conditions of the previous age group and will, in turn, affect the health of patients as they age into the next age group. For this reason, comprehensive care of any given patient requires knowledge of current medical concerns, as well as those that have gone before and those that will come, and a willingness to help patients to help themselves achieve longer, healthier lives.

What are the general guidelines for adult visits?

Form a therapeutic alliance with the patient. All meaningful change will come from the patient. It is the role of the physician to provide the necessary tools for all patients to be as healthy as possible. It is not the physician's role to make the patient change.

Listen fully, look carefully, test sparingly. The history will provide the overwhelming majority of the necessary information. The physical examination will add small but important additional pieces of information. Screening tests have an important but very limited role in adult care and should be ordered with careful consideration of their role in patient management.

Counsel patiently. Behavior change is incremental and slow. Do not assume that the absence of change means the patient did not hear what you said. Repetition, understanding, encouragement, and patience will provide the best results.

What are the general medical issues of adults ages 25 to 39?

Although this grouping is arbitrary, these adults are generally healthy with limited acquired medical morbidity. They share many health concerns with adolescent patients and represent a natural continuum with that population. For these patients the history is by far the most critical element of the healthcare maintenance visit.

What is included in the history for a well 25- to 39-year-old adult?

History of Present Illness. Although most patients will have no chief complaint, some will. A good open-ended question will allow patients to share those concerns. Examples of such questions might include "tell me what brings you in today" or "tell me what I can do for you today" or "do you have any health concerns that I should be sure to address?" Should you uncover specific medical concerns these should be developed more fully. In the absence of specific concerns, the attention should turn to the other elements of the history.

Past History. A review of the past history allows the physician to begin to develop an overall picture of the patient's health. It also allows the physician to gather information concerning health maintenance issues. There are a number of good models for structuring the past history. One such model includes the following elements (tailored to the patient in question):

Medical problems—medical conditions now or in the past of which the patient is aware
Surgical problems—including childhood surgeries such as tonsillectomy and any adult surgeries
Hospitalizations and emergency care
Medications—including prescription, over-the-counter, natural, herbal, and other complementary/alternative medicinal preparations
Allergies—including which medications and the reaction that occurred
Toxic habits—tobacco, alcohol, and illicit drug use (including quantity when present)
Obstetrical/gynecologic/sexual history—including menstrual and pregnancy history for women and a sexual history for both men and women
Psychiatric history—including psychological concerns for which the patient may not have sought care
Health care maintenance—including a review of age-appropriate and gender-appropriate health maintenance issues

Family History. A review of medical conditions that occur in the patient's family allows the physician to develop a broader understanding of health concerns that may arise in the future for this patient. A general family history should encompass three generations: up one generation (parents), down one generation (children, if any), and the index generation (siblings, if any). Basic information in the family history includes age, whether the person is alive or dead, and important medical conditions for each person. For persons who are dead, the age and cause of death should be noted as well as any additional medical conditions that may have been present.

Social History. The social history is a rich and varied component of the medical history. It may contribute to a broader understanding of the patient (e.g., hobbies, education, family status) and may also yield important information that may impact the health of the patient (e.g., high-risk occupations, incarceration, travel to endemic disease areas, exercise, and diet patterns).

Review of Systems. The well visit is often an excellent opportunity to review with patients "minor" complaints that they would not necessarily bring to the physician's attention. The review of systems allows for a broad, systematic but reasonably focused recapitulation of common complaints that may be indicative of broader medical issues.

What is included in a physical exam for a well 25- to 39-year-old adult?

The physical examination is largely directed by health concerns raised during the review of the patient's history. For the general population (i.e., those with no identifiable risk factors) the USPSTF recommends blood pressure, height, weight, and calculation of the body mass index (BMI).

What screening is recommended for a well 25- to 39-year-old adult?

The USPSTF recommends very limited screening for this age group. For the general population, only total cholesterol in men beginning at age 35 and Pap smear in women (every one to three years starting within three years of first sexual activity or age 21, whichever comes first). For appropriate risk groups the USPSTF also recommends STD (gonorrhea, chlamydia, HIV, viral hepatitis, syphilis) and PPD screening.

What vaccinations should be reviewed for a well 25- to 39-year-old adult?

As with younger patients, you should review vaccination status. In this age group particular attention should be paid to hepatitis B, Td, varicella, and rubella. These last two are of particular concern for women of childbearing age. For high-risk groups, offer patients hepatitis A, pneumococcal, and influenza vaccines.

What counseling should be done with a well 25- to 39-year-old adult?

Appropriately document issues uncovered during the history and counsel patients concerning risk reduction. In addition, the USPSTF recommends specific counseling concerning tobacco cessation, problem alcohol use, alcohol and drug use while driving (or engaged in similar activities), dietary issues (including fat/cholesterol intake, caloric balance, calcium intake for women, and folic acid for women of childbearing age), regular physical activity, seat belt use, firearms, smoke detectors, high-risk sexual activities, contraception/condom use, and dental health.

What are the general medical issues of adults ages 40 to 64?

This age group is marked by the increasing prevalence of acquired disease such as hypertension, diabetes, cancer, and hypercholesterolemia. This age group is also marked by an increasing prevalence of morbidity and mortality associated with these common disease processes. These disease processes are common, often asymptomatic early, and the natural disease course can be modified with appropriate medical intervention. In addition, screening tests exist with sufficient sensitivity and specificity to adequately identify the disease. These tests are generally acceptable to patients and of reasonable cost for the healthcare system as a whole. For this reason healthcare maintenance in this age group includes several screening protocols designed to identify patients with modifiable disease.

What is included in the history of a 40- to 64-year-old adult?

The elements of the history remain the same as previously noted. Given the disease processes of greatest concern in this age group, pay particular attention to elements of the history that point to increased risk for cardiovascular disease, diabetes, elevated cholesterol, cancer (especially lung, breast, colon, and prostate), and such high-risk behaviors as tobacco use and excessive alcohol use.

What is included in the physical examination of a 40- to 64-year-old adult?

Patients in this age group will often have medical conditions that dictate a more comprehensive physical examination. For patients with medical problems, the healthcare maintenance physical examination should include all necessary components of the physical examination necessary to assess the patient's status in regard to these illnesses. For the general population (those without underlying disease) the elements of the exam are the same as for younger adults noted above. In addition, routine examination of eyesight may be important in this age group.

What screening is recommended for a healthy 40- to 64-year-old adult?

In the general population, the USPSTF recommends cholesterol (men 35 to 65; women 45 to 65), fecal occult blood testing or flexible sigmoidoscopy (men and women 50 and older), and mammograms (women 50 and older). The American Diabetes Association recommends screening for diabetes beginning at age 40 (fasting blood glucose ≥126 on two occasions or random blood glucose ≥200). The American Cancer Society and the American Urologic Society recommend screening for prostate cancer beginning at age 50 (digital rectal examination and prostate specific antigen). There are currently no recommended screening tests for lung cancer. Screening consists of identification of smokers (and counseling concerning smoking cessation).

What vaccinations should be reviewed for a 40- to 64-year-old adult?

Recommendations concerning vaccinations are the same as for the previous age group.

What counseling should be done for a 40- to 64-year-old adult?

Recommendations for this age group are similar to those above. Women in this age group are likely to reach menopause and should receive counseling concerning symptom reduction, bone density preservation, and postmenopausal gynecologic care.

What are the general medical issues of adults 65 and over?

As previously noted, this group is not homogenous but most recommendations apply to all patients over the age of 65. Many patients in this age group, especially the "young elderly," are remarkably healthy and active with a significant life expectancy.

One common mistake in caring for older patients is the false assumption that issues important to younger adults no longer apply. Many older patients remain sexually active. Many continue to drive. An increasing number of people over the age of 65 are continuing to work (either in their primary job or perhaps in a new area). Elderly patients may misuse alcohol or other drugs. In fact, many of the common assumptions concerning the "elderly" are either incorrect or significantly limited in their applicability. The key to a complete history is to remember that it should be *complete*.

What history should be obtained for adults 65 and older?

Elements of the history previously discussed remain important. Many patients in this age group reach retirement. This may require living on a fixed income that may not be sufficient to maintain previous expenditures. For patients in this age group Medicare insurance provides important but by no means comprehensive medical coverage.

For many patients in this age group, though not all, declining function may limit their ability to safely perform the many activities of daily living. Safety around the home takes on increasing importance. The ability to see, to hear, and to function cognitively may diminish with age. Patients may not recognize these limitations themselves and, therefore, you may need to obtain portions of the history from others.

Nutrition is a significant concern among older patients and a brief review of the patient's eating and drinking habits may be helpful.

Most patients in this age group will have specific medical problems for which they are followed and the history should include a brief synopsis of these medical conditions. Make note of medications the patient may be taking, because many older patients take a large and potentially confusing array of medications. Explore the possibility of medication side effects and interactions and review the necessity of medications carefully.

Describe the physical examination in adults 65 years and older.

The physical examination in this age group is likely to be considerably more complete because of the increase in underlying health issues. For the general population the USPSTF recommends blood pressure, height, and weight measurements, as well as vision and hearing examinations.

What screening is recommended for adults 65 years and older?

The USPSTF–recommended screening in this age group includes fecal occult blood or flexible sigmoidoscopy and mammogram with or without a clinical breast examination. Consider discontinuing Pap smears after 65 years of age for women who have been screened regularly and are otherwise at low risk. The American Cancer Society and the American Urologic Society recommend that screening for prostate cancer continue in males who are otherwise healthy and can be expected to live at least 10 more years. The role of cholesterol screening in this population is not clear.

What vaccinations should be reviewed with adults 65 years and older?

Give special consideration to pneumococcal and influenza vaccines in this age group. This age group experiences significant morbidity and mortality related to these infections. In addition, patients in this age group may require a Td booster. For patients at high risk the USPSTF recommends hepatitis A, hepatitis B, and varicella.

What counseling should be performed with adults 65 years and older?

Issues previously mentioned continue to pertain to this population. Tobacco cessation has been shown to be helpful even in this age group. If resources are available, intensive fall-prevention programs have been shown to be effective in patients at increased risk. Consider discussing this issue in this age group.

Patients who have not already done so should be encouraged to consider end-of-life planning. This is much more effectively done well before any need for such plans arises. Issues should include a will, a living will, and/or designation of a healthcare proxy.

KEY POINTS

- **A thorough history provides the foundation for comprehensive healthcare maintenance.**
- **The physical examination and use of diagnostic studies are limited in the general population and directed by the patient's history.**
- **Healthcare maintenance is best understood in the context of age-appropriate physical, cognitive. and psychosocial development.**

CASE 51–1. A 45-year-old woman and her 50-year-old husband present to your office for well visits. She has mild hypertension controlled with hydrochlorothiazide and is otherwise well; she has no significant family history or social history. He has no significant current medical complaints or past history but does have a family history of colon cancer in an older sibling (diagnosed at the age of 58).

A. Describe the most significant cancer-related risks for the woman. What screening would you recommend?
B. Describe the most significant cancer-related risks for the man. What screening would you recommend?

CASE 51–2. A 5-year-old boy is brought to your office for a preschool well visit. His past history is unremarkable; growth and development have been normal to this point.

A. Describe the major age-appropriate developmental tasks this child should be able to demonstrate.
B. Assuming that he was on schedule for vaccinations at 2 years old and he has received no vaccinations since, what vaccinations will he require today to complete his preschool vaccination series?

USEFUL WEBSITES

Centers for Disease Control and Prevention. *http://www.cdc.gov*
The United States Preventive Services Task Force recommendations and updates. *http://www.cdc.gov.mmwr/preview/mmwrhtml/rr5102al.htm*

52

Liver and Biliary Tract Disease

▶ ETIOLOGY

What are the causes of liver disease?

The causes of liver disease vary. Infections such as acute or chronic viral hepatitis and liver abscesses can damage the liver, as can injury by substances such as ethanol, hepatotoxic medications, and organic solvents. Systemic illnesses including hereditary hemochromatosis, Wilson's disease, autoimmune disorders, hyperlipidemia, and congestive heart failure can result in abnormal function of the liver and abnormal liver tests. Many conditions that cause acute liver injury can also result in chronic liver disease and cirrhosis. Malignancies, both primary and metastatic, can result in damage to the liver that will reflect in both its functional capacity and abnormal liver tests.

What are the causes of biliary tract disease?

Blockage of the bile ducts or the cystic duct results in cholecystitis, cholangitis, and obstructive jaundice. Most often this blockage is a result of gallstones, but intrinsic or extrinsic neoplasms, adenopathy, or primary sclerosing cholangitis may also cause blockages. Cholecystitis results most frequently from obstruction of the cystic duct by gallstones. This condition is a painful and potentially serious inflammation of the gallbladder commonly leading to gangrene of the gallbladder in diabetics and other immunocompromised individuals. Acute cholangitis is a life-threatening infection most often resulting from obstruction of the common bile duct by stones or tumor. Primary sclerosing cholangitis is an idiopathic disorder of unknown etiology. It is frequently associated with inflammatory bowel disease leading to inflammation and subsequent scarring of the extrahepatic and intrahepatic ducts.

▶ EVALUATION

Describe a relevant history.

Liver disease may be relatively asymptomatic or result in nonspecific symptoms including malaise, weakness, anorexia, abdominal pain, changes in bowel habits, weight loss, fever, and pruritus. In contrast, biliary tract disease is usually more specific and manifested by right upper quadrant or epigastric abdominal pain, nausea, fever, and jaundice; all of which can also be symptoms of liver disease. A history of dark urine and clay-colored stools often signifies liver or biliary tract dysfunction that can produce an elevated serum bilirubin.

Note both the occupational and social history of the patient. The occupational history should determine if the patient has had any exposure to potentially hepatotoxic agents such as organosolvents. The social history should elicit lifestyle choices, such as significant amounts of alcohol ingestion, intravenous drug use, or promiscuous sexual practices, which predispose one to hepatitis B and hepatitis C. A patient who has received blood products in the past is also at higher risk of hepatitis B and hepatitis C, though this risk has dropped substantially in the last 10 to 20 years because of more complete testing of donated blood. Travel history, along with any potential exposure to unsafe water or food sources, is necessary to assess the likelihood of hepatitis A or parasite exposure. A medication history, including nonprescription and prescription medications, will disclose the possibility of those that are potentially hepatotoxic. The family medical history may give clues regarding inherited disorders including Wilson's disease and hemochromatosis. By investigating a complete review of systems, items such as hyperlipidemia and inflammatory bowel disease may become apparent as causes of abnormal liver function.

What should I look for on physical exam?

Evaluate vital signs closely because fever, tachycardia, hypotension, and tachypnea frequently are signs of an acute, serious infection or shock. Jaundice and scleral icterus are usually obvious if they are present. In liver disorders the degree of jaundice reflects the severity of the liver dysfunction and in biliary tract disorders the degree of obstruction. Jaundice becomes apparent at a total bilirubin level of approximately 2.5 mg/dL. Purpura and petechiae often represent clotting abnormalities secondary to deficient production of clotting factors by the liver. Palmar erythema and spider angiomata frequently are present in chronic liver disease. Generalized muscle wasting is significant for long-standing hepatic dysfunction and typically is accompanied by ascites and lower extremity edema, which signify portal hypertension. The presence of prominent superficial veins of the abdomen, a caput medusa, and splenomegaly are signs of portal hypertension. Carefully assess liver size and consistency; an inflamed liver is often enlarged and firm, while a cirrhotic liver is usually shrunken and nodular. A tender liver edge signifies acute inflammation of the liver. Note gallbladder inflammation by palpating in the right midclavicular line along the liver edge and asking the patient to inhale deeply. This procedure may elicit a positive Murphy's sign, which is an expression of pain by the patient as the tender gallbladder meets your hand.

Which initial basic laboratory tests should I order?

Whenever you suspect hepatitis or cirrhosis of any cause, multiple laboratory tests are indicated. The recommended tests include:

- A full liver function profile, which includes liver enzymes, bilirubin, and serum albumin
- A hepatitis profile, which evaluates for the presence of antibodies to the various forms of viral hepatitis
- A complete blood count (CBC) and a prothrombin time/INR.

This combination of tests will not only indicate the degree of acute hepatocellular damage that is present but will also identify the functional capacity of the liver and the likelihood of acute or chronic infection. Increases in the levels of aspertate transaminase (AST) and alanine transaminase (ALT) reflect hepatocellular damage. The ratio of AST to ALT is typically greater than two in alcoholic liver disease and usually less than one in other types of hepatitis. An elevated bilirubin and prothrombin time/INR along with a depressed albumin level indicate a decrease in the functional capacity of the liver.

Where may the results of the aforementioned tests lead?

If the direct (conjugated) component of the bilirubin is high, accompanied by elevations in the alkaline phosphatase and gamma glutamyl transpeptidase (GGT), suspect intrahepatic or extrahepatic obstruction to the outflow of bile. This obstruction can be from cholestasis or obstruction of the hepatobiliary tree by stones, tumors, or scarring of the ducts as in primary sclerosing cholangitis.

In the common benign hereditary condition of Gilbert's syndrome, the level of the indirect (unconjugated) bilirubin is elevated with consistently normal values of all other liver parameters. The CBC may show an elevated white blood cell count consistent with an acute inflammatory or infectious process. If you suspect obstruction of the common bile duct, you will need to obtain an amylase and lipase to determine the presence of pancreatitis.

Of those patients who present with metabolic liver disease, the most common disorders are steatohepatitis, hereditary hemochromatosis, and Wilson's disease. To investigate for these, order a fasting lipid profile, serum ferritin and transferrin saturation, and a ceruloplasmin level. In patients with primary biliary cirrhosis, antimitochondrial antibodies are present more than 90% of the time. Those patients with autoimmune hepatitis characteristically have elevated levels of smooth muscle antibodies, antinuclear antibodies, and liver-kidney microsomal antibodies.

Which imaging test might be helpful?

Ultrasonography is highly useful in delineating many types of liver and biliary tract disorders. It can detect dilation of the biliary tree and gallbladder, as well as the majority of stones present in the gallbladder or common bile duct. Ultrasound will visualize liver cysts, abscesses, and most solid masses including hepatocellular carcinoma. Computed tomography (CT) with intravenous contrast is useful to evaluate disease of the liver parenchyma and to enhance space-occupying lesions. Magnetic resonance imaging (MRI) can visualize vascular structures within the liver without the use of iodine containing contrast. If preliminary testing, as outlined in the previous sections, indicates a potential obstruction of the biliary tree, endoscopic retrograde cholangiopancreatography (ERCP) can delineate the anatomy more precisely, allow for endoscopic extraction of obstructing stones, and lend the opportunity for relief of some distal common bile duct strictures. Magnetic resonance cholangiopancreatography (MRCP) affords a noninvasive approach to visualizing the biliary tree but does not allow for intervention. If you suspect cholecystitis but ultrasound is either normal or inconclusive, an HIDA scan can confirm a diagnosis of acute cholecystitis by showing the absence of tracer uptake by the gallbladder.

▶ TREATMENT

What treatment steps are appropriate for patients with acute hepatitis?

Management of the patient with acute hepatitis is supportive. Maintaining adequate hydration is essential, either by intravenous replacement of fluid or control of nausea and vomiting by medications. The patient should avoid any potentially hepatotoxic substances, including alcohol and many medications. Vitamin K supplementation is useful in those with a prolonged prothrombin time. In severely ill patients manifesting signs of fulminant hepatic failure, intensive care unit admission and early consideration for liver transplantation is indicated.

List appropriate treatment steps for patients with chronic hepatitis and cirrhosis.

Identifying the etiology of the disorder is paramount in the treatment of chronic liver disorders to tailor treatment to that particular cause.

Chronic hepatitis B and hepatitis C respond to interferon and antiviral medications. Alcoholic liver disease responds favorably to discontinuation of alcohol intake. Liver disease from hemochromatosis responds to lowering the total body iron load through episodic therapeutic phlebotomy. Copper-chelating agents such as penicillamine or trientine and zinc salts can lessen the effect of Wilson's disease on the liver. Autoimmune hepatitis responds to prednisone and azathiaprine. In treating primary biliary cirrhosis, ursodeoxycholic acid has shown to delay the progression of the disease. For those patients diagnosed with steatohepatitis, weight loss and control of frequently accompanying hyperlipoproteinemia are the treatments of choice. Note that in chronic hepatitis or cirrhosis a liver biopsy is usually performed to clearly diagnose the cause and the extent of the underlying disorder.

What treatment is appropriate for acute cholecystitis or cholangitis?

Broad-spectrum intravenous antibiotics covering enteric gram-negative organisms, gram-positive organisms, and anaerobes (*Enterobacteriaceae,* enterococci, *Bacteroides,* and *Clostridium*) are essential to treating acute cholecystitis and cholangitis. In many cases, antibiotics and intravenous hydration are sufficient in clearing acute cholecystitis with the consideration for eventual elective cholecystectomy. It is wise to obtain surgical consultation early in the course of the illness. In cases of ongoing fever, pain, leukocytosis, or peritoneal signs, urgent cholecystectomy is indicated—particularly in diabetics who are prone to develop gangrene of the gallbladder. In patients with acute cholangitis, adequate biliary drainage must be ensured through ERCP or surgical intervention to remove or somehow bypass the obstruction. If untreated, cholangitis is fatal. Chronic cholelithiasis without symptoms requires no intervention.

KEY POINTS

- **Treatment of acute hepatitis is supportive.**
- **Treatment of chronic hepatitis and cirrhosis requires establishment of a precise etiology for optimal therapy.**
- **Cholangitis manifested by jaundice, right upper quadrant pain, and fever is a medical emergency requiring urgent imaging studies and gastroenterology consultation.**
- **Patients with acute cholecystitis benefit from urgent surgical consultation to optimally time cholecystectomy if it becomes necessary.**

CASE 52–1. **A 26-year-old woman presents with symptoms of malaise, weight loss, and a transient episode of jaundice associated with fever and vomiting occurring four months prior.**

A. The most appropriate laboratory tests to order are:
   Complete blood count, antinuclear antibody, and basic metabolic profile
   Liver function panel, hepatitis profile, and complete blood count
   Urinalysis, thyroid-stimulating hormone, and serum uric acid
   Serum ferritin, ceruloplamin level, and antimitochondrial antibodies
B. If the patient's hepatitis profile is significant only for a positive hepatitis C virus antibody, what further testing is appropriate?

CASE 52–2. **An 82-year-old man presents to the emergency department with a 24-hour history of increasing right upper abdominal pain and fever. His urine has been dark-colored over the last two to three days, and he is nauseated. A recent hospitalization for chest pain revealed single vessel coronary artery stenosis. He underwent a successful angioplasty and stenting. During that hospitalization he was diagnosed with type 2 diabetes mellitus.**

A. The most important initial imaging study for this man will be:
   Chest x-ray
   Flat and upright abdominal x-rays
   Intravenous pyelogram
   Ultrasound of the liver and gallbladder
B. If an ultrasound of the liver and gallbladder is obtained and the findings are consistent with acute cholecystitis and cholelithiasis, what are the appropriate steps to be taken?

CASE 52–3. A 62-year-old woman taking simvastatin for the last three months in order to lower her cholesterol presents to your office for advice after she was found to have an ALT and AST three times the upper limits of normal on recent blood testing. These tests were not done prior to initiation of therapy but she did have normal levels of these tests on an evaluation done three years prior for unrelated reasons.

A. You should recommend:
   A hepatitis profile
   Stopping the simvastatin and repeating the ALT and AST in three to four weeks
   An ultrasound of the liver and gallbladder
   Stopping her weekly glass of wine and repeating the ALT and AST in two months

B. If her liver enzymes remain elevated after three to four weeks off of the simvastatin, what is your next step in investigation of the cause?

REFERENCES

Ahya SN, Flood K, Paranjothi S: The Washington Manual of Medical Therapeutics, 30th ed. Philadelphia: Lippincott Williams & Wilkins, 2001, pp 376–392.

Johnston DE: Special considerations in interpreting liver function tests. Am Fam Physician 59:2223–2230, 1999.

Kaplowitz N: Liver and Biliary Diseases, 2nd ed. Baltimore: Williams & Wilkins, 1996.

Nordling MK, Rao G: Common Hepatobiliary Conditions. FP Essentials, edition no. 294, AAFP Home Study. Leawood, KS: American Academy of Family Physicians, 2003.

USEFUL WEBSITE

Centers for Disease Control and Infection, National Center for Infectious Diseases: Viral Hepatitis. Available at *http://www.cdc.gov/ncidod/diseases/hepatitis.*

53

Menopause

What is menopause?

Menopause is the permanent cessation of menstruation that occurs after 12 months of amenorrhea, associated with the loss of ovarian follicular function.

What is surgical menopause?

Surgical menopause is the abrupt cessation of ovarian function second to bilateral oophorectomy.

What is meant by perimenopause?

Perimenopause is the period preceding menopause that begins with the first break in cyclicity and is characterized by menstrual irregularity in both cycle length and amount of flow, accompanied by increasing months of amenorrhea. In perimenopause the anovulatory cycles become more prevalent and cycle length increases.

When does perimenopause usually begin, and how long does it last?

The Massachusetts Women's Health Study, one of the largest studies ever to investigate the age of onset and duration of perimenopause, longitudinally followed more than 2500 women and identified that the median age of onset of perimenopause was 47.5 years. The median age of last menstrual period was 51.3 years.

Menstrual cycle changes are the starting point of the clinical definition of perimenopause. We consider women with regular cycles who begin to experience a break in cyclicity but who have not gone more than 3 months without menstruating to be in early perimenopause. As women progress toward menopause they experience more missed cycles. After 3 to 11 months of amenorrhea, a woman is considered to be in late perimenopause. After the twelfth month of amenorrhea a woman has reached menopause.

The period during which a woman transitions from having regular reproductive cycles through the perimenopausal transition to menopause is called the "climacteric." The duration of perimenopause is two to eight years.

What factors affect the time sequence of perimenopause and menopause?

Women who are older at the onset of perimenopause are likely to have a shorter transition to menopause. Smokers are likely to begin the perimenopause earlier, and have shorter transitions than non-smokers. Nulliparous women also tend to reach perimenopause earlier than those with children.

What takes place physiologically during perimenopause and menopause?

After age 35, fertility declines sharply. During perimenopause the depletion of primary follicles happens more precipitously. In perimenopause the intermenstrual intervals shorten significantly, usually by three to seven days. This shortening is caused by an accelerated follicular phase secondary to lower progesterone levels. The follicular stimulating hormone (FSH) levels rise in response to altered folliculogenesis and reduced inhibin (hormones that inhibit pituitary production of FSH) secretion. In perimenopause the estradiols are "irregularly irregular" and often reach levels above those seen during reproductive years. There is a hyperestrogenic but hypoprogestegenic environment that probably accounts for the increased incidence of endometrial hyperplasia, carcinoma, uterine polyps, and leiomyoma observed in women during the perimenopause. With transition to menopause, estradiol levels fall markedly as FSH and luteinizing hormone (LH) levels increase.

In early perimenopause women may experience an increase in menstrual flow correlated with luteal phase insufficiency or anovulatory cycles. As menopause approaches, however, estrogen levels fall, the flow becomes lighter, and the length increases. Ovarian follicle loss accelerates until the supply is depleted.

Why do women experience menopause?

It is estimated that there have been about 5000 generations of humans. Only in the last five generations has the average life expectancy advanced into the menopausal range. It seems that women's capacity to reproduce and rear their offspring into their own reproductive years is what was expected physiologically. With advances in public health and medicine, the life expectancy is now 86 for women who reach menopause. These women will spend, on the average, more than one third of their lives in a postmenopausal state.

What are the long-term risks of menopause?

One of the major long-term risks of menopause is osteoporosis. This may occur in the late stages of menopause as a result of the effect on bones of the loss of estrogen.

What is premature menopause?

Premature menopause is defined as menopause before the age of 40 (not by surgical means).

What is the cause of premature menopause?

The cause of premature menopause is not clearly understood but we believe that some women either have a genetic predisposition or some type of autoimmune phenomenon. A biopsy of an ovary of a woman experiencing premature menopause reveals a large lymphocytic infiltrate.

What happens if a woman has bleeding after going 12 months without a menstrual period?

After becoming menopausal, this bleeding is classified as "post-menopausal bleeding" and must be evaluated. Although there are common benign reasons for postmenopausal bleeding, you should evaluate with a pelvic or vaginal ultrasound and an endometrial biopsy.

► EVALUATION

What are the common signs and symptoms of perimenopause that extend into menopause?

Signs and symptoms of perimenopause are menstrual changes with irregular cycles, menorrhagia, and spotting. Many women also experience vasomotor disturbances (hot flashes and night sweats), sexual dysfunction, and reduced libido. There are also a number of mood, cognitive, and somatic symptoms including irritability, anxiety, memory loss, fatigue, and insomnia. These signs and symptoms vary greatly in intensity, duration, and frequency.

Is there a difference between hot flashes and hot flushes?

No. Various books, journal articles, and the lay press use these terms interchangeably. Hot flashes/flushes are feelings of intense heat over the trunk and face, with flushing of the skin and sweating. They often occur before the cessation of menses. They are caused by an increase in pulsatile release of gonadotropin-releasing hormone from the hypothalamus, which affects the adjacent temperature-regulating area of the brain.

Are there any laboratory or diagnostic tests that can determine whether someone is in perimenopause?

A low FSH in the early follicular phase (days two to five) is inconsistent with a diagnosis of perimenopause. However, in menopause the serum FSH and LH levels are markedly elevated. Pap smear vaginal cytology will reveal findings consistent with a low estrogen effect with predominately parabasal cells, indicating a lack of epithelial maturation.

What will I find on physical exam?

In a postmenopausal woman the physical exam (when the woman has not been treated with postmenopausal hormone replacement therapy) will reveal a decreased vaginal introital diameter; the mucosa will appear pale and smooth with loss of the usual vaginal rugae; the cervix and uterus will feel small; and the ovaries are usually not palpable.

▶ TREATMENT

How should I treat women during the perimenopausal period?

The perimenopausal period may require no treatment. However, women who have significant symptoms such as hot flashes, night sweats, insomnia, vaginal dryness, mood swings, or depression may require some hormonal intervention. They may be treated with low-dose combined oral contraceptives. These would typically include 20 micrograms of ethinyl estradiol with 1 mg of norethindrone acetate, taken for 21 days per month. Low-dose oral contraceptives tend to eliminate the vasomotor symptoms and restore regular cyclicity along with abbreviating many of the other symptoms associated with this transitional time. The unintentional pregnancy rate of women in their forties rivals that of adolescence, and this therapy provides an additional contraceptive benefit. Use progestin-only formulations for women experiencing marked menorrhagia during this time, especially for women at high risk for thromboembolic disease or those who smoke. For women experiencing menorrahagia, a nonhormonal strategy to reduce menstrual flow includes the use of nonsteroidal anti-inflammatory agents. When menorrhagia persists and hormone therapy has not been beneficial, consider endometrial ablation.

Should patients start taking calcium in perimenopause?

Yes, at this time it is advisable to administer calcium 1000 mg per day and vitamin D 400 IU daily.

What are the benefits and risks of postmenopausal hormone therapy?

The consistent benefits shown by both observational and randomized clinical trials show that estrogen therapy is very effective in controlling vasomotor and genitourinary symptoms. By reducing bone turnover and resorption rates, estrogen slows age-related bone loss. There is a 4–6% increase in bone mineral density of the spine and a 2–3% increase at the hip maintained through treatment.

The risks associated with postmenopausal hormone therapy include endometrial cancer if estrogen is used alone in women. With the addition of progesterone these risks are eliminated. The risk of venous thromboembolic disease was at least doubled in postmenopausal women on hormone replacement therapy (HRT). For women who undergo HRT for more than five years there is an increased risk of breast cancer of approximately 35% (80 additional cases per 100,000 woman)—more in estrogen–progesterone regimens than estrogen alone. There is currently no evidence that HRT helps prevent cardiovascular disease. Gallbladder disease also seems to increase in HRT. Cognitive decline and dementia thought earlier to be protected somewhat by HRT has shown no actual benefit at this time.

One benefit, however, is that colorectal cancer seems to be diminished significantly in women who undergo HRT, a 20–35% reduction over a five-year period.

Are there other ways to treat menopause?

Although the Women's Health Initiative is a very large study, it focused on the most commonly used estrogen–progesterone combination, conjugated equine estrogen 0.625 mg and medroxyprogesterone 2.5 mg daily. It is unclear whether or not the benefits and risks evidenced by the Women's Health Initiative are extrapolated to the other combination HRT prescription products available that vary in estrogen type or dose and vary in progesterone dose.

When is the use of contraceptives during perimenopause or HRT during menopause contraindicated?

The use of oral contraceptives and HRT would be relatively contraindicated in cigarette smokers, and contraindicated in patients with significant liver disease, a history of thromboembolic phenomenon, active breast cancer, or unexplained vaginal bleeding.

When do you transition a woman who was previously on low-dose oral contraceptives and wishes to stay on hormone replacement therapy?

A woman may be transitioned from oral contraceptives to HRT either at the age that her mother went into menopause, or you may arbitrarily assign a duration of four or five years from the onset of perimenopause.

It is very important to individualize HRT for the patient and to educate the patient about the risks and benefits, given the controversy that has occurred since 2001. Since the late 1990s there has been a tremendous amount written in the lay press, and most women in this phase of life are aware of the controversy.

One rational approach is to use a lower-dose estrogen–progesterone (0.45 mg, 1.5 mg) combination for five years to control the menopausal symptoms, at which time a selective estrogen receptor modulator or bisphosphonate may be administered.

What are selective estrogen receptive modulators (SERMs)?

There are estrogen receptors in numerous tissues including the uterus, breast, vaginal mucosa, brain, and skin. An ideal estrogen receptive modulator would give the benefits of an estrogen to protect bone without increasing the risk of breast cancer. This ideal medicine would also help prevent vaginal atrophy and vasomotor and affective symptoms. At this writing there is currently one selective estrogen receptive modulator (SERM) available in the United States. It does prevent bone loss and probably has a benefit in prevention of cardiovascular disease, but it also increases thromboembolic disease and vasomotor symptoms; it does not cause an increased risk of breast cancer. It is hoped that future additional SERMs will have a more ideal profile.

What are other alternatives to hormone replacement therapy for the management of menopausal symptoms?

Other medications that have been demonstrated to help alleviate vasomotor symptoms include selective serotonin reuptake inhibitors, clonidine, and gabapentin. Vaginal atrophy and dryness can be alleviated with the use of topical estrogens or an estrogen ring. Depression may be treated with typical antidepressant medications, and insomnia may respond to sedating antihistamines (diphenhydramine) or low-dose sedating tricyclic antidepressants (e.g., amitriptyline).

What are the alternative medicine approaches?

There are no controlled studies that show phytoestrogens, which have been popularized in the early 2000s, have a significant benefit on prevention of menopausal symptoms. The herb "black cohosh" has been shown to be moderately effective in prevention of vasomotor instability.

Should androgens be given to women?

Testosterone is sometimes given to postmenopausal women. Indeed, the addition of androgens in the therapeutic regimen has been demonstrated to improve women's enjoyment of and ability to have intercourse and to increase libido. Sexual well-being can be enhanced with the restoration of testosterone to physiologic levels.

What treatments are available to treat osteoporosis that accompanies menopause?

Osteoporosis is seen most commonly in slender, fair, Caucasian women. The gold standard testing for diagnosis is a nuclear medicine DXA scan. Ultrasound of the heel is also an appropriate screening method for osteoporosis.

There are several treatments to help prevent osteoporosis in women in their postmenopausal years. The foundation of treatment is calcium in a 1000-mg supplement in divided doses per day plus vitamin D 400 IU per day until age 70, at which time it is recommended the vitamin D dose be increased to at least 600 IU per day. Bisphosphonates, calcitonin, PTH, and SERMs, all used to treat osteoporosis in women, have been shown to have preventive effects.

Is there such a thing as male menopause?

Men do not have a readily identifiable marker such as menses. "Andropause" has been described in the literature. This condition is marked by decreased libido, decreased muscle mass, decreased energy, and erectile dysfunction, all related to decreased testosterone production.

What should I be aware of in evaluating and managing menopause?

It is critical that you approach the patient in menopause with understanding and sensitivity, remembering that women may have a variety of menopausal symptoms. Keep in mind that women undergoing the transition through perimenopause and throughout menopause can experience multiple changes including menstrual cycle changes, vasomotor instability, sexual dysfunction, depression, and significant insomnia. This is often related to changes in their life with regard to children achieving adulthood and moving away, and with male partners that may be experiencing their own physiologic changes. The student and physician must be aware of the changing physiology. Discuss these problems openly with the patient, and attempt to address each symptom the patient is experiencing. The patient will greatly appreciate your understanding and sensitivity during this time.

KEY POINTS

- **Menopause begins after the cessation of menses for 12 months.**
- **Perimenopause begins with the first break in regular cyclicity and lasts about four years.**
- **The treatment for symptomatic perimenopause is low-dose oral contraceptives.**
- **Symptoms of perimenopause and menopause include vasomotor instability, mood changes, insomnia, and vaginal dryness.**
- **The principal long-term consequence of menopause is osteoporosis.**
- **Treatment for menopause should be individualized.**

CASE 53–1. **A slender, fair, 64-year-old Caucasian woman, whose last menstrual period was 13 years ago, presents with chronic fatigue secondary to awakening four times per night, nocturia, vaginal dryness, dyspareunia, loss of libido, and midthoracic back pain. She notes that her clothes do not seem to fit as well, in that she seems somewhat "hunched over." She has never taken any menopausal medicines (hormones). She has not had any doctor visits in more than five years, has had no past surgeries, and has a negative FH. Physical exam findings reveal normal vitals, mild kyphosis, a 3-cm loss in height, and small vaginal introitis. Otherwise the exam is normal.**

A. Describe your differential diagnosis.
B. What tests are most appropriate?
C. Given the available history and physical information, which treatments would be most appropriate?

REFERENCES

Barbieri RL, Berga SL, Chang RJ, Santoro NF (eds): Managing the Perimenopause. Crofton, Md: Association of Professors of Gynecology and Obstetrics, 2001.

Barbieri RL, Lobo RA, Walsh BW, Santoro NF (eds): Improving Quality of Life During Menopause: The Role for Hormone Replacement Therapy. Crofton, Md: Association of Professors of Gynecology and Obstetrics, 2002.

Kasper DL, Braunwald E, Fauci AS et al. (eds): Pre-Publication Prospectus—Harrison's Principles of Internal Medicine, 16th ed. New York: McGraw-Hill, 2004.

Tierney LM, McPhee SJ, Papadakis MA (eds): Current Medical Diagnosis & Treatment 2003, 42nd ed. New York: Lange Medical Books/McGraw-Hill, 2003.

USEFUL WEBSITE

The North American Menopause Society website has an outstanding scientific review section, which can be accessed at *http://www.menopause.org.*

54

Nutrition and Obesity

NUTRITIONAL DEFICIENCY

▶ ETIOLOGY

What underlying physical problems can cause vitamin deficiency?

Any physical condition that impairs digestion or absorption of nutrients can cause a vitamin deficiency. A review of the physiology of digestion and absorption is helpful. Patients with poor or no teeth may have difficulty eating a balanced diet. Likewise, patients with any reason for difficulty chewing or swallowing are also at risk for nutritional deficiencies.

The absorption of vitamin B_{12} is dependent on *intrinsic factor* (IF), which is made in the parietal cells of the stomach. If a patient has had extensive ulcer disease and part of the stomach removed, there may be insufficient IF for adequate vitamin B_{12} absorption in the ileum. The other water-soluble vitamins are absorbed in the proximal small intestine; thus, if part of the small intestine is impaired (e.g., with Crohn's disease) or surgically absent, the patient may experience vitamin deficiency.

Vitamins A, D, E, and K are fat soluble vitamins, and depend on a functioning pancreas and bile duct for absorption in the small intestine. Patients with chronic pancreatitis or other conditions resulting in steatorrhea may have deficiencies of the fat-soluble vitamins. It is difficult to obtain adequate vitamin D from the diet, despite the fact that many dairy products are fortified. The role of UV light in activating provitamins in the skin is important in vitamin D metabolism. Patients who do not have much exposure to sunlight or who cannot tolerate lactose in their diets are at risk for vitamin D deficiency.

Describe the special role of folate in the diet.

Folate is important in cell reproduction and division, protein metabolism, and prevention of birth defects, including neural tube defects and possibly heart defects. The U.S. Preventive Services Task Force recommends folate supplementation in all women who are planning and are capable of pregnancy. This recommendation is endorsed by the American Academy of Pediatrics (AAP), which specifies that all women should include 400 micrograms of folic acid in their diets each day. Folic acid supplementation decreases the level of homocysteine, elevated serum levels of which have been associated with coronary artery disease. There is conflicting evidence as to whether treating coronary artery disease with folic acid improves outcomes.

▶ EVALUATION

What signs and symptoms point to nutritional deficiency?

The signs and symptoms of a nutritional deficiency depend on the missing nutrient and the length of the deficiency. Interpreting these signs and symptoms can be more complex if the patient is deficient in more than one nutrient. The nutrient inadequacy may be a progressive, continuous process that can eventually lead to depletion of body nutrient reserves. The development of a nutritional deficiency disease occurs in five stages: nutritional inadequacy, tissue depletion, biochemical changes, functional changes, and anatomic lesions. Biochemical changes, or lesions, occur in selected tissues throughout the body depending on the nutrient that is inadequately supplied. These biochemical changes eventually will result in functional alterations such as loss of appetite, easy fatigability, and gastrointestinal disturbances. As the nutritional deficiency continues, anatomic lesions develop, along with gross clinical signs and symptoms like glossitis, cheilosis, and dermatitis.

There are two categories of nutritional deficiency:

Primary nutritional deficiency is caused by the failure to ingest an essential nutrient. Patients may miss essential nutrients because of poor food habits; lack of money to purchase an adequate diet; lack of knowledge of adequate nutrition; or excess consumption of highly refined foods or beverages. Dietary interventions that do not supply the correct nutrients, such as inadequate parenteral-enteral nutrition/total parenteral nutrition (PEN/TPN) formulas, may also contribute to a deficiency.

Secondary nutritional deficiency is caused by failure to absorb or utilize an essential nutrient because of an environmental condition or physical state, not the lack of consuming the nutrient. Secondary nutritional deficiency is categorized into six areas of concern:

- Interference with ingestion (e.g., mouth lesions; lack of taste acuity)
- Interference with digestion and absorption (e.g., lack of hydrochloric acid in the stomach for absorption of B_{12}; gastric surgery; nonabsorbable fat ingestion)

- Interference with utilization (e.g., diabetes mellitus; alcoholism)
- Increased nutrient requirement (e.g., the increased need for protein and calories in a person with decubitus ulcer; lactation)
- Increased nutrient destruction (e.g., achlorhydria; some drugs)
- Increased nutrient excretion (e.g., diarrhea; diuretics)

What are the common presenting signs of an eating disorder?

The presenting signs of an eating disorder can be subtle, especially when the eating may be disordered and not fully meeting the DSM-IV criteria for an eating disorder of anorexia, bulimia, or mixed variety of both. Factors to consider:

- Significant weight loss
- Distress at addressing any topic related to food or diet
- Extreme interest in food, but not in eating it (such as cooking lots of foods, but not eating them)
- Nutrient deficiencies
- Depression with weight loss
- Normal weight, but with signs of purging such as alkalosis, dehydration, hypokalemia, or dental enamel erosion

How should I evaluate unintended weight loss in adults?

An unintended weight loss of at least 5% of the usual body weight over a 6-month to 12-month period is cause for evaluation. The most common causes of unintended weight loss in adults are cancer, gastrointestinal disorders, dementia, or depression. Evaluation of the problem involves a complete medical history including review of systems, mental status, and depression screening, as well as a physical examination. Symptoms or signs may point to the origin of disease in the case of malignancy or gastrointestinal disorder. Celiac disease is a common malabsorption syndrome (with an incidence of 1 in 250 people) in which the ingestion of gluten causes a patient to develop an autoimmune inflammatory disease resulting in damage to the intestinal mucosa and impaired absorption. These patients often present with chronic diarrhea, anemia, or fatigue, and may have a history of type 1 diabetes or family history of celiac disease.

Relevant laboratory tests to evaluate weight loss include a CBC (evaluate for anemia, infection, inflammation); blood chemistries; urinalysis (looking for protein, blood, ketones, or infection); serologic tests (HIV if indicated, serologic tests for celiac disease including endomysial antibodies); TSH; and screening for common malignancies such as colon cancer, cervical cancer, or breast cancer. Some experts recommend radiographic evaluation of the upper GI tract to help rule out malabsorptive or maldigestive causes. Pay particular attention to medications that may impair the appetite or absorption of food, especially with elderly patients.

▶ TREATMENT

Who is at risk of nutritional deficiency?

Many individuals within the medical care system are likely to be at risk for a nutritional deficiency. Those most vulnerable are individuals who are immunocompromised, chronically ill, or frail.

How should I treat these deficiencies?

The missing nutrient(s) should be administered through oral or parenteral supplementation. *Note:* If a person is not deficient in a nutrient, the addition of that nutrient to a person's diet will not accomplish more or better results from the nutrient's function. For example, if a person is deficient in zinc, then wound healing will be poor, but if a person is *not* deficient in zinc, increased intake of zinc will not speed or improve the healing process. See Table 54–1 for specific nutrients, function, and deficiency signs.

WEIGHT MANAGEMENT

What do I tell a patient who is gaining weight through middle age about obesity prevention?

The primary reason that a person gains weight is that his energy intake exceeds energy expenditure. To gain or lose 1 pound (lb) requires a caloric excess or deficit of 3500 kilocalories (kcal). Maintaining energy balance becomes harder with age because although we become more sedentary, we continue to enjoy a plentiful supply of foods. Only 50 extra kcal per day adds up to an excess of 3500 kcal in 10 weeks, resulting in the usual American weight gain of 5 lb in a year. Thus, an individual must increase physical activity and/or moderate food intake to make up the 50 kcal/day. This adjustment can be difficult, considering that energy needs decrease about 2–5% per decade of life. A little more activity and smaller portions, or fewer added fats, or fewer high-calorie foods make a big difference in maintaining healthy weight. The increased activity should be anything the person likes to do and will do regularly. The current guideline for physical activity is for at least 30 minutes per day for weight maintenance, and at least 1 hour per

Text continued on p. 382

TABLE 54–1

Summary of Major Nutrients

Nutrient	Major Dietary Sources	Major Functions	Signs of Deficiency	Usual Causes of Deficiency	Effects of Excess
Protein (Pro) (Supplies 4 kcal/g)	Fish, chicken, beef, other animals, lentils, seeds, legumes, dry beans, dairy products, eggs, nuts	Building material (amino acids [AA]) for growth, maintenance, and repair of all cells; regulates fluid balance between blood andcells; provides energy. Essential AA are threonine, typtophan, histidine, lysine, leucine, isoleucine, methionine, valine, and phenylalanine.	Kwashiorkor (protein malnutrition); decreased immune response; edema; stunted growth and development; poor musculature; maramus (protein-energy malnutrition)	Poor intake of protein especially high-quality protein; too few calories so that protein used for energy; malabsorption; genetic diseases of protein/aminoacids (such as PKU)	Reduced calcium retention; weight gain/obesity
Carbohydrates (CHO) (Supplies 4 kcal/g)	Cereal grains, dry peas and beans, bread, pasta, vegetables, fruits, dairy products, sugar, jellies, other sweets	Provides energy for body processes and physical activity; aids in use of fat and spares protein; provides energy. Many vitamins and most fiber are carried in CHO.	Growth retardation; weight loss	Poor intake; malabsorption; genetic diseases of CHO (such as glycogen/storage diseases)	Weight gain/obesity; increased blood triglycerides

continued

Table 54–1. Summary of Major Nutrients *continued*

Nutrient	Major Dietary Sources	Major Functions	Signs of Deficiency	Usual Causes of Deficiency	Effects of Excess
Fat (Supplies 9 kcal/g)	Saturated fats: meat, dairy fats (such as ice cream, sour cream, butter), bacon, sausages; unsaturated fats: avocado, oils (such as corn, safflower, vegetable); monounsaturated fats: olive oil, canola oil; Omega 3 & 6 fatty acids: fish, shellfish, nuts	Supplies concentrated source of energy; carries fat soluble vitamins; supplies essential fatty acids (linoleic, linolenic, arachidonic acids); membrane structures and transport processes of cells	Flaky and scaly skin, poor growth, hair loss; impaired wound healing and immune functioning	Poor intake; malabsorption; extreme diets or supplement feedings for long periods of time (such as IVs or TPN without fats)	Increased blood cholesterol and/or triglycerides; weight gain/obesity
Water	Water, beverages, fruits, nearly all foods contain some water	Provides medium for most of body's reactions; helps move materials to and waste from cells; helps control body temperature; lubricates joints in body	Dehydration, death	Poor intake; medications; diarrhea; vomiting; high temperatures	Excess retention of fluid related to imbal ance of minerals; overconsumption is rare but can result in death
Folate (folic acid, folacin, pteroylpoly-glutamates) 400 mcg/day recommended prepregnancy	Dark green leafy vegetables, whole grains, legumes, nuts, organ meats, orange juice, fortified cereal products	Assists in red blood cell maturation; cofactor for synthesis of purine and pyrimidine; coenzyme in metabolism of nucleic and AA	Megaloblastic anemia; gastrointestinal upsets; poor growth; maternal deficiency linked to neural tube defects in fetus	Poor intake; malabsorption	Masks deficiency of vitamin B_{12}

Niacin (includes nicotinic acid amide, nicotinic acid, nicotinamide)	Liver, meat, bran cereal, fish, poultry, whole grains, peanuts, fortified cereal products	Part of coenzymes for oxidation/reduction reactions; release of energy and biosynthesis of fatty acids	Pellagra; pigmented dermatitis; inflammation of mucous membrane; diarrhea; weakness; depression	Poor intake; malabsorption; consumption of processed grains that have niacin removed; hemodialysis	Flushing, burning and tingling around the face, neck and hands; liver damage; gastrointestinal distress
Pantothenic Acid	Liver, egg yolks, meat, fish, poultry, whole grains, fresh vegetables, oats, yeast, broccoli	Component of coenzyme A; functions in release of energy from CHO, Pro and Fat; coenyzme in fatty acid metabolism	Fatigue; malaise; insomnia; abdominal cramps, burning parasthesias; impaired coordination; depression	Poor intake; malabsorption; incomplete PEN/TPM formulas	Not known
Biotin	Liver, meat, fruits	Coenzyme for carboxylation reactions; plays a role in CHO and fat metabolism; coenzyme in synthesis of fat, glycogen, and AA	Dermatitis; neuritis; appetite loss; nausea; vomiting; glossitis; insomnia; thin hair; depression	Incomplete PEN/TPM formulas	Not known
Water-Soluble Vitamins					
Vitamin B_1 (Thiamine)	Lean pork, wheat germ, whole/enriched cereals, legumes, bread products	Assists in use of CHO and fat for energy; promotes growth, appetite and muscle tone; promotes normal functioning of nervous system; coenzyme in metabolism of CHO & branched chain AA	Beriberi; changes in nerves; excessive water retention; loss of appetite; depression; muscle tenderness; high-output cardiac failure; polyneuritis	Poor intake; malabsorption; hemodialysis	None reported

continued

Table 54–1. Summary of Major Nutrients *continued*

Nutrient	Major Dietary Sources	Major Functions	Signs of Deficiency	Usual Causes of Deficiency	Effects of Excess
Vitamin B_2 (Riboflavin)	Dairy products, liver and other organ meats, meat, fish, dark green vegetables, fortified grain products	Functions as part of energy release; essential for growth; part of flavin coenzymes required in cellular oxidation	Cheilosis; photophobia; angular stomatitis, magenta tongue, seborrhea; corneal vascularization	Poor intake; malabsorption	None report
Vitamin B_6 (Pyrodoxine) B_6 comprises group of 6 related compounds: pyridoxal, pyridoxine, pyridoxamine, and 5′ phosphates (PLP, PNP, PMP)	Liver, pork, poultry, whole and fortified grain products, bananas, legumes, lentils, fortified soy-based meat substitutes	Cofactor for many enzymes in metabolism of protein and amino acids, functions in hemoglobin synthesis	Anemia; irritability; convulsions (in infants) skin lesions; changes in nerves; smooth red tongue (glossitis); weight loss	Poor intake; malabsorption; aging (increase need with age)	Unstable walking, numb feet, poor coordination of hands
Vitamin B_{12} (Cobalamin)	Liver, beef, poultry, fish, eggs, brewer's yeast (not present in plant foods); other prophylactic IM dose: 5–50 mg/ month; low IM dose: 100–250 mg/week; high IM dose: up to 500 mg/week	Maintenance of nervous tissue and blood formation; nucleic acid synthesis; recycling of tetrahydrofolate	Megaloblastic anemia (pernicious anemia); permanent damage to nervous system; peripheral neuropathy; weight loss; glossitis	Deficiency of hydrochloric acid in stomach (as occurs with aging); strict vegetarians; high intakes of folate can mask deficiency of B_{12}	None reported

Vitamin C (Ascorbic Acid)	Citrus fruits, tomatoes, potatoes, cabbage, broccoli, strawberries, spinach	Cofactor for reactions requiring reduced copper or iron metalloenzynes and as protective antioxidant	Scurvy; easy bruising; slow wound healing; degeneration of skin, teeth, gums and blood vessels	Smokers have increased need, poor intake	Gastrointestinal dis-turbances; kidney stones; excess iron absorption
Fat-Soluble Vitamins					
Vitamin A (includes provitamin A such as retinols, carotenoids)	Liver, dairy products, fish; carotene (provitamin) carrots, dark leafy green vegetables, sweet potato, cantalope, apricots, broccoli	Maintenance of skin and mucous membranes; component in visual process; particular adaptation to darkness; immune function	Night blindness; xerophthalmia, keratomalacia; Bilot's spots; follicular hyperkeratosis; reduced immunity; poor growth	Poor intake; malabsorption with steatorrhea; liver diseases	Loss of appetite; headache; vomiting; blurred vision with eventual eye damage; liver toxicity
Vitamin D (also called calciferol)	Fortified dairy products, fish, oils, eggs; sunlight (15 min/day for 3–4 days/week)	Mineralization of bones and teeth; intestinal absorption and regulation of calcium and phosphorus	Rickets (children); osteomalacia (adults); costochondral beading; muscle weakness and twitching; low serum calcium	Poor sunlight exposure; poor intake; with aging poor utilization; glucocoriticoid therapy may need additional D	Poor growth; weight loss; poor appetite; calcium deposits in soft tissues
Vitamin E (also called α-tocopherol)	Nuts, fats and polyunsaturated vegetable oils, margarine, seeds, whole grains	Antioxidant; prevents peroxidation of polyunsaturated lipids; free radical scavenger	Hemolytic anemia of newborn; increased fragility of red blood cells; nerve and muscle disturbances in severe malabsorption	Malabsorption	Interferes with vitamin K (so some risk of bleeding especially in trauma); hemorrhagic toxicity; monitoring needed for individuals on anticoagulant therapy & E supple ments

continued

Table 54–1. Summary of Major Nutrients *continued*

Nutrient	Major Dietary Sources	Major Functions	Signs of Deficiency	Usual Causes of Deficiency	Effects of Excess
Vitamin K	Green leafy vegetables, liver, vegetable oils & margarines, cabbage family	Synthesis of prothrombin and clotting factors II, VII, IX and X	Bleeding (especially in newborns); ecchymosis; epistaxis	Bacteria that produce vitamin K destroyed in gut	Not known; monitoring needed for individuals on anticoagulant therapy with K intake
Minerals					
Calcium	Dairy products, fish with small bones, dark, leafy green vegetables (mustard greens, kale); corn tortillas, calcium-set tofu	Structure of bones and teeth; nerve transmission; muscle contraction; essential role in blood clotting	Stunted growth; bone loss; rickets; osteomalacia; osteoporosis; tetany; possibly hypertension	Poor intake; poor consumption vitamin D and poor sunlight exposure; lack of physical activity; high phosphorus intake	Decreased absorption of other minerals; kidney stones; hyper-calcemia, mild alkali syndrome, renal insufficiency
Chloride	Table salt, seafood, meat	Acid-base balance; consituent of gastric juice; major anion of extracellular fluid	Rare; mental apathy, muscle cramps, usually accompanies sodium depletion	Rare in U.S. (occurred in recent history in babies whose formula did not have chloride)	None reported
Chromium	Fish, cheese, meat, poultry, whole grain cereals, beer	Insulin cofactor; glucose and energy metabolism	Insulin resistance; glucose intolerance	Unknown	None reported

Cobalt	Organ and muscle meats, dairy products	Constituent of B_{12}	Only as B_{12} deficiency; pernicious anemia	Those associated with B_{12}	None reported
Copper	Liver, shellfish, nuts, whole grains, cereals, legumes, cocoa products	Absorption and use of iron; enzyme cofactor; myelin sheath of nerves	Anemia; kinky hair; neutropenia; disturbance of bone formation	Usually genetic	Wilson's disease (genetic); iron deficiency anemia; chronic renal failure
Fluoride	Fluoridated drinking water, fluoridatec dental products, seafood	Structure of bone and teeth enamel; reduce dental caries	Dental caries	Unfluoridated water or dental products	Mottled teeth; enamel & skeletal fluorosis
Iodine	Iodized salt; seafood, salt water fish	Constituent of thyroid hormone	Goiter; cretinism	Lack of iodine in food or soil that grows food	Rare; goiter may be caused by too much; elevated thyroid stimulating hormone (TSH) concentration
Iron	Liver, lean meats, legumes, egg yolk, fortified cereals and breads	Constituent of hemoglobin; involved in oxygen and electron transport	Microcytic hypochromic anemia; fatigue; decrease immune response	Poor intake; blood loss	Liver and pancreas damage; large dose at one time shock and death; gastrointestinal distress

continued

Table 54–1. Summary of Major Nutrients *continued*

Nutrient	Major Dietary Sources	Major Functions	Signs of Deficiency	Usual Causes of Deficiency	Effects of Excess
Magnesium	Bran cereals, nuts, legumes, green leafy vegetables, meat	Part of protein synthesis; helps muscles contract and nerve impulse transmission	Rare; behavioral disturbances, tremor, spasms, neuromuscular irritability	Rare	Rare; diarrhea; fatigue; disturbances of nervous system (usually from pharmacological agents, not food sources)
Manganese	Nuts, legumes, whole grain cereals	Involved in formation of bone & enzymes in AA, cholesterol, & CHO metabolism	Rare; dermatitis; weight loss	Rare	Rare; inhaled manganese linked to CNS disorders/ neurotoxicity
Molybdenum	Whole grain cereals, legumes, nuts	Oxidation/reduction process; enzyme factoring catabolism of sulfur AA, and purine & pyridines metabolism	None	None	Not known
Phosphorus	Dairy products, eggs, meat, whole grain cereals, soda pop	Structure of bone and teeth; component of phospholipid; acid-base balance; energy metabolism	Rare; demineralization of bone; weakness; poor growth; parasthesia of hands and feet	Rare in U.S.	May cause deficiency of calcium; skeletal porosity; interference with calcium absorption

Potassium	Fruits (particularly bananas and citrus juices), dairy products, potatoes, vegetables	Major component of intracellular fluid; regulates acid-base and water balance; maintains heart and nerve failure	Muscle weakness; rapid irregular hear rate; paralysis and death	Medications such as diuretics especially with poor intake	Electrolyte imbalance; muscle weakness; disturbed heart function; death
Selenium	Organ meat, seafood, plants from selenium-containing soil	Antioxidant; consistuent of glutathione oxidose	Rare; cardiac myopathy; muscle tenderness	Rare	Rare; hair and nail brittleness and loss
Sodium	Table salt, processed foods in most foods except fruits	Maintains water balance; influences muscle contraction and nerve irritability	Rare; muscle cramps and reduced appetite	Rare; restricted diet with excessive medication	In some individuals retention of fluids and hypertension
Sulfur	Protein foods such as meat, dairy, legumes	Consistent of co-enzyme A, amino acids, hair, and cartilage	No dietary deficiency with adequate protein	Rare	Rare
Zinc	Meat, seafood, dark meat of poultry, whole grains, legumes	Component of multiple several enzymes and proteins; involved in the regulation of gene expression	Growth failure; impaired wound healing, taste changes, decrease immune response	Poor consumption of protein foods; phytate consumption that inhibit absorption	Fever, nausea, vomiting diarrhea; reduced copper status

day for weight loss. Stress to your patients that the activity counts as it occurs throughout the day and does not have to happen all at one time.

What do I tell patients who complain that they can't gain weight?

There isn't much sympathy for those who can't gain weight in a society that has many individuals who struggle with the opposite problem. The mechanics are the same in weight gain as in weight loss—energy balance between energy expenditure and food intake within the genetic range of the individual. As with weight loss, it is hard to implement the changes needed for weight gain. Some of the following suggestions have helped patients with gaining weight so that food intake is greater than energy expended:

- Eat small, frequent meals.
- Increase the calories of frequently consumed foods without increasing volume. For example, use high-protein milk in the place of water in hot cereals or soups. High-protein milk is the same volume (1 cup) with nonfat dry milk added to boost the calories.
- If using liquid supplement, take it about two hours prior to a meal so that it does not replace the meal.

Although fat has the most calories per gram, it is usually not an effective addition to the diet of those who want to gain weight. Fat tends to fill and satisfy the person too quickly, so that he or she does not obtain the extra calories that are needed (Box 54–1).

▶ TREATMENT

What is a realistic goal for weight loss in an overweight/obese individual?

At this point it is not clear that there is a realistic attainable goal for weight loss. The current guidelines suggest that an average of no more than 2 lb per week is reasonable. Remember, though, that this

BOX 54–1

Caloric Density of Macronutrients

Fat	9 kcal/g
Protein	4 kcal/g
Carbohydrates	4 kcal/g
Alcohol	7 kcal/mL

might be too much weight loss within the parameters of a caloric differential of 3500 kcal to lose 1 lb. That means that in order to net the 7000 kcal deficit for a 2-lb weight loss in one week, a person must increase his physical activity by 1000 kcal or decrease his food intake by 1000 kcal per day or some combination of both. Most literature on behavior change views these significant changes in lifestyle as unsustainable. A small amount of weight lost per week is discouraging to the obese person, while a large amount is potentially unattainable and unsustainable. Remind your patient that even a 10-lb weight loss can reduce negative health effects of obesity while reinforcing improvements in exercise and diet.

How do I efficiently debunk fad diets?

If fad diets worked in the long run, we would be a skinny country. But we have tried every variation of fad dieting, and we are most definitely not a skinny populace. What works over the long term is negative energy balance: physical activity that exceeds kcal consumed. Additionally, you must realize that there is a genetically determined weight range for individuals, so that every person will not be healthy at 120 lbs. Energy balance within one's genetic range will determine what one's weight will be, not a transient fad diet plan.

Many current fad diets are based on the drastic reduction in consumption of one of the macronutrients (protein, carbohydrate, or fat). Current studies have not shown any clear advantage to diets deficient in a particular macronutrient when compared to diets focused simply on reducing overall energy intake. The currently popular low-carbohydrate diets may result in an initially larger weight loss because of the fluid loss that occurs during the first few weeks, combined with the temporary effect of ketosis on reducing the appetite. When the low carbohydrate dieters compare to conventional dieters at one year, however, there is no significant difference in weight loss

When are medication and surgery indicated in obese adults?

The FDA has approved effective weight loss drugs (Table 54–2). These agents are indicated as *adjunctive treatment* (i.e., in addition to diet and activity modification) in patients with a BMI of 30 or greater, or in patients with a BMI of 27 or greater who have other obesity-related risk factors or diseases, such as cardiovascular disease, diabetes, or degenerative joint disease in weight-bearing joints.

Weight loss (bariatric) surgery is indicated in patients with a BMI of 40 or greater, or a BMI of 35 or greater with comorbid conditions. Surgery should be reserved for patients in whom other therapy has failed and who have clinically severe obesity (according to National Heart, Lung, and Blood Institute [NHLBI] guidelines). Bariatric

TABLE 54–2

Weight Loss Drugs

Drug	Dose	Action	Adverse Effect
Sibutramine (Meridia)	10 mg po qd to start, may be increased to 15 mg or decreased to 5 mg	Norepinephrine, dopamine, and serotonin re-uptake inhibitor; suppresses appetite	Increase in heart rate and blood pressure
Orlistat (Xenical)	120 mg po tid before meals	Inhibits pancreatic lipase; decreases fat absorption	Decrease in absorption of fat-soluble vitamins; soft stools and anal leakage

surgery carries many potential complications, some of which are related to the degree of obesity and the underlying medical condition of the patient. The NHLBI recommends integrated programs that offer guidance on exercise, nutrition, and psychosocial concerns both before and after surgery.

What are some simple tips for adults and children who are fighting obesity?

Children

- Limit television—watching television puts children at increased risk of obesity, relating to inactivity and increased caloric density of foods. The AAP recommends no more than one hour per day of TV for children up to the age of 2, and no more than two hours per day for all other children.
- Avoid "dieting" in children—fad diets are ineffective and can be dangerous in children. Specific diets promote poor self-esteem in children.

Adults

- Move more . . . whenever and however you can.
- Eat slowly! It takes 20 minutes before your stomach knows you have started to eat.
- Never supersize anything! Supersizing adds between 500 and 1000 kcal to the meal.
- Enjoy what you are eating.
- Do not eat continuously throughout the day.
- Do not skip meals.

- Watch out for highly processed foods because the more processing food undergoes, the more calories are added.
- Make your calories count—eat foods that fill you up and taste good.

KEY POINTS

- **Nutrients must be sufficient to prevent deficiency diseases and promote health.**
- **Excessive nutrient intakes will not necessarily promote better health.**
- **Energy balance is the key for weight management: Excess energy (food) intake beyond energy expenditure (physical activity plus basal metabolic rate) results in weight gain. Excess energy expenditure beyond energy intake results in weight loss.**

CASE 54–1. **A previously healthy 50-year-old man presents to the office with unexplained weight loss of 50 lb over the last four months. He also notes fatigue and occasional episodes of diarrhea. He denies any change in diet and does not take any medications. His height is 72 inches, weight six months ago was 225 lb (100 kg) (BMI = 30), and his current weight is 175 lb (78 kg) (BMI = 24). Other vital signs are normal. His physical examination is normal.**

A. What are the most likely potential etiologies of his weight loss?
B. What further evaluation would you obtain?

CASE 54–2. **A 45-year-old woman complains of inability to lose weight. She has tried two different versions of a low-carbohydrate diet with initial successful losses of up to 20 lb over two months. However, both times she gained back more weight than she lost after stopping the diets for several months. Her current height is 65 inches, and her weight is 170 lb (80 kg) (BMI = 29).**

A. How would you help the patient set a reasonable goal for weight loss?
B. What changes would you recommend she make to attain that goal?

REFERENCES

Clinical Guidelines on the Identification, Evaluation, and Treatment of Overweight and Obesity in Adults: The Evidence Report. The National Institutes of Health, National Heart, Lung, and Blood Institute. NIH Publication Number 98-4083, 1998.

Manson JE, Skerrett PJ, Greenland P, VanItallie TB: The escalating pandemics of obesity and sedentary lifestyle. Arch Intern Med 164:240–258, 2004.

USEFUL WEBSITES

Children's Nutrition Research Center at Baylor College of Medicine *http://www.bcm.tmc.edu/cnrc/index.html*

Directory of U.S. Federal Government Nutrition sites *http://www.nutrition.gov*

CDC Chronic Disease Prevention: Improving Nutrition and Increasing Physical Activity *http://www.cdc.gov/nccdphp/bb_nutrition*

Facts about Dietary Supplements from the NIH Clinical Center *http://www.cc.nih.gov/ccc/supplements*

Tufts University Nutrition Navigator *http://www.navigator.tufts.edu*

55

Pregnancy

Prior to pregnancy, what issues should I cover with my patients?

At each clinic visit you will have the opportunity to intervene in your patients' healthcare and help educate them. Prior to conception, several issues should be addressed with each potentially fertile female patient. Discussions should focus on recognizing conditions that could harm the woman or her fetus as well as identifying applicable interventions that could improve outcomes for either or both. Methods of recognizing harmful conditions might include taking a brief medical and surgical history including medicines currently in use by the patient (be sure to ask about herbal or alternative therapies), a family history looking for genetic conditions, a past obstetric and gynecologic history, and a direct questioning about the patient's desires for childbearing (Table 55–1). Finally, you may wish to do a nutritional assessment.

▶ EVALUATION

How is pregnancy diagnosed?

You should always ask any potentially fertile female about the possibility of pregnancy before rendering treatment. Most patients will present seeking confirmation of a positive home pregnancy test (urine) or with a complaint of a missed period and/or having other symptoms of pregnancy such as breast tenderness or nausea. You may order pregnancy tests in a variety of forms—mainly urine or serum tests (looking for the β-HCG molecule, the presence of which is equated with the pregnant state generally). In certain situations, such as a possible miscarriage, the level of human chorionic gonadotropin (HCG) can be measured and compared to other HCG levels in the same patient to look for trends. There are some physical findings that are traditionally discussed, such as Hegar's (softening of the uterine fundus and isthmus) and Chadwick's (cervical cyanosis) signs, but these are often unreliable. Ultrasound is a tremendous tool for diagnosing and dating a pregnancy and for help in managing certain complications of pregnancy.

TABLE 55–1

Historical Questions to Ask Your Patients at a Preconception Visit

Questions	Interventions
Any family history of genetic disorders?	Screen for sickle cell disease (other hemoglobinopathies), cystic fibrosis (other congenital diseases like Tay-Sach's disease), mental retardation (such as fragile X), or muscular dystrophies
At risk for STDs?	Screen for HIV, syphilis, or hepatitis, and ensure up-to-date vaccinations
Encourage positive health habits	Maintaining or normalizing body fat (body mass index), exercising, maintaining good eating habits including supplementation with folic acid (400 μg per day for reduction in risk of neural tube defects) through the first trimester of pregnancy
Review medical and surgical history	Optimize preexisting medical conditions management (e.g., diabetes or hypertension)
Review medication use	Adjust any potentially teratogenic or mutagenic medicines such as coumadin or antiseizure medications

What should I cover with the initial obstetrical exam?

Once pregnancy is confirmed, the patient's initial exam serves as a general health review of all medical, surgical, and familial conditions as well as a complete physical exam and antenatal counseling. Certain lab tests are also ordered.

You may use one of the many standard antepartum forms available to cover with the patient all the important areas and to highlight areas for additional evaluation. One such form is the American College of Obstetricians and Gynecologists (ACOG) Antepartum Record (Forms A–D) that highlights the patient's basic demographics, menstrual history, past obstetrical history, past medical history, genetic counseling, and initial physical exam. The record also includes a visit-to-visit flow sheet with problem list and a lab flow sheet. Each doctor's office or clinic that provides obstetrical services has adapted some variety of this form to cover these areas. Familiarize yourself with the form that your particular clinic uses.

When should a patient present for the initial obstetrical exam?

There is no one best answer here, but current recommendations are that the exam should be completed by 12 weeks estimated gestational age (take the first day of the patient's last menstrual period and add 84 days). By completing the exam in this window of opportunity, you should be able to accurately date the pregnancy, complete the historical and physical parts of the exam, and start any interventions in a reasonable fashion. Dietary supplementation with iron and folate should begin as soon as possible.

What are the initial obstetrical labs that are ordered?

The initial labs that are ordered include blood typing (ABO and Rh) and screening for prenatal antibodies (these tests help identify patients at risk for isoimmunization); hemoglobin and hematocrit (to set a baseline and to help monitor for anemia); Pap smear (to ensure cervical health); sexually transmitted disease screening (to rule out chlamydia, gonorrhea, rubella, hepatitis B, HIV, and syphilis); and a check for rubella immunity. You will find most of these labs listed on the preprinted antenatal form and can track them there. If you suspect your patient might be at risk for either a disease of the hemoglobin or a congenital illness based on her race or ethnic origin, then you should order the appropriate screening and track it also.

Usually two additional tests are ordered: a urine culture and sensitivity to check for cystitis and asymptomatic bacteriuria (ASB), and a wet prep (saline mount) of a vaginal swab looking for bacterial vaginosis (BV). ASB and BV can lead respectively to pyelonephritis and premature rupture of the membranes—either of which can seriously complicate the pregnancy.

▶ TREATMENT

What is the schedule of visits for the routine obstetrical patient?

After the initial visit, the patient is traditionally seen every 4 weeks until 28 weeks, then every 2 weeks until 36 weeks, and then weekly until delivery.

What should I cover with the patient at each obstetrical visit?

At each visit, inquire about any problems the patient has had, perform the appropriate exam, and record the data on the antepartum form.

The estimated gestational age (EGA) is calculated at each visit and recorded along with the patient's weight, blood pressure, and fundal height. The fundal height is accurate between 20 and 36 weeks to a plus/minus 2-week tolerance. It is measured from the top of the symphysis pubis in the midline to the top of the fundus. Also at each visit some effort should be made to listen to the fetus's heart tones. These are auscultatable as early as 8 weeks with the electronic fetal stethoscope, and should definitely be present at an EGA of 12 weeks if the patient's dates are accurate. As the patient progresses into the second and third trimesters, examine her for fetal presentation (is the fetus head up [breech] or head down) and, if appropriate, for cervical dilation or other signs of labor. Although some physicians have stopped checking urine for protein and glucose at each visit, this is still done by many.

Update the patient's lab flow sheet, answer any questions she has, and recheck her dating criteria to make sure you have an accurate EGA.

Of what basic precautions should each patient be aware during her pregnancy?

At least once during each pregnancy either you or a qualified counselor from the office should go over some or all of the following items with each patient and document her awareness of these issues:

Toxoplasmosis prevention—patient shouldn't handle cat feces and should avoid raw or partially cooked meats.

Exercise—pregnancy ends in labor, and good aerobic noncontact sport cardiovascular exercise plays an important role in health and well-being.

Travel restrictions—avoid traveling after 36 weeks (in case labor begins), and while traveling stretch the legs frequently (for instance take a 10-minute stretch break every 2 hours of traveling time) to avoid blood clots.

Heat—don't exercise to the point of overheating or heat exhaustion and avoid exposure to extreme heat sources such as hot tubs and saunas.

Intercourse during pregnancy—in an uncomplicated pregnancy, vaginal intercourse is safe and limited only by the patient's comfort level.

Substance abuse—the risk of alcohol, tobacco, and illicit drugs should be discussed and documented with the patient.

Safety—wearing and continued use of seat belts and shoulder harnesses.

Occupation—question the patient about her job and any workplace exposures that might endanger her baby's health and development.

Weight gain and nutrition—a gain of 25 to 35 lbs. in a pregnant woman with a single fetus is adequate. The hospital's dietitian could counsel her on caloric and nutritional supplementation as needed.

What other counseling might occur later on?

Counseling is an ongoing and never-ending process. There are two specific types of counseling: the trimester-dependent version and that which occurs at every visit. See previous text for information on counseling during the first trimester. Second trimester counseling would include mainly the labs that are performed during the second trimester—the triple screen, which looks for fetuses with trisomies (e.g., Down syndrome) and diabetes screening.

Counseling during the third trimester includes advising the patient on childbirth preparation (selecting a doctor for her baby, desire for instruction in labor and delivery plans, and breastfeeding preparation) and introducing the patient to the technique of fetal movement monitoring (as an indicator of fetal well-being).

General counseling about the warning signs of rupture of membranes, pregnancy-induced hypertension (PIH), and preterm labor (PTL) is conducted frequently. Remind the patient that if she experiences any leaking of fluid or any of the signs of PIH or PTL, she should contact her physician immediately.

What other labs are ordered later in the pregnancy?

The two key labs needed are the 24- to 28-week screening for gestational diabetes as well as perineal culture for group B strep (a major cause of neonatal infectious morbidity and mortality).

What are the leading causes of morbidity and mortality in the pregnant patient?

PTL with subsequent preterm delivery, PIH, hemorrhage, and deep venous thrombosis (DVT) and its sequelae, including pulmonary embolism, are the major complications seen in pregnancy. You might be able to reduce or more effectively deal with both PTL and DVT by educating and counseling the patient about the warning signs and the necessary steps the patient should take to deal with the signs.

More than 10% of all births in the United States are delivered preterm (delivery prior to 37 weeks EGA). Counsel the patient to present for evaluation when contraction frequency exceeds a certain level (six to eight contractions every hour), or when she experiences persistent repetitive back or pelvic pain, or leak of fluid.

Pregnancy-induced hypertension occurs in 6–8% of all pregnancies. Warn patients to report for evaluation when they have any symptoms of PIH. Symptoms include persistent headaches or visual disturbances, shortness of breath, epigastric and/or right upper quadrant pain, and a sudden change in edema (particularly of the hands and face). At each visit the patient's weight and blood pressure are monitored and may provide some clues. If the blood pressure exceeds 140 systolic or 90 diastolic after an EGA of 20 weeks or if the patient has significant proteinuria, then further laboratory investigation is warranted to try and complete the work-up for PIH.

Counseling on prevention of DVT and on presenting for symptoms of DVT (shortness of breath, leg edema [especially unilateral], or leg pain) is critically important because pulmonary embolism and death are complications of a DVT.

Hemorrhage is rarely preventable primarily, but should always be reported to the physician as it may herald placentation abnormalities (e.g., placenta previa) or preterm labor.

KEY POINTS

- **Anticipatory guidance is critical to successful pregnancy outcomes.**
- **Use of a standardized flow sheet will help to minimize errors of omission.**
- **Always consider the diagnosis of pregnancy in potentially fertile women.**
- **Correctly dating a pregnancy is crucial.**

CASE 55–1. **A 28-year-old woman presents to the emergency room complaining of painless vaginal bleeding. She is sexually active, not using contraception, and cannot remember when her last menstrual period was. Her vital signs are stable and a pregnancy test is positive.**

A. What is the next step in her management?
B. What is your differential diagnosis?
C. What tests would you order?

CASE 55–2. **A 22-year-old newlywed presents with her husband and wants to talk about preconception counseling.**

A. What medicine should you ensure she is taking?
B. What other factors should you review with them?

REFERENCE

American Academy of Pediatrics and the American College of Obstetricians and Gynecologists: Guidelines for Perinatal Care, 5th ed. Elk Grove Village, Ill: AAP, 2002.

56

Perioperative Care

► ETIOLOGY

What constitutes perioperative care?

Perioperative care refers to the process of assessing patient safety prior to surgical intervention by identifying key historical facts, physical exam findings, laboratory tests, and other studies that will help you and your surgeon stratify risk and permit correction/stabilization of any abnormalities.

► EVALUATION

What is the primary method of evaluating perioperative risk?

The combination of the type of surgery and the underlying condition of the patient determines perioperative risk. A detailed medical history is the single most important element in the perioperative assessment. It accounts for greater than 50% of all diagnoses associated with perioperative complications.

What cardiovascular factors should be assessed?

First and foremost, does your patient have known cardiac disease, such as coronary artery disease (CAD), heart failure (HF), hypertensive cardiomyopathy, a symptomatic arrhythmia, pacemaker, or an implantable cardioverter/defibrillator? Does he/she have cerebrovascular or peripheral vascular disease, which may be markers for underlying CAD? If he/she has known cardiac disease, is it active or stable?

What questions should be asked for a patient that has no known cardiac history?

For a patient with unknown CAD, determine if there are other risk factors such as smoking, diabetes mellitus, dyslipidemia, hypertension, or age 70 or older. It should be noted there is little evidence that hypertension alone presents a risk unless severe (class III, systolic >180 mmHg or diastolic > 110 mmHg). Also, age itself is not a risk but a marker for other underlying diseases. Further stratification of cardiac risk (MI, HF, death) by procedure and by clinical predictors is described in Box 56–1 and Box 56–2, respectively.

Under what circumstances would I postpone surgery in a cardiac patient?

You would postpone elective surgery in a patient with a recent (less than one month) myocardial infarction (MI), unstable or severe angina, uncompensated HF, critical aortic stenosis, third-degree heart block, or significant ventricular or symptomatic arrhythmia.

What noncardiac risks should be assessed in the history?

Other important medical conditions to ask your patient about and to look for in chart review are histories of chronic obstructive

BOX 56–1

Cardiac Risk* Stratification for Noncardiac Surgical Procedures

High (Reported cardiac risk often greater than 5%)

Emergent major operations, particularly in the elderly
Aortic and other major vascular surgery
Peripheral vascular surgery
Anticipated prolonged surgical procedures associated with large fluid shift and/or blood loss

Intermediate (Reported cardiac risk generally less than 5%)

Carotid endarterectomy
Head and neck surgery
Intraperitoneal and intrathoracic surgery
Orthopedic surgery
Prostate surgery

Low (Reported cardiac risk generally less than 1%)**

Endoscopic procedures
Superficial procedures
Cataract surgery
Breast surgery

*Combined incidence of cardiac death and nonfatal myocardial infarction.
**Do not generally require further preoperative cardiac testing. Adapted with permission from Eagle, et al.

BOX 56–2

Clinical Predictors of Increased Perioperative Cardiovascular Risk (Myocardial Infarction, Heart Failure, Death)

Major

Unstable coronary syndromes

- Acute or recent myocardial infarction* with evidence of important ischemic risk by clinical symptoms or noninvasive study
- Unstable or severe angina (Canadian class III or IV[†])

Decompensated heart failure
Significant arrhythmias

- High-grade atrioventricular block
- Symptomatic ventricular arrhythmias in the presence of underlying heart disease
- Supraventricular arrhythmias with uncontrolled ventricular rate

Severe valvular disease

Intermediate

Mild angina pectoris (Canadian class I or II)
Previous myocardial infarction by history or pathological Q waves
Compensated or prior heart failure
Diabetes mellitus (particularly insulin-dependent)
Renal insufficiency

Minor

Advanced age
Abnormal EKG (left ventricular hypertrophy, left bundle-branch block, ST-T abnormalities)
Rhythm other than sinus (e.g., atrial fibrillation)
Low functional capacity (e.g., inability to climb one flight of stairs with a bag of groceries)
History of stroke
Uncontrolled systemic hypertension

EKG = electrocardiogram
*Recent MI is >7 days but <30 days; acute MI is <7 days (American College of Cardiology National Database Library, 2004)
[†]Campeau L. Grading of angina pectoris. Circulation 54:522–523,1976.
Adapted with permission from Eagle, et al.

pulmonary disease (COPD), asthma, malignancy, thyroid disease, primary adrenal insufficiency, secondary adrenal suppression from corticosteroid use, mitral valve prolapse, chronic renal disease, and bleeding disorders. Elective surgery would be cancelled in patients with an acute exacerbation of COPD, unexplained dyspnea or cough, or an upper respiratory tract infection.

Other than predisposing conditions, what other respiratory risk factors should be considered?

The number one predictor of pulmonary complications (pneumonia, delayed ventilator weaning, unexpected intubation, and pulmonary embolism) is the surgical site. Surgeries closest to the diaphragm (upper abdomen and thorax) pose the greatest risk.

How can a history of a bleeding disorder be assessed?

The best screening test for bleeding is a history of excessive bleeding with previous minor trauma, surgery, or dental extractions. Easy bruising or heavy menses may also predict a bleeding disorder. Medical illnesses that increase the risk for operative and postoperative bleeding include liver, renal, and collagen vascular diseases. Is there a family history of bleeding or clotting disorders?

What questions should be asked about the patient's medication use?

A detailed review of the patient's medications is of paramount importance. Be sure to ask about medications that patients often do not think of as medication, such as aspirin, oral contraceptive pills, and over-the-counter drugs. Medication use can also be a clue to a diagnosis that was missed in the medical history or forgotten by the patient. Does the patient take vitamin and herbal supplements? Some medications will need to be stopped, others reduced, and still others increased to optimize outcomes (Table 56–1). Is there a history of allergies to medications or has the patient had a problem with sedatives or anesthetics in the past? Is there a family history of malignant hyperthermia?

What other aspects of the history may factor into preoperative risk assessment?

Does your patient smoke cigarettes? Smokers should stop eight weeks or more before surgery to decrease anesthesia complications as well as general morbidity. Stopping for less than eight weeks or merely reducing use is associated with a much greater incidence of postoperative pulmonary complications because of decreased sputum clearance. Is your patient dependent on alcohol? What is your assessment of his or her nutritional status? Patients with poor dentition, a chronic illness, depression, low-income, social isolation, frailness, and advanced age should be evaluated carefully for evidence of poor nutrition. Are they ambulatory and active? Patients with poor functional capacity have an increased risk of perioperative complications. Those unable to walk four blocks or climb two flights of stairs without symptomatic

TABLE 56–1

Perioperative Adjustment of Common Medications

Drug/Class	Number of Days to Stop Before Surgery
ASA	7
NSAIDs/Cox-2 inhibitors	3
Oral contraceptives[a]	28
Estrogen (HRT)	30
Herbal remedies	14
Antihypertensives[b]	Continue
Pulmonary metered-dose inhalers[c]	Continue
Diabetes (oral)[d]	Hold morning of; resume after regular diet post-op
Lipid-lowering	Hold morning of; resume after regular diet post-op
L-thyroxine	Hold morning of; resume after regular diet post-op
Coumadin[e]	INR <1.5 on day of surgery
Corticosteroids	Increase at time of surgery if chronic use; stress doses if taken during last 6 months

[a]Unless risk of unplanned pregnancy exceeds that of DVT
[b]Diuretics should not be given on day of surgery
[c]Unless asymptomatic and with clear lungs, may need to increase to optimize care
[d]Control blood glucose with insulin. Note: Patients on daily insulin at home are at higher risk for perioperative complications than those who do not need insulin.
[e]Prosthetic valve—change to heparin several days before surgery; atrial fibrillation—stop 2 to 3 days pre-op and restart when taking po postoperatively on day of surgery.

limitations are at nearly two times the risk for serious perioperative complications.

What components of the physical exam should be performed?

First, review the vital signs: blood pressure, pulse, respirations, and temperature. Hypertension should be controlled (see earlier section of this chapter). Is the patient's pulse regular and normal in rate? Are respirations normal? How does the patient's weight compare to previous measurements? Weight loss of 5% in the last month or 10% over the previous six months may indicate malnutrition. Does the patient have an active infection? Are there conditions of the oropharynx (such as loose teeth or problems opening the jaw) that might cause problems with intubation? Diminished breath sounds, prolonged expiration, wheezes, rhonchi, and rales can predict postoperative pulmonary complications in patients with COPD better than a chest x-ray or spirometry. Asthmatics should be free of wheezes with peak flows above 80% predicted. If a heart murmur is found in a patient without known valvular heart disease (VHD), further investigation is required. In someone with known VHD, endocarditis prophylaxis may be needed or an echocardiogram indicated for worsening aortic stenosis or other possible valvular abnormality. Is there a carotid bruit, which can be a sign of underlying cerebrovascular disease? Is the abdomen free of hepatosplenomegaly? Is there a mass or pulsatile enlargement of the aorta (abdominal aortic aneurysm)? Unexpected clubbing or peripheral edema would be suspicious for pulmonary or cardiac disease. Check for any hematomas, hemarthroses, or evidence of arthritis. Decreased mobility increases the risk of postoperative thrombotic disease. Is there superficial thrombophlebitis (frequently associated with varicose veins)? This is associated with an increased incidence of deep vein thrombosis and would necessitate an ultrasound of the deep veins? Does the skin exam reveal petechiae or ecchymotic areas that could indicate an underlying bleeding tendency?

What general lab tests are necessary in preoperative assessment?

The information in the history and exam is essential in directing appropriate testing. Generally, lab work performed in recent months does not need to be repeated in stable patients. Although nonselective testing is generally not effective, a complete blood count (CBC) tends to be a common preoperative test except in cases of minor surgery. Surgery would be delayed in patients with hemoglobin below 9 g/dL because this degree of anemia is associated with increased surgical mortality. Also, a patient's age can influence testing. Men over 45 and women over 55 with two or more atherosclerotic risk factors should have an EKG. Pathologic Q waves on the EKG put the patient at intermediate risk for cardiac mortality. Individuals 45 and older should also be screened for diabetes. Patients 75 or older should have a basic metabolic profile. A creatinine greater than 2 mg/dL confers increased perioperative risk. Further testing is based on the history and physical exam.

What specific history-based testing should be performed?

Patients with angina should be evaluated with an EKG and exercise treadmill test (ETT) or cardiac stress imaging for those unable to exercise. Individuals with minimal, intermediate, and those with no cardiac risk but who have poor functional capacity and are undergoing high-risk surgery should have an ETT. Patients having major vascular surgery are more likely to have underlying heart disease and should have more extensive cardiac testing with stress imaging. Diabetic patients need their glucose, electrolytes, and serum creatinine measured and an EKG. Those with thyroid disease should have a recent thyroid-stimulating hormone (TSH) documented. Unexplained murmurs require evaluation with an EKG and echocardiogram. Findings for bleeding risk should prompt a CBC (with a platelet count), prothrombin time (PT/INR), and partial thromboplastin time (PTT). Patients with risk factors or evidence of malnutrition should have a serum albumin measured and total lymphocyte count performed. A low serum albumin (less than 3.2 g/dL) or low total lymphocyte count (less than 3000 per μL^3) can be indicators of poor nutrition. All women of childbearing age should be screened for pregnancy.

What postoperative plans should be made prior to surgery?

One should anticipate the degree of postoperative pain and outline a treatment plan with the patient prior to surgery. Nutrition should be optimized. Malnourished patients and those without anything by mouth for 3 to 5 days preoperatively should receive enteral tube feedings or parental nutrition for 7 to 15 days before surgery. Proton pump inhibitors (PPIs) or H_2-blockers may be needed to decrease postoperative gastric/duodenal ulceration. It may be useful to prepare your patient to use incentive spirometry to help prevent or treat postoperative atelectasis and early fever. Starting patients with ischemic heart disease or risk factors for CAD on a β-blocker (if no contraindications, e.g., asthma, reactive airway disease, or bradycardia) weeks or even days before surgery and continuing it during the postoperative period significantly reduces myocardial infarctions and mortality. Perioperative supplemental oxygen during surgery and for two hours postoperatively reduces surgical wound infections. Systemic antibiotic prophylaxis is routinely given for head and neck surgery when the aerodigestive tract is opened, many abdominal surgeries, hysterectomies, joint and aortic valve replacement, and revascularization of lower extremities.

What postoperative physical exam components should be assessed?

Always check vital signs first including pain level. Postoperative fevers are divided into early (less than 48 hours) or late (greater than 48 hours). A postoperative fever is one greater than 38°C. Early postoperative fevers are usually noninfectious and often indicate atelectasis. One caveat is that a temperature greater than 39°C in the first 48 hours represents a necrotizing wound infection until proven otherwise. Late postoperative fever is often secondary to wound infection, urinary tract infection, or deep vein thrombosis (DVT). Often patients have tubes and drains that provide a portal of entry for infection. Listen for new murmurs (acute bacterial endocarditis), which should prompt blood cultures, an EKG, and an echocardiogram. Beware of drug fevers, signaled by temperature elevation related to start of a medication. These can be common with cephalosporins or in someone receiving repeated IM injections, especially hydroxyzine.

What are some common postoperative problems?

Other postoperative problems to watch for include wound dehiscence; an early sign is serosanguinous drainage day 3 to 5 postoperatively. Declining blood pressure or rising pulse may indicate blood loss or inadequate fluid replacement either during surgery or postoperatively. Pulmonary embolism (PE) is a common concern and may be heralded by dyspnea. Often the respiratory rate is normal but the heart rate may be elevated. Always keep in mind that normal oxygen saturation does not rule out PE. If the patient is symptomatic or you are suspicious of a PE, a spiral CT of the lungs is indicated.

What are risk factors to keep in mind in regard to postoperative DVT and PE?

Patients with a history of DVT or PE in the past, previous lower extremity or pelvic surgery, a high-risk surgical site (abdominal, pelvis, lower extremity), older patients, or trauma cases are at risk for thromboembolic disease. Additional risk factors are underlying HF, past MI, prolonged immobilization, paralysis, malignancy, clotting disorders, obesity, varicose veins, estrogen and oral contraceptive use, and pregnancy. These patients should receive DVT prophylaxis with low-molecular weight heparin 12 to 24 hours after surgery. Sequential compression devices and T.E.D. hose are possible adjuncts.

Why is pain an important concern during the postoperative period?

Pain is often invisible unless the patient is prompted using a visual analog scale. Up to 75% of hospital patients on intramuscular opioids do not receive adequate pain relief. Certain conditions, such as unstable angina, have increased morbidity when there is a lack of adequate pain control. Postoperative pain can cause detrimental psychological effects, such as an increased stress response. This, in turn, can lead to adverse physiological effects, such as elevation of catecholamines, systemic and coronary vasoconstriction, and metabolic shifts to a catabolic state (protein wasting, immunosuppression, and hypercoagulability). Pain from abdominal or thoracic surgery can compromise pulmonary function and be involved in the pathogenesis of postoperative ileus.

KEY POINTS

- **The condition of the patient combined with the type of surgery determines risk.**
- **Two thirds of diagnoses that place patients at increased risk for perioperative complications can be identified by the history and physical exam alone.**
- **Preoperative testing and imaging are guided by the history and physical exam.**
- **Smoking should be stopped at least eight weeks before surgery.**
- **Perioperative β-blockers save lives.**
- **A medication history is a key aid in identifying perioperative risk.**

CASE 56–1. A 50-year-old male, apparently healthy, presents for a preoperative exam prior to having an open cholecystectomy. He is scheduled for surgery in two weeks. During the history, you discover that his father and brother died of MI at ages 55 and 45, respectively. He has smoked one pack of cigarettes per day since age 17. He is asymptomatic but sedentary and unaware of his cholesterol level. On exam, he has an elevated body mass index (BMI) of 30 and a mildly elevated blood pressure of 140/92.

A. For what perioperative complications is your patient at risk?
B. What single laboratory test or study would be the best predictor of perioperative risk?
C. Should the patient stop smoking?
D. During his evaluation you determine that he has mild hypertension. Would you start him on a new medication (antihypertensive) before surgery?

CASE 56–2. **You are called to see a patient of yours in the emergency room who fell and fractured her right hip. Pending your evaluation, orthopedics has tentatively scheduled her for surgical repair that day. She is a 70-year-old woman with COPD. Albulterol and ipratropium bromide inhalers are her only routine medications. A few months ago, she did require a steroid taper for a COPD flare. She is active despite her COPD and has no history of angina or CAD. She gardens in the summer and plays doubles-tennis year round. She stopped smoking 20 years ago. There is no history of easy bruising. Her exam is remarkable for an elevated body mass index (BMI) of 28, unlabored respirations, a normal room air O_2 saturation, slightly decreased breath sounds, and a few scattered faint wheezes.**

A. Should your patient proceed with surgery as planned?
B. What potential postoperative complications concern you?
C. What preoperative medications would you give her?
D. What postoperative medications does your patient need?

REFERENCES

Carpenter RL: Optimizing postoperative pain management. Am Fam Physician 56:835–844, 1997.

Eagle KA, Berger PB, Calkens H et al.: ACC/AHA guideline update for perioperative cardiovascular evaluation for noncardiac surgery: executive summary. Circulation 105:1257–1267, 2002.

King MS: Preoperative evaluation. Am Fam Physician 62:387–396, 2000.

Norton LW, Stiegmann GV, Eiseman B: Surgical Decision Making. Philadelphia: WB Saunders, 2000.

Smetana GW: Preoperative pulmonary evaluation. N Engl J Med 340:937–944, 1999.

USEFUL WEBSITES

American College of Cardiology Foundation *http://www.acc.org/clinical/guidelines/perio/update/periupdate_index.htm*

American Academy of Family Physicians. This site has updated guidelines available for stratifying risk. *http://www.aafp.org*

57

School/Behavioral Problems—ADD/ADHD

▶ EPIDEMIOLOGY

How common are school behavior problems?

It is estimated that about 19% of children have some form of behavior problems or learning disabilities in school. The main players include learning disabilities (7–10%), ADHD (9%), emotional disturbances (5%), chronic illnesses (5%), and mental retardation (2–3%).

ATTENTION DEFICIT HYPERACTIVITY DISORDER/ ATTENTION DEFICIT DISORDER (ADHD/ADD)

▶ ETIOLOGY

What causes ADHD?

The cause of ADHD is multifactorial, without a known cause. The development of ADHD is found in the nature of the individual, and the nurturance he/she received. Some have attempted to link ADHD to maternal alcohol consumption during pregnancy, psychiatric issues surrounding the home environment, television watching, and laxity of rules.

▶ EVALUATION

What is the differential diagnosis?

The differential diagnosis of ADHD can be broken down into four categories. (1) *General medical* causes include vision or hearing, medication effects, asthma, enuresis/encopresis, hypothyroid, and lead toxicity. (2) *Neurologic* causes include learning disabilities, tic disorders, seizure disorders, developmental delays, brain injury, and sleep disorders. (3) *Psychiatric* causes include these disorders: oppositional defiant, conduct, anxiety, depression, obsessive compulsive, and substance abuse. (4) *Environmental* causes include parental psychopathology, family dysfunction, poor parenting, child abuse/neglect, and learning environment problems.

What should I ask about when seeing an ADHD patient?

The first step of the evaluation is a thorough history. The history helps you narrow your differential diagnosis. Pertinent questions include: (1) Is there a family history of learning disabilities, mental retardation, metabolic diseases, or degenerative neurologic diseases? (2) Did the child have any delays in reaching developmental milestones? If the child had developmental delay, the diagnosis of ADHD is less likely. (3) Does the child have any learning disabilities? Learning disabilities that go undiagnosed can cause children to become frustrated with their schoolwork. (4) Has the child ever been checked for vision or hearing disabilities? Vision and hearing difficulties cause children to cognitively develop slower than other children, causing frustration and attention deficit. (5) What is the family living situation like? (6) Are there any major causes of stress at home?

What should I do on a physical exam?

Special attention should be placed on observing the child at play while you are getting the history from the parent. Then focus on the eyes, ears, height, weight, head circumference, and neurologic exam. If there is no apparent organic cause for the behavior problems the next step is to evaluate the cognitive function of the child to assess if there is any learning disability or mental retardation. Children with ADHD can have below normal, normal, or even above normal IQs. At the same time, it is wise to do behavior-rating scales from both the school and home to assess the core ADHD symptoms that affect the child.

Should I be worried about anything else?

Approximately 40% to 50% of children with ADHD have at least one other psychiatric illness. The comorbid illnesses are oppositional defiant disorder (35%), conduct disorder (26%), anxiety disorder (26%), and depressive disorder (18%).

▶ DIAGNOSIS

How do I diagnose ADHD?

The diagnosis of ADHD is a clinical diagnosis of exclusion. It is the role of the physician to rule out any organic or other psychiatric cause for the behavior. There is no laboratory test for ADHD. The American Association of Psychiatry set forth guidelines in the DSM-IV to make the diagnosis of psychiatric illness uniform. Following are the criteria for the diagnosis of ADHD.

A. Criteria for the diagnosis of inattention is to have six or more of the following symptoms for at least six months:

- Fails to give close attention to details and/or makes careless mistakes.
- Difficulty sustaining attention on tasks or play activities.
- Doesn't seem to listen when spoken to directly.
- Doesn't follow through on instructions and fails to finish schoolwork and chores.
- Has difficulty organizing tasks and activities.
- Doesn't like or avoids engaging in tasks that require sustained mental effort.
- Often loses things necessary for tasks or activities (school assignments, pencils, books).
- Easily distracted by extraneous stimuli.
- Forgetful in daily activities.

B. Criteria for the diagnosis of hyperactivity-impulsivity is to have six or more of the following symptoms for at least six months:

- Fidgets with hands or feet or squirms in seat.
- Leaves seat in classroom or in other situations in which remaining seated is expected.
- Runs about or climbs excessively in situations in which it is inappropriate.
- Difficulty playing in leisure activities quietly.
- Is often "on the go" or often acts as if "driven by a motor".
- Talks excessively.
- Blurts out answers before questions have been completed.
- Difficulty waiting turn.
- Interrupts or intrudes on others.

In addition to meeting the criteria above, the child must show signs of hyperactivity and inattention before the age of 7 and for at least six months in duration and in two or more settings (school and home). He or she must be significantly impaired in social, academic, and occupational functioning. Finally, the physician must make sure that no other pervasive developmental or psychiatric disease is causing these symptoms.

▶ TREATMENT

What are some nonpharmacologic treatment options?

Psychosocial interventions encourage the child to participate in sports or other recreational activities that may promote self-esteem and improve positive relationships with peers and adults. The *behavioral interventions* include the use of positive rewards to encourage appropriate behaviors and reduce problem behaviors. The *educational interventions* are changes in academic work that breed success. Focus is placed on developing areas of strengths, adaptations are made for special needs, and knowledge and skill deficits are remediated.

What are the pharmacologic options for treatment?

There are currently many different medications available to treat ADHD. They have different half-lives, release mechanisms, and different side effect profiles. The most common drugs used are Ritalin (methylphenidate), Adderall (amphetamine-dextroamphetamine), Concerta (a purified form of methylphenidate), and Strattera.

The side effects of the stimulant medications include insomnia, appetite suppression, stomach pain, headache, decreased growth velocity, hypertension, and the worsening of tics (involuntary muscular movements).

OPPOSITIONAL DEFIANT DISORDER (ODD)

How do I diagnose ODD?

Oppositional defiant disorder is a condition that is usually a comorbid condition with another psychiatric disease. However, it can present by itself. The DSM-IV criteria for the diagnosis of ODD is the observation of a pattern of negativistic, hostile, and defiant behavior lasting at least six months, during which four (or more) of the following are present:

Often loses temper.
Often argues with adults.
Often actively defies or refuses to comply with adults' requests or rules.
Often deliberately annoys people.
Often blames others for his/her mistakes or misbehavior.
Is often easily annoyed by others.
Is often angry and resentful.
Is often spiteful or vindictive.

In addition to meeting the criteria above, the behavior must cause clinically significant impairment in social, academic, or occupational functioning. The physician must also rule out other psychiatric or organic causes for the behavior. Finally, these behaviors must be evident before the age of 18; otherwise the diagnosis is antisocial personality disorder.

CONDUCT DISORDER

How do I diagnose conduct disorder?

Conduct disorder is a condition that is usually a comorbid condition with another psychiatric disease. However, it can present by itself. The DSM-IV criteria for the diagnosis of conduct disorder is the repetitive and persistent pattern of behavior in which the basic rights of others or major age-appropriate societal norms or rules are violated, as manifested by the presence of three (or more) of the following criteria in the past 12 months, with at least one criterion present in the past 6 months:

Often initiates physical fights
Has used a weapon that can cause serious physical harm to others.
Has been physically cruel to people.
Has been physically cruel to animals.
Has stolen while confronting a victim (mugging, purse snatching, armed robbery).
Has forced someone into sexual activity.
Has deliberately engaged in fire setting with the intention of causing serious damage.
Has deliberately destroyed others' property.
Has broken into someone else's house, building, or car.
Often lies to obtain goods or favors or to avoid obligations ("cons" others).
Has stolen items of nontrivial value without confronting a victim (shoplifting, forgery).
Often stays out at night despite parental prohibitions, beginning before age 13.
Has run away from home overnight at least twice while living at home.
Is often truant from school, beginning before age 13.

In addition to meeting the criteria above, the behavior must cause clinically significant impairment in social, academic, or occupational functioning. The physician must also rule out other psychiatric or organic causes for this behavior. Finally, these behaviors must be evident before the age of 18; otherwise the diagnosis is antisocial personality disorder.

What is the difference between a learning disability and mental retardation?

When a learning disability is present, a child has a very difficult time with a particular subject or life skill. However, they can perform all other subjects and skills at normal or often above normal levels. The etiology of learning disabilities is multifactorial and often difficult to determine. These disabilities could stem from perinatal insults, developmental insults, physical abnormalities (eyes, ears, limbs), genetic predisposition, or a number of other causes.

Mental retardation is defined by having an IQ of less than 70. There are different severities of mental retardation, but the intellectual deficit is over the entire range of cognition (unlike learning disabilities). Children with mental retardation are also significantly below average in two of the following: communication, home living, self-care, social skills, community involvement, self-direction, health and safety awareness, functional academics, and leisure and work skills.

KEY POINTS

- **To be diagnosed with ADHD, the child has to be under the age of 7, have symptoms longer than six months, and show symptoms in two or more settings.**
- **Learning disabilities are evident in a particular subject or skill. Mental retardation is difficulty with all subjects and skills.**
- **In children with ADHD, look for other comorbid psychiatric illnesses; 40% to 50% of the children will have them.**
- **Conduct disorder comprises actions that are illegal and cause harm. ODD features actions of annoyance to others but no physical harm or illegality.**

CASE 57–1. **A 6-year-old boy is brought into the clinic by his mother at the request of the school. The teacher had informed the mother that the child is having difficulty in class. He often gets up out of his chair and begins to play with toys during class. When he is engaged in class, he often offers the answer without first raising his hand and isn't good about waiting his turn. The teacher notes that he is unable to complete an art project because he is easily distracted by other kids in the room. The mother confirms these behaviors also occur at home. During the interview you observe the child acting very busy in the room, looking into cabinets and removing items. He interrupts his mother while she is trying to talk to you. On exam, his vitals are normal and there are no abnormalities noted.**

A. What is your differential diagnosis?
B. What other questions would you like to ask the mother to make your diagnosis?
C. Do any further labs or tests need to be done at this time?
D. What are the treatment options for this child?
E. What are the side effects of the treatments?

CASE 57–2. **An 11-year-old boy is brought into the clinic by his mother for behavior problems. He has been in trouble at school off and on for the past year. His mother informs you that the school teacher is becoming tired of his short temper and refusal to follow directions. He often tries to annoy other classmates on purpose and then blames them for what happened. His vital signs are temperature 36.5°C, blood pressure 100/82, respirations 20, heart rate 96. Exam is normal.**

A. What could be the cause of this child's symptoms?
B. What other questions need to be asked?
C. Is there any lab work that needs to be drawn?
D. How would you treat this child?
E. What is the prognosis?

REFERENCES

Herrerias C, Perrin J, Stein M: The child with ADHD: Using the AAP clinical practice guidelines. Am Fam Physician 63:1803–1810, 2001.

Phillips D, Longlett S, Mulrine C et al.: School behavior problems and the family physician. Am Fam Physician 59:2816–2824, 1999.

Smucker W, Hedayat M: Evaluation and treatment of ADHD. Am Fam Physician 64:817–829, 2001.

USEFUL WEBSITES

National Institute of Mental Health. *http://www.nimh.nih.org*

American Academy of Pediatrics. *http://www.aap.org*

58

Seizures

▶ ETIOLOGY

What is a seizure?

Seizures are individual discrete events resulting from abnormal rhythmic neuronal discharges in the brain. Seizures are symptoms of brain dysfunction, which may range from a minor transient dysfunction in an otherwise normal brain (e.g., hyponatremia or drug withdrawal) to temporarily or permanently altered brain tissue. Epilepsy, or seizure disorder, refers to an enduring tendency to seizures and is characterized by the spontaneous recurrence of seizures.

What types of seizures exist?

There are two main categories of seizures: (1) *generalized*, involving the whole cerebral cortex and leading to loss of consciousness; and (2) *partial* (or focal), originating in one region of the brain without loss of consciousness. Partial seizures are subdivided into *simple* partial seizures, originating in a small region of cortex and causing specific symptoms but no alteration of consciousness, and *complex* partial seizures, originating in a larger region and leading to alteration but not loss of consciousness.

How frequently are seizures seen?

Approximately 5% to 10% of the population will have at least one seizure. However, age-specific incidence rates are highest in childhood and decline to a steady level in 20- to 60-year-olds.

▶ EVALUATION

Describe the history-taking when caring for a patient who has had a seizure.

First, verify that a seizure occurred. Next, determine the circumstances under which the seizure occurred. If necessary, use specific questions to elicit pertinent information.

Was the episode preceded by localized sensory or motor phenomena, nausea, or light-headedness?

Any type of warning or aura before a seizure indicates a focal-onset seizure. In contrast, generalized seizures are not associated with a warning.

Did the patient lose consciousness?

If the patient did not obviously lose consciousness during the episode, it was either not a seizure or was a partial seizure or absence type generalized seizure.

If not, was consciousness altered?

By definition, simple partial seizures are not associated with altered consciousness but complex partial seizures are.

If consciousness was altered but not lost, did the episode include staring and unresponsiveness, lip smacking, picking at the clothes, hand wringing, or other motor manifestations?

During a typical complex partial seizure, the patient will appear "out of touch" for 30 to 90 seconds, and will display automatisms such as lip smacking, etc.

Did the patient have generalized stiffness (tonic contraction) or rhythmic muscle movements (clonic contractions)?

A typical generalized tonic-clonic seizure begins with a loss of consciousness and a tonic phase, which consists of generalized stiffening of the body and extremities. The tonic phase will merge with the clonic phase of high amplitude rhythmic jerks.

How long did each component of the episode last?

Typical absence seizures usually last less than 15 seconds, partial and generalized seizures usually last about 30 seconds to 3 minutes, and pseudoseizures often last more than 10 minutes.

How quickly did the patient return to normal after the spell ended?

Simple partial seizures and absence seizures are not typically associated with postictal confusion. Complex partial seizures are commonly associated with postictal confusion and sleepiness. The postictal state following generalized tonic-clonic seizures is characterized by transient stupor, confusion, and sleepiness that lasts minutes to hours.

Ask about possible risk factors and predisposing events. Risk factors for seizures include a history of febrile seizures and a family history of seizures. Predisposing events include prior head trauma, stroke, tumor, or vascular malformation. Possible precipitating events include sleep deprivation, electrolyte or metabolic abnormalities, systemic disease, acute infection, alcohol, and use of either medications or illegal drugs.

What should I look for during the physical examination?

Perform a complete general physical examination to look for signs of systemic disease, infection, and trauma. Look for signs of head and other trauma, alcohol or illicit drug use, chronic liver or renal disease, and disorders associated with cerebrovascular disease. Identification of a neoplasm that has a high predisposition to CNS metastasis is particularly relevant.

Perform a thorough neurological examination focused on finding deficits suggesting a cerebral lesion. Abnormalities in the visual fields suggest lesions in the optic pathways or occipital lobes. A contralateral superior visual field defect helps identify temporal lobe–originating seizures. Abnormal or asymmetrical findings on motor examination or deep tendon reflexes suggest lesions in the frontal (motor) cortex. If nystagmus or ataxia is present, consider possible drug toxicity.

Which laboratory testing is appropriate?

A complete blood count and standard chemistry battery (e.g., electrolytes, magnesium, calcium, glucose, creatinine, liver enzymes) are indicated in a patient presenting with an unexplained seizure. An electroencephalograph (EEG) is required in the evaluation of patients with suspected epilepsy. The first EEG results are abnormal in about 25% of patients with seizures. Because the results will still be normal after as many as seven EEGs in 40% of patients with definite seizures, a normal EEG does not exclude the diagnosis of epilepsy. If a routine EEG does not reveal abnormalities, consider ordering an EEG after a night of sleep deprivation.

Order magnetic resonance imaging (MRI) in all patients with partial seizures. All adults with unexplained new-onset seizures should undergo a brain imaging study to determine whether an underlying structural lesion is responsible. Invasive testing is rarely required.

How do I distinguish seizures from other problems?

A careful history, neurologic examination, EEG, and, if necessary, neuroimaging usually clarify the diagnosis. Because the differentiation between seizures and disorders that may mimic seizures is often based primarily on history, the importance of obtaining an eyewitness account cannot be overemphasized. Conditions that can mimic seizure include syncope (cardiac, vasovagal, reflex), transient ischemic attacks and stroke, migraine (classic, common, basilar), vertigo, sleep disorders (terrors, myoclonus, hallucinations, paralysis, walking), and pseudoseizures secondary to psychiatric disease (hysteria, Munchausen syndrome, conversion disorder).

What tools are available to help me make the diagnosis?

See Figure 58–1.

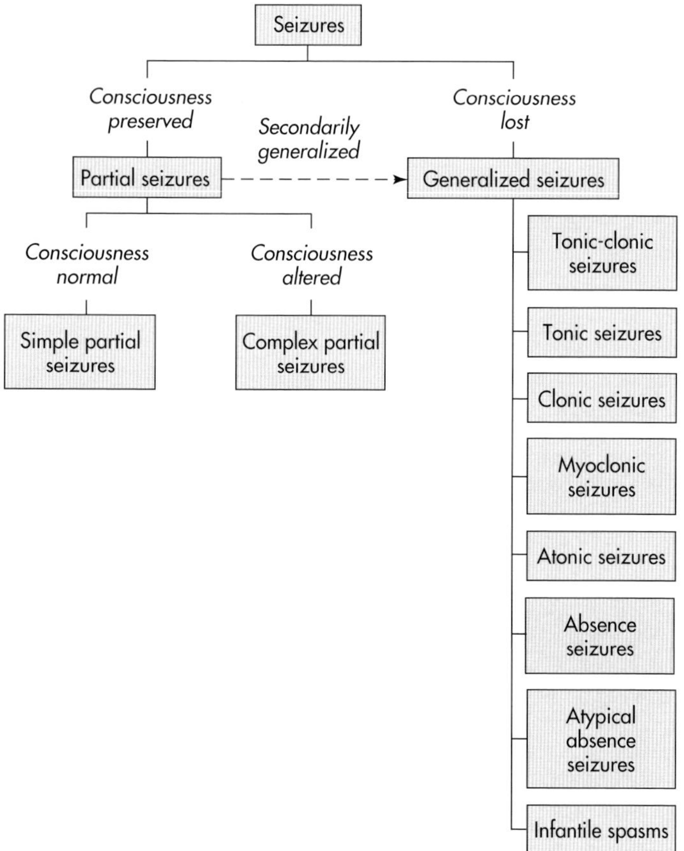

Figure 58–1. Flowchart of International League Against Epilepsy (ILAE) seizure classification. From: Dreifuss FE, Bancaud J, Henriksen O et al.: Proposal for the revised clinical and electroencephalographic classification of epileptic seizures. Epilepsia 22:489–501, 1981.

▶ TREATMENT

How are seizures managed?

- In a patient presenting acutely with an unexplained seizure, first determine whether there is an acute medically or surgically amenable cause of the seizure.
- Treat the patient who is still seizing upon emergency department arrival for *status epilepticus*. Continuous seizure activity lasting more than 30 minutes, or intermittent seizure activity without return of consciousness between episodes lasting more than 60 minutes, can cause permanent brain injury. Because most seizures typically stop within 3 minutes, seizures that last more than 10 minutes, or long enough for the patient to get to the emergency department, should be treated as status epilepticus.
- Educate patients with seizure disorders about how to avoid injury during seizures. Teach patients who have warning signs before their seizures to take immediate precautions to protect themselves from falling.

Describe medical therapy for the patient with seizures.

Expect most patients to respond well to one or more antiepileptic drugs (AEDs). However, not all seizures need to be treated with AEDs. For example, seizures secondary to a metabolic derangement are generally responsive to treatment of the underlying metabolic disorder. Also, patients who present with a first unexplained generalized tonic-clonic seizure and have a normal neurological examination, EEG, and MRI have a 70% chance of no recurrence and may elect to not be treated until after they have had a second seizure. In general, optimal treatment is based on accurate classification of seizure type and epilepsy syndrome. *Conventional AEDs* have been available for many years. This group includes phenobarbital, primidone, phenytoin, carbamazepine, and valproate. The drug of choice for most generalized-onset epilepsy syndromes is valproate. The most responsive of the generalized seizures are absence seizures, which usually respond to valproate or ethosuximide.

KEY POINTS

- **History, neurological examination, and EEG may help with diagnosis of seizures.**
- **Conditions like syncope, stroke, migraine, vertigo, sleep disorders, and pseudoseizures secondary to psychiatric disease may mimic seizures.**
- **When taking care of a patient with a seizure, determine whether there is an acute medically or surgically amenable cause of the seizure.**

CASE 58–1. **A 35-year-old man is experiencing nausea and light-headedness, which began after an upper airway infection two weeks ago. He says that people told him he begins lip smacking immediately for a short duration. The patient says he is not aware of this, but feels strange and tired sometimes during the day. His personal history revealed a history of febrile convulsion during childhood. His physical was normal.**

A. What might be the possible diagnosis?
B. Which factors might affect the patient?
C. Would you order a test?

CASE 58–2. **A 60-year-old woman was brought by her relatives to the emergency service. The patient was reported to have fallen unconscious to the ground and displayed rhythmic muscle movements for two minutes. She has been in a deep sleep for the past hour.**

A. What is the differential diagnosis for this patient?
B. What physical findings and history are you expecting of this patient?
C. What is your medical treatment strategy for this patient?

REFERENCES

Berg AT, Testa FM, Levy SR, Shinnar S: Neuroimaging in children with newly diagnosed epilepsy: a community-based study. Pediatrics 106(3):527–532, 2000.

Deckers CLP, Genton P, Sills GJ, Schmidt D: Current limitations of antiepileptic drug therapy: a conference review. Epilepsy Research 53:1–17, 2003.

Dreifuss FE, Bancaud J, Henriksen O et al.: Proposal for the revised clinical and electroencephalographic classification of epileptic seizures. Epilepsia 22:489–501,1981.

Markand ON: Pearls, perils, and pitfalls in the use of the electroencephalogram. Seminars in Neurology 23(1):7–44, 2003.

Steinhoff BJ, Hirsch E, Mutani R, Nakken KO: The ideal characteristics of antiepileptic therapy: an overview of old and new AEDs. Acta Neurologia Scandinavica 107:87–95, 2003.

Wheless JW: Acute management of seizures in the syndromes of idiopathic generalised epilepsies. Epilepsia 44(Suppl.2):22–26, 2003.

USEFUL WEBSITES

Epilepsy Foundation. Epilepsy: A report to the nation. *http://www.efa.org/epusa/nation/nation.html*

Fountain NB: Seizure. Best Practice of Medicine. April 2001. *http://merck.praxis.md*

59

Substance Abuse

What are the basic facts of substance abuse?

The etiology of substance abuse is extremely varied. Some common causes are genetic predisposition, chronic marital and family stress, situational stressors (e.g., unemployment), physical and mental illness, social influences, and peer pressure. Substance use problems take on many forms including misuse, abuse, and dependence. Alcohol, prescription drugs, illegal drugs, and other substances (e.g., glue, gasoline, propellants) can all be used for their stimulating or sedating effects. The highest rates of illicit drug use are found in the 16- to 20-year-old age group (35.6%), with marijuana as the most commonly abused drug. Alcohol is the third leading cause of preventable mortality, contributing to 100,000 deaths annually. The 18- to 29-year-old age group includes the highest prevalence of problem drinkers. Substance abuse can be found in families of all socioeconomic, racial, and ethnic groups.

The impact of the substance on the individual and the family depends on the type of drug, length of use, amount being used, and any comorbid conditions. Physicians need to regularly include substance abuse screening in their encounters with patients. Denial is often a complicating factor when working with these individuals and families, so physicians must provide a safe, nonjudgmental environment so patients can share their struggles. Successful intervention with these patients is based on: (1) the individual's desire to stop, (2) effective detoxification, (3) treatment of dual diagnoses, (4) inpatient or outpatient treatment, and (5) relapse prevention.

▶ EVALUATION

What issues are important to consider during initial screening?

It is important to identify the individual's level of substance use.

Substance misuse: Occasional excessive use of a legal or illegal substance.

Substance abuse: A maladaptive pattern of substance use occurring within a 12-month period leading to impairment in social, occupational, or interpersonal functioning or legal problems.

Substance dependence: A maladaptive pattern of substance use occurring within a 12-month period, leading to significant impairment or distress and characterized by either tolerance (need for markedly increased amounts of the substance or marked diminished effect with continued use of the same amount of substance) or withdrawal (even if withdrawal does not happen because the patient uses a substance to relieve or avoid withdrawal symptoms).

A common and simple way to screen for alcohol use is to use the ***CAGE*** mnemonic (one positive response indicates high risk for abuse):

C: Have you ever felt that you ought to *cut* down on your substance usage?
A: Have you ever been *annoyed* by people criticizing your substance use?
G: Have you ever felt *guilty* or bad about your substance use?
E: Have you ever had to use the substance first thing in the morning to get your day going, steady your nerves, or to treat a hangover (*eye opener*)?

How do I screen for abuse of other substances?

It is important to ask patients if they use any substances that are illegal (e.g., cocaine, methamphetamine, designer drugs) or in a manner for which the medicine was not prescribed (e.g., benzodiazepine abuse). Three questions that are believed to be helpful are:

Have you used street drugs more than five times in your life?
In the last year, have you ever used drugs more than you meant to?
Have you felt you wanted or needed to cut down on your drug use in the last year?

A positive response to any of these questions signals a need for a more thorough evaluation.

What are the stages of readiness for change? How are they important?

If the care provider can identify the patient's stage of readiness for changing the problem behaviors, he or she will be better able to intervene at the appropriate level. The goal should be to help the patient progress to the next stage. The stages of change are:

Precontemplation: Has not considered that a substance use problem exists.
Contemplation: Has wondered whether or not the use is a problem and considered changing use-related behaviors.

Preparation: Is beginning to formulate a plan to stop or otherwise change substance use behaviors.
Action: Has begun making behavioral/situational changes.
Follow-up: Continued implementation/alteration of plan, despite possible setbacks.

How do I know if the patient has an alcohol problem?

Evaluate current drinking patterns: Does the patient drink alcohol? How many days per week? How much is consumed each time? (A typical drink is 1.5 ounces of hard liquor, 5 ounces of table wine, or 12 ounces of regular beer.) What is the maximum number of drinks consumed on any given day in the last month?

Current guidelines state that an adult male less than age 65 is at risk for alcohol-related problems if he has 14 or more drinks per week, or more than 5 on a given day. Both males over age 65 and females in general are at risk if they have 7 or more drinks per week or 4 or more drinks during any given day.

What else do I need to assess when working with alcohol and substance abusers?

It is important to screen patients for comorbid psychological disorders. Depression, bipolar disorder, schizophrenia, anxiety, victims of abuse, marital and family dysfunction, and post-traumatic stress disorders are common comorbid conditions. These conditions, if left untreated, hamper substance treatment efforts.

▶ TREATMENT

What does substance abuse treatment involve?

While a majority of patients with addictions resolve their substance problems independent of formal treatment plans or professional help, some people choose or appear to need formal treatment of one kind or another. Treatment for substance use problems depends on an understanding of the etiology, as well as an assessment of the level of problem severity. Some professionals in the field believe that substance abuse is a disease over which the person has little or no control. Consequently, these disease model proponents typically prescribe treatment involving a medical exam, medical management of detoxification, total abstinence, and a 12-step treatment program (e.g., Alcoholics Anonymous).

How do 12-step programs approach treatment of addiction?

Programs such as Alcoholics Anonymous are organized according to 12 treatment steps that the alcoholic/addict must take in order to recover fully. Core beliefs of this approach include that the alcoholic/addict will always be "one drink away" from the downward spiral of addiction, the necessity of relying on a higher power, and the philosophy that recovery is a "one day at a time" proposition. The disease model also addresses the effect of addiction on the family members of alcoholics/addicts. Most communities in the United States have 12-step groups and many formal treatment programs incorporate this approach to some degree.

Describe the concept behind the non-disease model.

Other addiction specialists treat these problems from a psychological/behavioral point of view. The Moderation Management and Rational Recovery movements are two related examples of this type of approach. The idea is that not everyone who recognizes that alcohol and/or drug use is a problem is a full-blown alcoholic/addict. Most people whose alcohol or drug use is a problem (perhaps the majority mentioned earlier who quit without formal treatment) can choose to not use alcohol or drugs, or even to moderate their use in order to minimize the negative impact.

Moderation Management (MM) is a behavioral change program and support group for people concerned about their drinking and who desire to make positive lifestyle changes. It is billed as an approach for people who don't consider themselves "out-of-control alcoholics," but do recognize a need to moderate or discontinue their drinking behavior. MM promotes early self-recognition of risky drinking behavior, when moderate drinking is a more easily achievable goal. The MM movement provides information and support groups to those who are intent on changing their problematic behavior. Rational Recovery (RR) has a similar philosophy. The core beliefs of RR include that planned abstinence is a skill, anyone can learn to be abstinent, and that psychosocial problems are likely a result of the addiction and not the cause.

What medications can be used for the treatment of substance abuse?

As an adjunct to psychological treatment of substance abuse, medication can be beneficial. Currently, nalmefene (Revex) and naltrexone (ReVia) are the most effective agents for minimizing the craving for alcohol's sedative effects. Disulfiram (Antabuse) has been found to decrease frequency of use but is no better than placebo in attaining abstinence. Benzodiazepines are commonly used to treat withdrawal symptoms during detoxification. Methadone, naltrexone, suboxone, and subutex have all been used to treat opiate addictions. The comorbid conditions described earlier should be adequately treated with antidepressant, antianxiety, and mood stabilizing agents.

KEY POINTS

- **Substance abuse is common; therefore, regular screening is necessary.**
- **Provide nonjudgmental, medically-based education and support.**
- **Check the patient's stage of readiness for changing behaviors.**
- **Negotiate behavior change progress and treatment with the patient.**

CASE 59–1. **A 53-year-old man is brought to the emergency department by his wife and son. He is combative, hallucinating, and disoriented. His wife states that he has had a drinking problem for the past 25 years (approximately six to eight beers a day). She tells you that his father died of cirrhosis the previous week, prompting her husband to finally decide to stop drinking. He had his last drink a day and a half ago.**

A. What is the most likely problem for this patient?
B. What should be done for this patient medically?
C. What is the most appropriate treatment plan for this patient upon discharge from the hospital?

CASE 59–2. **A 20-year-old male is brought to the hospital by his parents. They report that they found him two hours ago very agitated and hallucinating, and when he started to have convulsions they brought him to the ER. You note that his body temperature is 38.8°C, and his skin is clammy. He is continuing to have hallucinations with intermittent convulsions. He has increased heart rate with intermittent irregular heartbeat, increased respiratory rate, elevated blood pressure, dilated pupils, loss of coordination, and collapse. There is no alcohol noted on his breath.**

A. What is most likely the cause of this person's symptoms?
B. What should be done medically to treat this patient?
C. What is the most appropriate treatment plan for this individual when he leaves the hospital?

REFERENCES

Brown RL, Rounds LA: Conjoint screening questionnaires for alcohol and other drug abuse: Criterion validity in primary care practice. Wisconsin Medical Journal 94:135–140, 1995.

McGinnis J, Foege W: Actual causes of death in the United States, JAMA 270(18): 2208, 1993.

National Institute on Alcohol Abuse and Alcoholism (NIAAA), Alcohol Health & Research World 18(3): 243, 1994.

National Institute on Drug Abuse (NIDA), 1997 National Household Survey on Drug Abuse.

Roberts L, McCrady B: Alcohol problems in intimate relationships: Identification and intervention. National Institute on Alcohol Abuse and Alcoholism, 2003.

USEFUL WEBSITES

Alcoholics Anonymous (AA). *http://www.alcoholics-anonymous.org*
Moderation Management. *http://www.moderation.org*
Narcotics Anonymous/Nar-Anon Family Group. *http://www.na.org*
Rational Recovery. *http://www.rational.org*

60

Sexually Transmitted Diseases

▶ ETIOLOGY

What are the causes of genital ulcers?

The most common causes of genital ulcers are genital herpes, syphilis (caused by *Treponema pallidum)*, and chancroid (caused by *Haemophilus ducreyi*). Genital herpes generally causes a very tender ulcer, as does chancroid, while the ulcers of syphilis are not painful. Other ulcer-causing infections, though occurring rarely in the United States, include granuloma inguinale, caused by *Calymmatobacterium granulomatis,* and lymphogranuloma venereum (LGV), caused by *Chlamydia trachomatis.* LGV more commonly manifests itself as enlarged tender inguinal lymph nodes, however.

What are some other symptoms of syphilis?

Patients infected with syphilis may present in one of three stages. In the primary infection stage (usually several days to a few weeks following initial infection), they will experience the painless genital ulcer or chancre. If they exhibit secondary syphilis (six to eight weeks following healing of the chancre), they may develop rashes on the skin, lymphadenopathy, and/or mucocutaneous lesions. In the case of tertiary syphilis (arising months to years following initial infection), patients may exhibit gummatous lesions, cardiac, ophthalmologic, or neurologic abnormalities. Patients may enter a latent phase in which no symptoms are apparent even though they are still infected.

What are the causes of urethritis and cervicitis?

In the case of these conditions, patients may have noticeable mucopurulent discharge, dysuria, or may be asymptomatic (especially females). The two predominant causes of such symptoms are *Neisseria gonorrhoeae* and *Chlamydia trachomatis.*

What is pelvic inflammatory disease (PID)?

Pelvic inflammatory disease (PID) is an infection of the upper female genital tract. It is most often caused by *N. gonorrhoeae* and *C. trachomatis,* but has also been associated with genital flora (such as *Gardnerella vaginalis, Ureaplasma urealyticum, Mycoplasma hominis,* and gram-negative rods). Symptoms vary among patients, from mild pelvic pain to fever, nausea and vomiting, discharge, abnormal vaginal bleeding, and severe abdominopelvic pain. PID has also been associated with subsequent infertility, often caused by scarring of the uterus and fallopian tubes, so it is very important to recognize and treat it.

What causes genital warts?

Genital warts are caused by the human papillomavirus (HPV), which is the same virus that is associated with cervical cancer. There are more than 30 serotypes of this virus, but only a few of them (16, 18, 31, 33, 35) are associated with cervical cancer. Genital warts may be found on the external genitalia, cervix, vagina, anus, or mouth.

What are the causes of other sexually transmitted diseases (STDs) not necessarily manifested by genital symptoms?

Other sexually transmitted infections include human immunodeficiency virus (HIV), hepatitis B, and hepatitis C. Diagnosis and treatment of these diseases is outside the scope of this chapter, but should be considered if another STD diagnosis is made on a patient.

▶ EVALUATION

What historical factors are important to elicit from the patient?

Ask the patient about recent change in sexual partners, history of prior infections, new lesions, fevers, use of condoms, and dyspareunia. If the patient is female, ask about menstrual history, especially last menstrual period.

What physical examination should be performed when evaluating for STDs?

Examine the mouth and oropharynx for lesions. Perform a thorough abdominal exam, including a search for inguinal lymphadenopathy. Examination of the external genitalia for ulcers, warts, and discharge is also important. In women, perform a careful pelvic examination looking for vaginal and cervical lesions. During the bimanual exam, assess for cervical motion tenderness and adnexal masses. In both male and female patients, a rectal examination should be performed in suspected cases of STDs.

What tests might be done to determine the underlying cause of a genital ulcer?

Important tests include serology for syphilis (RPR testing), darkfield exam of the ulcer exudate for *T. pallidum,* and culture of the ulcer for herpes and *H. ducreyi* (if chancroid is prevalent in the area).

What tests might be done to determine the underlying cause of cervicitis, urethritis, or PID?

A specimen may be taken from the cervical os or the meatus of the penis using a swab and culture medium to evaluate for gonorrhea and chlamydia. In females, a wet mount and KOH prep of vaginal secretions should be performed to evaluate for bacterial vaginosis and candidiasis.

How is pelvic inflammatory disease diagnosed?

It is difficult to diagnose PID, because there is a wide range of symptoms in patients with the disease. The minimum criteria for clinical diagnosis are uterine or adnexal tenderness, and cervical motion tenderness. Additional findings that support the diagnosis of PID include temperature above 38.3°C, abnormal cervical or vaginal mucopurulent discharge, white blood cells on wet prep of vaginal secretions, laboratory diagnosis of gonorrhea or chlamydia, and elevated c-reactive protein or erythrocyte sedimentation rate. Finally, more specific evidence may be found by utilizing more invasive tests. For example, an endometrial biopsy may be done, which would reveal endometritis on histopathology; a laparoscopy may be performed; or a transvaginal ultrasound or MRI may be ordered (if positive for PID, thickened and fluid-filled tubes or a tubo-ovarian complex would be noted).

How is the diagnosis of genital warts made?

The diagnosis is made by physical exam with warts present. No further testing is necessary.

▶ TREATMENT

What are the recommendations for treatment of the most common genital ulcers?

See Table 60–1.

TABLE 60–1

Treatment of Common Genital Ulcers

Diagnosis	Treatment Options
Chancroid	Azithromycin 1g x 1 OR ceftriaxone 250 mg IM OR ciprofloxacin 500 mg bid x 3d OR erythromycin 500 mg tid x 7d
Genital herpes, first episode	Acyclovir 400 mg tid OR famciclovir 250 mg tid OR valacyclovir 1 g bid x 7–10d
Genital herpes, recurrent episode	Acyclovir 400 mg tid OR acyclovir 800 mg bid OR famciclovir 125 mg bid OR valacyclovir 500 mg bid or 1 g qd for 5d
Genital herpes, suppressive therapy	Acyclovir 400 mg bid OR famciclovir 250 mg bid OR valacyclovir 500 mg qd
Primary and secondary syphilis	Benzathine penicillin G 2.4 million units IM (single dose)
Latent syphilis of unknown duration	Benzathine penicillin G 2.4 million units IM (3 doses, given at one week intervals)
Tertiary syphilis	Benzathine penicillin G 2.4 million units IM (3 doses, given at one week intervals)

What is the treatment of urethritis and cervicitis?

See Table 60–2.

It is important to note that if gonorrheal infection is diagnosed, there is a strong probability of coinfection with chlamydia, so the patient should be treated for both.

What if the patient is pregnant?

Quinolones and doxycycline are contraindicated if the patient is pregnant. Stick with macrolides and cephalosporins. Pregnant

TABLE 60–2

Treatment of Urethritis and Cervicitis

Diagnosis	Treatment Options
Gonorrhea	Ceftriaxone 125 mg IM OR cefixime 400 mg po OR cipro 500 mg po OR ofloxacin 400 mg po OR levofloxacin 250 mg po (all are one-time doses)
Chlamydia	Azithromycin 1 g po one time OR doxycycline 100 mg po x 7d OR erythromycin base 500 mg po qid x 7d OR ofloxacin 300 mg po bid x 7d OR levofloxacin 500 mg qd x 7d
Persistent urethritis	Metronidazole 2 g po one time PLUS erythromycin base 500 mg po qid x 7d OR erythromycin ethylsuccinate 800 mg qid x 7d

women should undergo repeat testing ("test of cure") three weeks after they have completed treatment.

What are the treatment options for pelvic inflammatory disease?

If a parenteral route of treatment is chosen, one may use cefotetan 2g IV twice a day OR cefoxitin 2g IV four times a day PLUS doxycycline 100mg by mouth or IV twice a day. An alternative choice is clindamycin 900 mg IV three times a day PLUS gentamicin 2mg/kg IM or IV three times a day. If choosing an outpatient regimen, use ofloxacin 400mg by mouth twice a day OR levofloxacin 500mg by mouth four times a day for 14 days, with or without metronidazole 500 mg by mouth twice a day for 14 days. The alternative is ceftriaxone 250mg IM or cefoxitin 2g IM plus probenecid 1g by mouth (administered at the same time) for one dose, plus doxycycline 100mg by mouth twice a day with or without metronidazole 500mg twice a day for 14 days. Although outpatient treatment of PID is increasingly more common, inpatient regimens should be considered for severe cases and for patients judged to be compliance risks.

How do you treat genital warts?

Treatment should be made after discussing options with the patient. Options include patient-applied and provider-applied local treatments (Table 60–3).

TABLE 60–3

Treatment of Genital Warts

Patient-Applied Treatments	Provider-Applied Treatments
Podofilox 0.5% gel or solution applied to warts bid x 3d, then rest for 4 days (may repeat up to 4 cycles)	Cryotherapy with liquid nitrogen—may require multiple treatments (every 1–2 wk)
Imiquimod 5% cream applied to warts 3 nights per week for up to 16 wk	Podophyllin resin 10–25% applied to warts—may be reapplied in 1 wk if necessary
	Trichloroacetic acid (TCA) or bichloroacetic acid (BCA) 80–90% applied to warts. If excess solution applied, add talc or liquid soap to remove unreacted acid; may reapply in 1 wk if necessary.
	Surgical removal
	Laser removal or intralesional interferon

What if a patient with genital warts is pregnant?

Serotypes 6 and 11 are associated with respiratory papillomatosis in infants. Therefore, removal of warts is highly recommended. In severe cases of HPV infections, as well as herpes outbreaks, caesarian section might also be considered. Keep in mind, however, that imiquimod, podophyllin, and podofilox should not be used during pregnancy.

KEY POINTS

- **If a diagnosis of chlamydia is made, the patient should be treated for concurrent gonorrheal infection. The sexual partner should seek treatment as well.**
- **The diagnosis of pelvic inflammatory disease is based on a constellation of symptoms and signs; it is very important to diagnose and treat this condition in order to prevent future problems with fertility.**
- **If a sexually transmitted disease is diagnosed, it is important to test for other concurrent STDs as well, including HIV, syphilis, and hepatitis.**

CASE 60–1. A 19-year-old college student presents with a complaint of burning while urinating and clear to white urethral discharge over the past week. He has no genital ulcers or warts visible. He goes on to state that he has had some increasing tenderness in the area of his right testicle and an occasional low-grade fever for the past two days. While he denies inguinal tenderness, there is some mild right inguinal lymphadenopathy. When discussing his social history, the patient states he had an unprotected sexual encounter approximately two weeks ago.

A. What organisms should be considered while evaluating this patient?
B. Why are his other symptoms important?
C. In reference to question A, how should this patient be treated?

CASE 60–2. A 24-year-old woman presents to your clinic with complaints of generalized abdominal tenderness and a fever of 38.5°C. Her social history includes several instances of unprotected sex and IV drug use. Upon examination, the patient nearly jumps off the table when assessment of cervical motion tenderness is performed. The patient also exhibits mild, but noticeable, adnexal tenderness as well.

A. What is the presumptive diagnosis and what exam sign is virtually diagnostic?
B. What tests should be performed relative to the presumed diagnosis?
C. Are there other tests that would be recommended in this patient?

REFERENCES

Centers for Disease Control and Prevention. Sexually transmitted diseases treatment guidelines 2002. MMWR 51(RR-6):1–77, 2002.

Miller KE, Ruiz DE, Graves JC: Update on the prevention and treatment of sexually transmitted diseases. Am Fam Physician 67(9):1915–1922, 2003

USEFUL WEBSITES

Center for Disease Control, Division of Sexually Transmitted Diseases. This site covers all STD epidemiology with an emphasis on HIV. *http://www.cdc.gov/nchstp/dstd/HIVSTDInfo.htm*

American Social Health Association. This site has good general information on STDs in a patient-friendly format. *http://www.ashastd.org/stdfaqs*

61

Thyroid Disease

▶ ETIOLOGY

What are the usual causes of hypothyroidism?

The majority of cases of hypothyroidism are caused by Hashimoto's thyroiditis. This condition is five to eight times more common in women and is an autoimmune disease in which autoantibodies are directed against the thyroid gland. This causes destruction of thyroid tissue and consequently results in a decreased production of thyroid hormone. Other frequent causes are surgical removal of the thyroid gland and radioiodine therapy, which is used for treatment of hyperthyroidism. Other causes include secondary dysfunction from pituitary or hypothalamic disease. Iodine deficiency, which is rare in the United States, is the most common cause of hypothyroidism worldwide.

What are the causes of hyperthyroidism?

The most frequent cause of hyperthyroidism is Graves' disease. This is another autoimmune disease caused by autoantibodies directed against the thyroid that stimulate production of thyroid hormone as well as its conversion to triiodothyronine (T3). In this condition, autoantibodies may also be directed against the eyes, causing proptosis (exophthalmos). Some thyroid nodules called adenomas occur either singly or together as a toxic nodular goiter and have an increased production of thyroid hormone, which may result in hyperthyroidism. Inflammation of the gland sometimes occurs after a viral infection; this is known as subacute thyroiditis. In this condition, the gland releases increased amounts of its stored thyroid hormone.

Are thyroid nodules a cause for concern?

They certainly can be. Although malignant thyroid nodules are the minority, a palpable nodule carries a 5–10% risk of malignancy, with nodules over 1.5 cm carrying a larger risk. Most commonly, thyroid nodules are colloid nodules (a larger nodule in a multinodular goiter), adenomas, or cysts. Although benign, adenomas can secrete hormone and cause hyperthyroidism.

▶ EVALUATION

What laboratory tests are most useful in evaluating the thyroid?

By far the most frequently ordered tests are the TSH (thyroid stimulating hormone) and the T4 (thyroid hormone). The T4 can be ordered in its unbound form, free T4, or bound and unbound forms together (total T4). Free T4 is the most helpful and easy to evaluate because it is the biologically active form. A free or total T3 can also be ordered. Occasionally in hyperthyroidism, the T3 is elevated and not the T4 (T3 thyrotoxicosis). Other tests that can be ordered include the antithyroid antibodies: antithyroglobulin and antithyroid peroxidase (also known as antimicrosomal) antibodies. These assays may assist in determining if the thyroid abnormality is autoimmune as in Grave's disease or Hashimoto's thyroiditis.

What are the signs and symptoms of high or low thyroid hormone?

Because thyroid hormone affects many organ systems, the symptoms are protean. In hypothyroidism one can see fatigue (99%), coarse dry skin (97%), coarse hair, constipation, thick tongue and facial edema, menstrual irregularities, cold intolerance (89%), slowed speech (91%), forgetfulness, mild weight gain, depression, and possibly bradycardia. Hyperthyroidism may give symptoms of weakness, tremor, heat intolerance, sweatiness, fatigue, anxiety, palpitations, anxiety, and weight loss. Additional signs include CHF, osteoporosis, atrial fibrillation and tachycardia, warm skin, lid lag, and—in Grave's disease—exophthalmos. Goiter is also quite common.

Which test should I order to monitor thyroid hormone replacement therapy?

The TSH will be the value that shows the earliest changes. A normal free T4 can be associated with an elevated TSH (subclinical hypothyroidism). This condition can be associated with elevations of blood pressure and cholesterol.

When is a thyroid scan (radioactive iodine uptake) or ultrasound of the thyroid useful?

While not the standard, there is a push toward ultrasound in the evaluation of the characteristics of a nodule and for follow-up of growth. This is especially true if a fine-needle aspiration (FNA) of a thyroid nodule was negative for malignancy and needs to be followed. These radiologic tests are not generally used when the thyroid is normal to palpation in a hypothyroid patient (frequent finding). Thyroid scans are useful in the evaluation of hyperthyroidism to help differentiate Grave's disease or subacute thyroiditis from a hyperfunctioning ("hot") nodule.

What tests are used in the basic evaluation of a thyroid nodule?

In a euthyroid (normal levels of thyroid hormone) patient, FNA, possibly with ultrasound, is standard. In a hyperthyroid patient (low TSH), a thyroid scan is ordered. If the nodule is "cold" (no increased uptake), FNA should be ordered. If the nodule is "hot," begin treatment (see next section).

▶ TREATMENT

What do I need to know to treat hypothyroidism?

Regardless of the etiology, thyroid hormone replacement with levothyroxine is the treatment. In adults this is usually initiated at a dose of 0.075 to 0.1 mg (about 1.7 micrograms/kg/day). A common stable dose in the adult is 0.1 to 0.15 mg daily. Care must be taken in the elderly because thyroid hormone can increase the metabolic demands on the heart and precipitate cardiac ischemia. The adage "go low, go slow" certainly fits here (0.025–0.05 mg/day). Once stable, a yearly check of the TSH is adequate.

If I change the dosage of thyroid hormone, when should I recheck the TSH?

It takes at least four weeks for the TSH to readjust, so wait a month after starting or changing the thyroid hormone dose before rechecking.

What are the methods of treating hyperthyroidism?

There are a lot of variables here, including the cause of the hyperthyroidism and personal preference of the patient and physician. If the hyperthyroidism is caused by a hyperfunctioning nodule, surgical removal or radioiodine are the treatments of choice. If the cause is subacute thyroiditis, anti-inflammatories (ASA, NSAIDs, or prednisone) and β-blockers to control heart rate, tremor, etc. are the mainstays of treatment until the condition resolves. If the diagnosis is Grave's disease, the options are surgical removal (unusual), antithyroid drugs, and radioiodine therapy. Approximately 70% of patients in the United States choose radioiodine.

What are the pros and cons of the antithyroid drugs and radioiodine therapy?

The downside to the antithyroid drugs (propylthiouracil and methimazole) are the low long-term resolution (20–30%) after one to two years of therapy, and possible side effects including agranulocytosis and aplastic anemia. Radioiodine therapy usually causes hypothyroidism and thyroid hormone replacement will need to be initiated; also, this treatment should not be used in pregnancy.

When should a thyroid nodule be removed?

If a nodule is malignant, partial or complete thyroidectomy is usually the procedure of choice. If benign, and not causing hyperthyroidism, the nodule would not need to be removed unless it caused local symptoms, e.g., cough, hoarseness, dysphagia. A nodule producing excess thyroid hormone and causing hyperthyroidism is usually treated with surgery or radioiodine therapy. Some physicians try to suppress nodules with levothyroxine, but this has questionable efficacy.

KEY POINTS

- **Signs and symptoms of thyroid dysfunction may affect many organ systems, so have a high index of suspicion and check a TSH if appropriate.**
- **Fine-needle aspiration is the recommended evaluation technique for a thyroid nodule in a euthyroid patient.**
- **Radioiodine therapy is the most frequent treatment for hyperthyroidism caused by Graves' disease.**
- **When changing the dose of levothyroxine, wait one month before checking the TSH.**

CASE 61–1. **A 53-year-old woman presents with recent nervousness, irritability, tachycardia, and weight loss. She has felt a lot of stress recently. Her vitals are: blood pressure 123/74, heart rate 104, weight 134 lb.**

A. What are some key points in the history to help narrow your differential?
B. What lab test(s) should be ordered?
C. If her TSH is low, what test should be ordered? What if it is high?
D. Would you be concerned if her heart rate was irregular and why?

CASE 61–2. **A 65-year-old man presents with a recent cough. On his exam you find a 1-cm nodule in the right lobe of his thyroid.**

A. What are important questions in addition to those concerning the symptoms of hyperthyroidism and hypothyroidism?
B. Laboratory evaluation showed a euthyroid state. What is the next step in evaluation?
C. What is the treatment of choice if the nodule is malignant?
D. What are some complications of thyroid surgery?

REFERENCES

Hueston WJ: Treatment of hypothyroidism. Am Fam Physician 64(10):1717–1724, 2001.

Welker MJ, Orlov D: Thyroid nodules. Am Fam Physician 67(3): 559–566, 2003.

62

Transient Ischemic Attack and Stroke

▶ ETIOLOGY

What is a transient ischemic attack?

A transient ischemic attack (TIA) is an ischemic neurologic deficit that rapidly resolves. It is an episode of a transient focal loss of cerebral function of occlusive vascular origin. Typically, the effects of TIAs last between 5 and 15 minutes; the temporal boundary between a TIA and stroke is 24 hours. TIAs affect an estimated 50,000 Americans annually. For one-third of these patients, a TIA is the precursor to an impending stroke.

What is a stroke?

A stroke is the sudden onset of a neurologic deficit owing to the acute loss of circulation to an area of the brain resulting in ischemia. Strokes are classified as hemorrhagic or ischemic; 20% are primary hemorrhages and 80% are ischemic. The ischemic brain tissue rapidly loses function because of lack of neuronal glycogen and rapid energy failure, but remains viable for hours. This period of viability allows a window of time for potential recovery, especially in the face of treatment options for ischemic strokes. Thus, there is a three to six hour "therapeutic window" during which intervention (in ischemic stroke) may lessen resulting brain damage. Strokes typically manifest with neurologic deficits such as weakness, numbness, or language deficits. The weakness and sensory deficits tend to be worst in the facial areas and progressively improve from the upper extremity to the lower extremity. With regard to hemorrhagic stroke, deficits are often caused by mass effect and the toxicity of blood on brain tissue.

Stroke is the most common cause of neurologic disability in the United States and the third leading cause of death, following cardiac disease and cancer-related deaths. Approximately 700,000 new and recurrent strokes occur each year in the United States. Nearly 30% of patients die within a year of their stroke. The direct and indirect cost of stroke in the United States is approximately $43 billion annually.

What causes TIAs and strokes?

Ischemic stroke is most often caused by embolic occlusion of the large cerebral arteries. Embolic sources include the carotid bifurcation, the aortic arch, or an arterial dissection; cardioembolic etiologies include atrial fibrillation, mural thrombus, myocardial infarction, dilated cardiomyopathy, valvular lesions including mitral stenosis, artificial (especially mechanical) valve, bacterial endocarditis, an atrial septal defect or patent foramen ovale, and left heart myxoma. Primary atherosclerosis within the cerebral arteries is much less common than the involvement of atherosclerosis in the coronary arteries. However, lacunar infarcts, which are small, deep, ischemic lesions, are most often caused by small artery disease, with hypertension and diabetes as the main risk factors. Ischemia caused by low or reduced flow is often seen in proximal artery stenosis in the face of severe hypotension and inadequate collateral blood flow. Hemorrhage typically is caused by rupture of cerebral artery aneurysms or small vessels within the brain tissue.

What are the risk factors?

Most of the risk factors involved are associated with atherosclerosis. Modifiable risk factors for both stroke and TIAs include hypertension, hyperlipidemia, diabetes, obesity, smoking, physical inactivity, alcohol consumption in excess of five drinks per day, and atrial fibrillation. Nonmodifiable risk factors include age, male sex, nonwhite race, presence of congestive heart failure or coronary artery disease, and a family history of stroke or ischemic heart disease. Identifying the modifiable risk factors and discussing possible interventions with the patient to decrease stroke risk can help decrease the morbidity and mortality associated with strokes.

▶ EVALUATION

What points in the history are important in evaluating TIA and stroke?

Questions may need to be addressed to possible witnesses (family, friends, neighbors) in addition to the patient to elicit a careful history. Because treatment options are based on a narrow "therapeutic window," it is important to get a clear understanding of the onset, duration, fluctuation, and intensity of the neurological deficit(s), and if any cardiac symptoms coincided with the neurologic event. It is important to ask about changes in behavior, speech, gait, vision, movement, and memory. Obtaining a history of previous strokes or

TIAs, recent surgery, and use of illicit drugs is important. Also secure a list of current medications.

What should the physical examination include in the evaluation of TIA and stroke?

A patient with a suspected TIA or stroke should have a complete physical examination, with special attention to a detailed neurologic exam. It is important to record a blood pressure in each arm, check peripheral pulses, and determine the respiratory rate and pattern. Carotid arteries should be examined for bruits; eyes should be examined fundoscopically for retinal plaques and pigmentation, and pupil reaction to light. It is important to perform a thorough cardiac exam, listening for unusual rates, rhythms, and murmurs or rubs that may indicate valvular disease, atrioseptal defects, or ventricular wall abnormalities, which may predispose a patient to embolic events.

The neurologic exam should be thorough, including cranial nerve testing, somatic motor reflex and strength testing, somatic sensory testing, a mini mental status examination, and a cerebellar exam with rapid alternating movements, gait assessment, and finger to nose or heel to shin tests. The symptoms exhibited by the patient may indicate areas of the central nervous system affected by a stroke (Table 62–1).

TABLE 62–1

Localization of Stroke

Symptom	Area Affected (Vessel Affected)
Hemiparesis	Contralateral parietal and frontal motor cortex (MCA)
Hemisensory loss	Contralateral somatosensory cortex (MCA)
Broca's (motor) aphasia	Dominant* frontal lobe (MCA)
Wernicke's (sensory) aphasia	Dominant temporal lobe (MCA)
Memory deficit	Temporal lobe (hippocampus), bilateral or dominant (PCA)
Aggressiveness, hypersexuality	Temporal lobe (PCA)
Unilateral neglect, apraxias	Nondominant parietal lobe (MCA)
Ataxia, dysarthria, nystagmus, intention tremor, scanning speech	Cerebellum (VA)
Cranial nerves 3 and 4	Midbrain (PCA)
Cranial nerves 5, 6, 7, 8	Pons (BA)
Cranial nerves 9, 10, 11, 12	Medulla (BA)
Dense sensory loss, spontaneous pain, dysesthesias, hemiballismus, choreoathetosis	Thalamus and subthalamus (PCA)

MCA = middle cerebral artery, PCA = posterior cerebral artery, BA = basilar artery, VA = vertebral artery
*Left side dominance is present in more than 95% of the population: 99% of right-handed people and 60–70% of left-handed people.

What lab tests and imaging studies should I order?

Lab studies should include a serum chemistry profile, a CBC, coagulation studies, syphilis serology, glucose level, erythrocyte sedimentation rate, and antiphospholipid antibodies. Screening for drugs and hypercoagulable states may be warranted, particularly in a younger patient (under 50 years of age).

Imaging studies should include, at the least, a noncontrast CT of the head to determine if a hemorrhage or possibly a tumor is present. An MRI shows areas of ischemia more accurately than does a CT, and within a couple of hours, compared to up to 48 hours with CT. Magnetic resonance angiography (MRA), conventional angiography, carotid duplex studies, and transesophageal echocardiography are additional studies that could provide insight into the etiology and treatment of the TIA or stroke.

▶ TREATMENT

What is the treatment for ischemic stroke?

Blood pressure and fluid status must be monitored carefully in a patient suffering an ischemic stroke. Hypertension should not be aggressively treated because a decrease in blood pressure may exacerbate the ischemic damage. Only if the systolic pressures rise above 220 should measures be taken to gradually decrease the blood pressure. Maintenance of fluid status with isotonic solution is important, as hypovolemia should be prevented. Mannitol may be used in cases of severe stroke to reduce the edema in the brain. In cerebellar infarctions or hemorrhage, a neurosurgery consult may be warranted if brainstem compression is suspected.

Thrombolysis may be considered if the duration of neurologic deficits has been less than three hours, and there is no evidence of hemorrhage on head CT. Tissue plasminogen activator (t-PA) administered within three hours of the onset of the deficit has been shown to improve clinical outcome in patients at three months. The risk of intracerebral hemorrhage within the first 36 hours is increased with thrombolysis, but overall mortality is not any higher, even with the increased risk of bleeding. Some contraindications to treatment with t-PA include:

- CT evidence of intracranial hemorrhage
- Rapidly improving deficit or minor symptoms
- Systolic pressures above 185 or diastolic pressures above 110
- A coagulopathy
- Recent surgery or invasive procedure
- History of hemorrhagic stroke

Within six hours of the onset of stroke, intra-arterial prourokinase has been shown to improve clinical outcome of patients with middle cerebral artery thrombosis.

The role of heparin in treatment of stroke is controversial, because objective clinical data are lacking. Generally it is used in the cases of atherothrombotic stenosis or occlusion, unstable TIAs, or posterior circulation deficits. Warfarin may be used for anticoagulation for cardiac sources of emboli, such as atrial fibrillation, with an International Normalized Ratio (INR) maintained between 2 and 3. In patients with prosthetic heart valves, a combination of aspirin and warfarin with an INR of 3 to 4 is recommended.

Antiplatelet agents, such as aspirin, clopidogrel, and dipyridamole, have been shown to reduce new stroke events by 25–30%. They all have proven benefits in acute stroke and reduction of risk of subsequent TIAs and strokes.

Carotid endarterectomy is recommended for patients with symptomatic carotid stenosis of greater than 70%. This is an elective, nonemergent procedure, and should not be carried out in the face of an evolving TIA or stroke.

What is the treatment for hemorrhagic stroke?

In treating a hemorrhagic stroke, the goal is to control impending complications. If a coagulopathy is present, it is important to rapidly correct the problem. In the case of an aneurysm rupture, early intervention, usually in the form of surgical isolation of the aneurysm, is necessary to decrease the risk of rebleeding. Vasospasm is common posthemorrhage, and can cause delayed ischemic stroke. Treatment with nimodipine, a calcium channel blocker, has been shown to decrease this risk. Symptomatic hydrocephalus can be treated with ventricular drains, shunts, and repeated lumbar punctures. In the case of intraparenchymal hemorrhage, measures should be taken to reduce the intracranial pressure by treating the edema and mass effect with mannitol, and in some cases corticosteroids. Urgent evacuation of hematomas may be necessary, particularly in the case of cerebellar hemorrhage.

What is the treatment for transient ischemic attack?

Treatment of the risk factors for atherosclerosis is paramount if atherosclerosis is thought to be the underlying etiology of the TIA. If the patient has carotid stenosis greater than 70%, a carotid endarterectomy is indicated, and has been shown to be superior to medical therapy in reducing subsequent stroke risk. If the stenosis is less severe, patients may use antiplatelet agents (aspirin, clopidogrel, and dipyridamole) as discussed above. Again, anticoagulation has a limited role depending on the etiology of the event.

KEY POINTS

- **Remember the "classic" causes of TIAs and strokes: ischemia caused by atherosclerosis (most common), emboli resulting from clot formation caused by atrial fibrillation, and septic emboli from infective endocarditis.**
- **In treatment of acute stroke, remember first your ABCs (airway management, breathing, and cardiac/circulation status).**
- **An initial CT study without contrast is warranted in the face of acute stroke to rule out hemorrhage or other mass lesions. A CT scan may be negative for 24 to 48 hours in ischemic stroke.**

CASE 62–1. **An 83-year-old woman with a history of type 2 diabetes mellitus, hypertension, hyperlipidemia, and obesity presents to the emergency department with aphasia.**

A. What additional information do you need in regard to this woman's history?
B. What imaging studies do you want to order?
C. What is the difference between Broca's aphasia and Wernicke's aphasia? Where would the lesion be in each case, and which artery is affected?

CASE 62–2. **A 62-year-old man presents with complaints of a "shade" descending over his right field of vision. The patient has had two recent episodes, one lasting about 5 minutes, and the other 10 to 15 minutes.**

A. What phenomenon is the patient describing?
B. What is the most likely diagnosis of this man's disorder?
C. What is this man's risk for developing a stroke in the future?

REFERENCES

Ezekowitz JA, Straus SE, Majumdar SR, McAlister FA: Stroke: Strategies for primary prevention. Am Fam Physician 68(12):2379–86, 2389–90, 2003.

USEFUL WEBSITES

Stroke, published by Lippincott Williams & Wilkins for the American Heart Association. *http://stroke.ahajournals.org*

American Stroke Association. *http://www.strokeassociation.org*

63

Trauma

▶ ETIOLOGY

What constitutes minor trauma?

Minor trauma in this chapter refers specifically to injuries that can be effectively evaluated and treated in a clinical office setting. While the range of injuries that may present in a family practice clinic is virtually limitless, there are some types of trauma that will be seen on a more frequent basis. General orthopedic injuries such as minor fractures, joint injuries, and their related conditions are most commonly seen. Head and facial trauma are also evaluated and treated in family practice clinics.

List some of the more common causes of minor trauma seen in the clinical office.

Like the presentations of trauma itself, the causes can be limitless. Sports and recreational activities generate many of these injuries. Work-related injuries commonly present in the office setting. Accidents (home-based, automobile) are yet another cause for people to present to their physician.

Under what circumstances should trauma be referred?

In dealing with all injuries, the physician needs to be aware of his or her limits in the evaluation and treatment of trauma. Foremost, any injury that represents a potential for mortality or permanent disability requires immediate hospitalization for more intensive evaluation. Injuries that have compromised neurovascular function should be immediately referred for hospitalization as well. Some injuries require evaluation and treatment modalities not available in most family practice settings. Examples include MRI for ligament injuries and trauma requiring surgical correction (severe fractures, certain ligament tears, and neurovascular repairs).

▶ EVALUATION & TREATMENT

What are some of the more common orthopedic injuries seen in the clinical setting?

The most commonly injured joints are the knee, shoulder, and ankle. The wrist and elbow are less commonly injured but patients with these injuries do occasionally present in the office.

What structures in the knee are susceptible to injury?

Four major ligaments, including the anterior cruciate ligament (ACL), posterior cruciate ligament (PCL), medial collateral ligament (MCL), and lateral collateral ligament (LCL), support the knee in all four directions of force. The knee also relies on a cartilaginous meniscus for cushioning and support. All of the supporting structures about the knee are vulnerable to injury from trauma.

How are these structures injured, evaluated, and treated?

ACL. Noncontact pivoting injuries commonly associated with a pop and immediate swelling (hemearthosis) can indicate an ACL injury. Lachman, pivot shift, and anterior drawer are effective in-office procedures, with an MRI required to confirm. Initially, stabilization and pain control can be done in a clinical setting, but in most cases ACL ruptures require reconstruction; therefore, a referral to an orthopedic surgeon is essential.

PCL. The PCL is most commonly injured by a direct blow to the anterior tibia with the knee flexed (dashboard injury) or hyperflexion with a plantar-flexed foot. Evaluation should include a posterior drawer test and distal neurovascular exam. Again, an MRI is required to confirm the injury. Initially, stabilization and pain control can be done in the office. Nonoperative treatment with stabilization and physical therapy is favored for most PCL injuries. If a bony avulsion fracture occurs, surgical repair is necessary. Chronic PCL deficiency can result in chondrosis of the patellofemoral joint.

MCL. Injury to the MCL occurs as a result of valgus stress to the knee, specifically a lateral blow while the knee is in slight flexion, which often produces an audible "pop." Valgus stress with the knee in 30 degrees of flexion will reveal increased laxity of the joint but, as with the other ligaments, an MRI is the best method to confirm the injury. Nonoperative treatment with a hinged knee brace is highly successful for isolated MCL injuries.

LCL. Injury to the LCL is uncommon but could occur with varus stress to the knee. Examination consists of placing varus stress to the knee in 30 degrees of flexion, producing increased laxity at the joint, with MRI as confirmation. Like the MCL and PCL, isolated LCL injuries are managed nonoperatively with knee stabilization.

Meniscus. The meniscus is a C-shaped cartilage that acts as a shock absorber, assisting in load distribution between the femur and the tibia. Injury can result from shearing, rotational force on the knee after which the patient has locking of the knee and/or pain with squatting. Injury can also occur with ligament injuries (commonly ACL and MCL). The medial meniscus is torn about three times more often than the lateral. Palpation of joint line for point tenderness and range of motion maneuvers while listening for audible clicks can indicate injury, although an MRI is required to confirm. Meniscal tears do not generally spontaneously heal and most problematic tears will require arthroscopic debridement or repair. Longitudinal tears in young people that involve the outer third (vascular zone) are the most likely to be reparable. Radial tears are commonly resected.

What is the nature of shoulder injuries?

The uniqueness of the anatomy of the shoulder can make it susceptible injury. The rather flat surface of the humeral head and its relation to the glenoid fossa makes the shoulder relatively unstable when compared to other joints. Like the knee, thorough history and physical exam is critical to establishing proper diagnoses of shoulder injuries. Humeral head dislocations, acromioclavicular separations, and rotator cuff injuries are three of the most commonly seen trauma-related shoulder injuries.

Describe the evaluation and treatment of shoulder injuries.

Dislocations. The shoulder is the most commonly dislocated joint in the body, with anterior dislocations being far more common than posterior dislocations. Dislocation generally results from excessive external rotation and hyperextension, such as getting hit in the arm while attempting to throw a ball. Inspection and palpation are the most useful. In addition, a distal neurovascular exam of the affected area should be done. X-ray can confirm anterior versus posterior dislocation as well as any associated bony injury (Hill-Sachs lesion). Immediate closed reduction is the treatment of choice with immobilization in a sling. Progressive range of motion is done with active rehabilitation to prevent stiffness in the shoulder and elbow. The recurrence rate is high as is the incidence of rotator cuff tears in patients older than 40.

Acromioclavicular (AC) Separation. This injury typically results from a direct force applied to the acromion, as in a fall on the point of the shoulder. The separation can vary in severity and is graded based on space between the two bones. Inspection and palpation of the joint should be performed, specifically feeling for AC separation. Evaluation with shoulder x-ray should be sought as well. Treatment of separation of the AC joint depends on the severity of the separation. Less severe injuries may be treated with a sling and physical therapy. More severe injuries such as those in which the clavicle is dislocated require surgery.

Rotator Cuff Injuries. Rotator cuff tears are most common in patients 50 and older, but can occur in young athletes as well. The mechanisms for injury include violent movements such as lifting or pulling, or sustaining a fall on an outstretched arm. Patients with tears complain of pain in the deltoid region and rotator strength is decreased. The most common place for a tear is the insertion of the supraspinatus. Observation and palpation can be very helpful, as can active and passive range of motion, specifically noting pain in certain directions. The supraspinatus sign is the most sensitive. It is done by abducting the arm to 90 degrees with the thumb turned toward the floor. This isolates the muscle and the patient with a tear will not be able to hold the arm in that position. MRI is also useful. The treatment of choice for tears of the rotator cuff is operative repair.

What is the evaluation and treatment of ankle sprains?

Ankle sprains are common in athletes and most often involve the anterior talofibular ligament. Injury can result from either excessive inversion or eversion of the foot at the ankle joint, but inversion injuries are generally more common. In addition to palpation of the ankle for point tenderness, range of motion and an anterior drawer test to assess the integrity of the talofibular ligament should be performed. Initial treatment of a suspected sprain includes elevation of the ankle, using ice and compression to reduce swelling, and rest. Immobilization may be useful for a short period (1–2 days), but early range of motion and light strengthening exercise is important. Surgical intervention is reserved for cases of recurrent or refractory ankle sprains that present with excessive instability.

What types of wrist injuries may present in a clinical situation?

Most injuries to the wrist result from falls on an outstretched hand. While sprains do often result, fractures are frequently seen in this type of fall. Assess for snuffbox tenderness via range of motion and palpation. This tenderness is a sign of possible scaphoid fracture. Radiographs in scaphoid fractures may be initially negative, but as callus formation occurs, the fracture will become visible on repeat films in approximately two weeks.

This patient should not be cast initially because of the soft tissue swelling that can result in neurovascular compromise. Conversely, the swelling may decrease, and the cast would become too loose to provide sufficient stability. A splint will still allow for the resolution of swelling while maintaining immobilization. In scaphoid fractures, a thumb spica should be used, in which the first metacarpophalangeal joint is included in the splint or cast. When the pain of the injury is increased with pronation or supination, this motion needs to be prevented with long arm immobilization as well. When pronation and supination are no longer painful, the cast can be changed to a short arm thumb spica.

What hand injuries are commonly seen in family practice?

The most common hand injuries are fractures of the digits and sprains of the interphalangeal joints. These injuries can be easily evaluated with in-office x-ray. In the case of sprains, ice and immobilization with a finger splint are indicated with care not to ice longer than 5 to 10 minutes to avoid frostbite. Simple fractures of the phalanges or metacarpals can be casted in the clinic. Compound or open fractures of phalanges should warrant immediate orthopedic consult as should markedly displaced fractures of the metacarpals. Trauma to the fingertips (commonly seen when fingers are closed in a door) can result in a subungual hematoma. These collections of blood beneath the nail exert pressure on the nail itself and on the underlying nail bed causing a remarkable amount of pain. These are easily treated using a fine-point cauterizing tool to bore a hole through the nail into the hematoma, releasing the pressure. In rare instances, a needle and syringe can be employed if the hematoma cannot be reached with the cautery tool. Anesthetic is rarely ever needed in cases of subungual hematoma.

What elbow injuries are commonly encountered in the office?

Subluxation of the radial head, also referred to as nursemaid's elbow, is a common injury in 2- and 3-year-olds. The injury occurs when an older sibling or parent applies traction to the arm while the forearm is pronated and the elbow is extended (as when lifting a child by one arm). This pulls the radial head distally, allowing it to become wedged in the annular ligament.

Reduction is performed by applying pressure to the radial head with the examiner's thumb and simultaneously supinating the forearm while flexing the elbow. A snap is felt as the radial head slides back into place. Parents should be warned prior to the reduction because this maneuver is uncomfortable for the patient and will typically produce some crying. Generally, children will be able to use the affected arm normally within minutes. If reduction is successful after one attempt and the patient is fully using the arm soon after, radiographs are not required. If reduction is unsuccessful or if the arm remains painful, x-rays are required.

Tendonitis of the tendons around the elbow is also a common complaint and results from overuse of the joint. Patients will present with pain and decreased range of motion. Recommendations are for rest from repetitive activities, icing the joint, and nonsteroidal anti-inflammatory drugs (NSAIDs) on a scheduled basis.

What is compartment syndrome? How does it relate to the previously discussed injuries?

Compartment syndrome is a medical emergency. It can be seen in patients who engage in repetitive activities such as running, but also often occurs in cases of fractures and ligament damage. Patients may note pain that has a gradual onset either during exercise or following an initial trauma; the pain is caused by increasing pressure in a muscular compartment. This pressure itself is from traumatic swelling caused by inflammation and vascular rupture into muscle fascial compartments. The anterior and posterior deep compartments of the leg are the most commonly affected areas. Inspection and palpation of the area where pain occurs is important. Perhaps one of the most important physical findings is pain with passive flexion and extension of the muscles of the compartment of interest. Intracompartmental pressure can be measured as well. In acute cases, an emergent fasciotomy is indicated. For cases of chronic and/or exertional compartment syndrome, rest, NSAIDs, and orthotics can be used.

How are common head and face injuries evaluated and treated?

Corneal Abrasion. Corneal abrasion is often the result of minor trauma to the eye or secondary to a foreign object scratching the eye's surface. The abrasion is confirmed by performing a fluorescein dye–Wood's lamp exam. The globe of the eye is anesthetized with a topical ocular anesthetic and a moistened fluorescein dye strip is lightly applied to the inferior palpebral conjunctiva, staining the cornea. On Wood's lamp exam, small defects are easily illuminated. Be alert for defects with a dendritic, branching pattern that can indicate an infectious etiology introduced to the eye during the trauma.

In most instances, patching the eye has not been shown to decrease patient discomfort and may increase the chance of secondary infection. Topical anesthetics are contraindicated in the management of corneal pain because of the possibilities of masking a worsening clinical course and inhibiting the protective corneal reflex. Simple corneal abrasions are managed by cycloplegia to reduce ciliary spasm and pain, a mild oral narcotic if needed, and a topical antibiotic to prevent secondary infection. Corneal abrasions generally heal phenomenally quickly. A follow-up fluorescein dye–Wood's lamp exam in 24 hours is necessary to confirm resolution of the abrasion. If the lesion has not resolved or improved significantly after 24 hours then ophthalmologic referral is necessary.

Nasal Fractures. Nasal fractures are common in the outpatient family practice clinic. Nasal bone radiographs are not routinely recommended in the acute setting because they are notoriously insensitive, especially for nondisplaced fractures, and rarely change the acute management. Nasal swelling, tenderness, and ecchymoses in the setting of trauma are enough to make the diagnosis of nasal fracture.

While most nasal fractures do not require immediate ENT referral, there are a few complications that require an urgent ENT evaluation. These complications include septal hematoma, cerebrospinal fluid (CSF) leak from nose, grossly deformed or open nasal fracture, and uncontrolled bleeding. Other concomitant facial or head injuries may also require urgent referral. A hematoma within the nasal septum, if not immediately surgically decompressed, can cause pressure necrosis of the septal cartilage resulting in substantial disfigurement. Nasal fractures can be associated with cribiform plate fractures causing a CSF leak. The presence of clear rhinorrhea after a nasal injury should alert the physician to this possibility. Bleeding can mask the presence of CSF.

CSF in this scenario can be detected by a filter paper halo test. A drop of blood mixed with CSF and placed on "filter paper" (e.g., a coffee filter, paper towel, or bed linen) should produce a halo beyond the blood drop border when the CSF migrates further under the influence of capillary pressure. Note that the presence of other fluids in the blood (saline, nasal secretions) also produces a halo.

The need for prophylactic antibiotics for patients with a suspected CSF leak is controversial. Nondisplaced, closed nasal fractures with controlled bleeding in the absence of septal hematomas and CSF leaks can be managed conservatively in the acute setting with cool compresses and analgesia, although they should be referred to ENT for a detailed exam a week or so after swelling subsides.

Facial Lacerations. Most facial lacerations around the margins of the face can be managed in the family practice clinic with careful, sterile irrigation and suturing using simple interrupted nylon sutures. Lacerations that extend to the bone (periosteum) or are longer than 4 to 5 cm may necessitate a referral to plastic surgery to minimize scarring. Lacerations that are more centrally located and longer than 2 cm or that overlap with facial structures (eyelids, nasolabial area) should also be referred to ophthalmology or plastic surgery to minimize the extent of structural damage and scarring. Additionally, keep in mind that facial sutures should be removed in approximately five days to reduce the scarring from the sutures themselves.

Traumatic Tooth Loss. Tooth loss due to minor trauma is a common presentation to many family practice clinics. While this is an injury that should always be referred to a dentist, there are some steps that can be taken in the clinic to help insure a better outcome. If the patient has possession of the tooth (whole and undamaged), it can be replaced in the socket following gentle irrigation with sterile water. Be observant for slivers of enamel that might have broken off or other foreign objects that can be imbedded in the gum tissue. If the tooth has been damaged through to the pulp, it is generally considered a loss but can be used by cosmetic dentists to mold a replacement. If the tooth has been lost, again gentle irrigation is indicated followed by packing of the socket with sterile gauze. Dental referral is still necessary for fitting with a prosthetic tooth or spacer. If the patient is a younger person who has lost a "baby" tooth, most dentists generally will not replace it and all that is generally required is irrigation and gauze to control the bleeding. More serious trauma, such as a fractured jaw with loss of teeth or severe disruption of soft oral tissue, warrants immediate referral to an oromaxillofacial surgeon.

KEY POINTS

- **Threatened mortality or loss of neurovascular function warrants immediate hospital evaluation.**
- **While surgical correction may be necessary, initial evaluation of simple (no neurovascular loss) orthopedic injuries can be performed in the family practice setting.**
- **More severe injuries of the head and facial region require specialist referral to prevent permanent scarring or dysfunction but initial stabilization can usually take place in the family practice clinic.**

CASE 63–1. **A 17-year-old high-school football player is brought to your clinic following a knee injury in which he was struck by an opposing player's helmet on the lateral side of the joint. He says he heard three loud pops and feels like the joint may buckle if he walks on it. He states pain is minimal. On examination, the area behind the right knee is swollen and ecchymosed. While he has good sensation in his foot, the distal pulses in his right foot are faint and the skin of that leg and foot is pale and dusky.**

A. What orthopedic structures are likely injured?
B. What other structure is also likely injured?
C. What is your evaluation strategy?
D. Would you perform any in-office testing?

CASE 63–2. **A 32-year-old mugging victim presents to your office approximately 30 minutes after the assault. He states two assailants struck him repeatedly on the head with heavy, hard objects before taking his watch. He currently has bruising about his eyes and at the base of his skull behind his ears (Battle's sign). His nose is bleeding but the blood appears watery, and he states that your office "doesn't smell like most doctors' offices do." No fluid is visible in the ear canals. He denies any loss of consciousness since the attack, but over the last several minutes has been feeling a compelling urge to go to sleep.**

A. What injuries has this patient definitely sustained?
B. What possible injuries need to be evaluated?
C. What type of evaluation needs to be performed?
D. What is your most urgent concern with this patient?

REFERENCES

Eachempati SR, Barie PS: Minimally invasive and noninvasive diagnosis and therapy in critically ill and injured patients. Arch Surg 134:1189–1196, 1999.

Smith BW, Green GA: Acute knee injuries: Part II. Diagnosis and management. Am Fam Physician 51:800, 1995.

USEFUL WEBSITES

American Academy of Family Physicians. This site has extensive journal and practice guideline resources covering injury and office-based trauma care. *http://www.aafp.org*

Beers MH, Berkow R (eds): The Merck Manual of Diagnosis and Therapy, 17th ed. Whitehouse Station, NJ: Merck & Company, Inc., 2004. This is a useful, all-inclusive, site with easy to use trauma guidelines. *http://www.merck.com/pubs/manual*

Case Answers

▶ ABDOMINAL PAIN

12–1, A. Learning objective: ***Take an appropriate history and physical examination.*** In taking further history, asking about the character of the pain, its severity, associated symptoms, and alleviating and exacerbating factors may help give you guidance. It also is important to ask about recent bowel movements, urinary symptoms such as frequency and dysuria, the date of the patient's last menstrual period, menstrual history and symptoms, and use of contraception. In performing a physical examination, you should carefully examine the abdomen and note if the right lower quadrant tenderness is over McBurney's point. In this patient, it also is important to do a pelvic and rectal examination to check for cervical motion tenderness, uterine size, pelvic and adnexal tenderness, and rectal tenderness.

12–1, B. Learning objective: ***Formulate a differential diagnosis.*** Appendicitis is the potential diagnosis of most concern. However, in a female patient of this age, there are other considerations that should be excluded including an ectopic pregnancy, ruptured ovarian cyst, pelvic inflammatory disease, and a urinary tract infection. Less likely considerations include gastroenteritis and irritable bowel syndrome.

12–1, C. Learning objective: ***Order appropriate diagnostic tests in the family physician's office.*** A complete blood count with differential may help confirm your suspicion of appendicitis if there is leukocytosis with a left shift. A urinalysis to look for signs of a urinary tract infection and a urine pregnancy test to rule out pregnancy also would be appropriate in this patient. If the diagnosis is still not clear or the patient continues to worsen, the patient may need admission to a hospital for more diagnostic tests or consultation with a surgeon or gynecologist.

12–2, A. Learning objective: ***Take an appropriate history and physical examination.*** Ask the patient to clarify her symptoms in regard to its location, duration of episodes, severity, associated symptoms, and alleviating and exacerbating factors. More careful questioning about her bowel movements is needed. (What does she mean by "diarrhea" and "constipation"? Is there blood or mucus in her bowel movements?) You should explore with her the relationship of these symptoms to her diet and also inquire about the presence of systemic signs such as weight loss or fever. In addition, you should ask about urinary symptoms, gynecologic history, and menstrual history and symptoms. You should perform a standard abdominal examination. The patient may not have any abnormality at the time of her examination. Pelvic and rectal examinations should also be performed.

12–2, B. Learning objective: ***Formulate a differential diagnosis.*** The patient most likely has irritable bowel syndrome. However, you must also consider other diseases such as inflammatory bowel disease; infectious gastroenteritis due to bacteria, viruses, or protozoa; malabsorption syndrome; lactose intolerance; and colorectal carcinoma. Ovarian cancer can also present with vague abdominal symptoms and deserves consideration.

12–2, C. Learning objective: ***Order appropriate diagnostic tests.*** Most experts agree that a complete blood count, erythrocyte sedimentation rate, thyroid stimulating hormone level, electrolytes, and a flexible sigmoidoscopy or colonoscopy are appropriate basic studies to rule out another serious disorder. Stool culture and ova/parasites may be sent if there is suspicion of a bacterial or protozoan infection. A colonoscopy should be recommended if any "red-flag" symptoms or signs such as anemia, weight loss, or hematochezia are present. A pelvic ultrasound may be ordered if there is a pelvic or adnexal mass present.

► ANEMIA

13–1, A. Learning objective: ***Understand the epidemiology of anemia.*** Iron deficiency anemia is the most likely cause in this menstruating young woman. Recent pregnancy may also contribute to anemia.

13–1, B. Learning objective: ***Do an appropriate evaluation of anemia.*** A CBC and peripheral smear will initially disclose the type of anemia (e.g., microcytic, hypochromic). Confirmation of iron deficiency can be assessed by checking total iron binding capacity, serum iron, and ferritin. A stool guaiac will help rule out gastrointestinal bleeding, an uncommon cause in a young, asymptomatic woman.

13–2, A. Learning objective: ***Understand the epidemiology of anemia.*** While the anemia of chronic disease (normocytic, normochromic) might be likely in this man, a careful evaluation for iron deficiency (microcytic and hypochromic), thyroid disease, and such conditions as B_{12} and folate deficiency (macrocytic) would be very important. Underlying cancer or occult disease could account for a variety of anemias.

13–2, B. Learning objective: ***Appropriate treatment of anemia.*** Treatment should be withheld in this individual until a clear etiology is established. Presumptive treatment with iron, B_{12} shots, or delaying a firm diagnosis are inappropriate. Treatment should be directed to the type of anemia unless the blood loss has been acute and the patient is unstable (e.g., if the patient has an active gastrointestinal bleed).

▶ ARTHRALGIA/JOINT PAIN

14–1, A. Learning objective: ***Learn to first classify if the joint pain is monoarticular or polyarticular, and know that the differential diagnosis will overlap for each.*** This patient is having acute, monoarticular joint pain. The main etiologies that should be considered are trauma, infection, and crystals.

14–1, B. Learning objective: ***Use the history to narrow the differential diagnosis using distribution, disease chronology, extra-articular manifestations, disease course, and patient demographics.*** In this patient, you already have an important piece of history: her prosthetic knee. She is at increased risk of a septic joint. Her diabetes also increases her risk. Even without this history, it is important to rule out a septic joint in this patient because a septic joint is rapidly destructive and requires immediate treatment. Also, ask this patient if she is having pain in any other joints, if the pain is getting worse, or if she has had any systemic symptoms of illness. Given her osteoporosis, you should inquire if she has had any falls lately. Trauma to the hip joint is often referred to the knee.

14–1, C. Learning objective: ***Learn the major categories in the differential diagnosis for monoarticular joint pain and polyarticular joint pain.*** As mentioned in the 14–1 (A) answer, there are three main etiologies to consider for monoarticular joint pain: trauma, infection, and crystals. Additional signs of trauma include cuts and bruises. An exam for infection may reveal a joint that is tender, erythematous, and warm. For gout, you may examine the entire body for tophi and may find extreme tenderness of the joint. See Box 14–1 for the differential diagnosis of polyarticular joint pain.

14–1, D. Learning objective: ***Know the diagnostic workup for joint pain.*** In this patient, a septic joint must be ruled out. Therefore, arthrocentesis is required (this is also therapeutic). The resulting fluid should be used for: Gram stain, culture, cell count, and differential and exam under a polarizing microscope. Blood cultures should also be collected.

14–2, A. Learning objective: ***Know the major indications of therapeutic joint injections.*** See page 69 for a list of indications.

14–2, B. Learning objective: ***Be able to describe and perform the lateral approach to knee injections.*** For a lateral approach, a line is drawn between the lateral and proximal borders of the patella. The needle is aimed at a 45-degree angle toward the joint and inserted near the intersection of the lines, and between the patella and the femur. Aspiration will insure proper placement into the joint capsule.

► LOW BACK PAIN

15–1, A. Learning objective: *Distinguish pertinent history and physical findings consistent with nonspecific back pain.* Mechanical low back pain is the diagnosis most consistent with this patient's presentation. In the absence of leg pain or neurological abnormalities, disk herniation is unlikely. Her history and physical exam do not suggest a serious underlying medical illness such as infection or cancer.

15–1, B. Learning objective: *Outline appropriate treatment for nonspecific low back pain.* Given the short duration of her symptoms, symptomatic treatment with NSAIDs would be appropriate, with reevaluation if she is not improved in two to three weeks. The majority of patients will resolve their symptoms spontaneously within four weeks without specific interventions. Patient education regarding the natural history of low back pain symptoms and encouragement to remain as active as possible are also important.

15–2, A. Learning objective: *Identify red flags for possible serious underlying medical diseases that can present as low back pain.* This woman has pain that is worse at night, which is unusual for mechanical low back pain. Her age and history of recent weight loss raise suspicion for an underlying disease such as cancer. Her back pain symptoms warrant further investigation.

15–2, B. Learning objective: *Describe appropriate diagnostic tests to further evaluate a patient with back pain that may be caused by a serious underlying medical condition.* A CBC and ESR should be done, and plain films of the lumbar spine would be appropriate to look for compression fracture or cancer. Abnormalities should be followed up with more specific testing. The physician should assess the status of this patient's cancer screening tests (e.g., mammography and colon cancer screening).

15–3, A. Learning objective: *Describe neurological findings consistent with nerve root compression from a disk herniation.* Low back pain associated with radiating leg pain below the knee in the acute setting may indicate nerve root compression from a disk herniation. Neurological exam of the lower extremities with close attention to asymmetry in reflexes, muscle strength, or sensation should be assessed. A positive straight leg raising test is also a sensitive finding suggesting disc herniation.

15–3, B. Learning objective: ***Describe the appropriate use of testing in the setting of acute low back pain.*** In the absence of serious neurological findings (such as seen in the cauda equina syndrome) or other "red flags," imaging studies are not indicated. Close follow-up and instructions to promptly report symptoms such as urinary incontinence or worsening leg weakness are appropriate. Imaging studies at this early stage of the patient's symptoms would not change his clinical management. This plan should be reassessed if his symptoms persist or worsen over the next two to three weeks.

15–3, C. Learning objective: ***Describe a treatment plan for a patient with acute low back and leg pain.*** Analgesia will be important given the severity of his symptoms. Acetaminophen, NSAIDs, and consideration of an opiate analgesic would be appropriate. Time off from work will be necessary initially; and avoiding heavy lifting and twisting for several months will speed recovery. Counsel the patient regarding the natural history of disk herniation and the treatment options available if symptoms do not improve. He will need to be followed closely over the next few weeks, and physical therapy should be considered.

▶ CHILDREN'S BEHAVIORAL PROBLEMS

16–1, A. Learning objective: ***Taking an accurate history.*** Additional information should include the family and social history, history of related behavioral problems, and prenatal and developmental history. Make sure to gather information from the father or other significant family members, interested caregivers, and the school.

16–1, B. Learning objective: ***Develop a broad differential diagnosis of school failure.*** Oppositional defiant disorder, ADHD, adjustment disorder, mood disorder, anxiety disorder, and problems with family dynamics or parenting skills should be considered.

16–2, A. Learning objective: ***Differentiating between normal and abnormal behavioral problems.*** If she has demonstrated these personality attributes consistently in the last three years and is otherwise progressing adequately developmentally, then chances are these behaviors do not indicate an underlying disorder.

16–2, B. Learning objective: ***Taking an accurate behavioral history.*** Is she capable of verbalizing at a level similar to her 4-year-old peers? Are her fine and gross motor skills intact? When she is in settings similar to a school environment—e.g., day care, religious school—how does she adjust over time?

► CHEST PAIN

17–1, A. Learning objective: *Accurate differential diagnosis of chest pain.* Assuming a normal physical examination, this patient sounds like she has gastroespoghageal reflux disorder (GERD).

17–1, B. Learning objective: *Cost-effective management of chest pain.* A presumptive diagnosis of GERD and treatment with a proton-pump inhibitor would be reasonable; patient education, smoking cessation, and follow-up are important.

17–2, A. Learning objective: *Knowing the cardiac risk factors.* This patient's risk factors include gender, age, history of smoking, hyperlipidemia, and hypertension.

17–2, B. Learning objective: *Cost-effective management of chest pain.* This patient should be considered to have unstable angina until proven otherwise. Troponin and cardiac enzymes should be drawn; an immediate EKG should be performed and aspirin and oxygen should be administered. If there is acute ST-elevation on the EKG, consider thrombolysis. Further management will hinge on this initial rapid assessment.

► COUGH & CONGESTION

18–1, A. Learning objective: *To generate a differential diagnosis of cough.* Because this is an acute illness the differential diagnosis includes URI, bronchitis, sinusitis, and exacerbation of chronic obstructive lung disease.

18–1, B. Learning objective: *To understand the role of testing in the evaluation of cough.* A peak flow measurement would help to evaluate this patient because he has tachypnea and wheezing. If hypoxia is suspected, oximetry can be performed.

18–1, C. Learning objective: *To be able to appropriately treat cough.* An inhaled β-agonist should be used to treat bronchospasm. Antibiotic usage is controversial in the setting of a patient presenting with acute exacerbation of chronic bronchitis. Those with mild or moderate disease may have no improvement with antibiotics. In more severe or prolonged presentations, the patient should be assessed for occult pneumonia and treated with amoxicillin/clavulanate, azithromycin, clarithromycin, a cephalosporin, or fluoroquinolone.

18–2, A. Learning objective: *Generate a differential diagnosis of rhinorrhea.* Given the chronic nature of the symptoms and appearance of the nasal mucosa, allergic rhinitis is the most likely etiology for this patient's complaints.

18–2, B. Learning objective: *Understand the diagnostic evaluation of nasal congestion.* If the etiology is in doubt, a nasal smear for eosinophils can be obtained.

▶ DIARRHEA

19–1, A. Learning objective: *Consider the causes of acute diarrhea.* As you review the office chart, remember that metformin can cause diarrhea, but there had not been a problem in the past or an increase in dosage. Infectious diarrheas are common. Her diet has changed with the move. The patient probably received antibiotics at the time of surgery and narcotics for pain relief. Are there any other new medications?

19–1, B. Learning objective: *Obtaining a history of an illness from a proxy (the nurse).* The patient appears well. Her blood pressure is normal with no orthostatic changes. No one else is ill with diarrhea at the nursing home and the staff has instituted enteric precautions. There is no blood in her stool. She is incontinent and is unable to get out of bed for physical therapy because of the soilage. She is not on any new medications. Yesterday the nursing home instituted their routine order for diarrhea, loperamide 2 mg four times a day. There has not been any improvement.

19–1, C. Learning objective: *Tests that are helpful in sorting out the diagnosis.* The diarrhea could be infectious and an antigen test of *Clostridium difficile* may be helpful and is 90% sensitive. Stool for occult blood may be negative in infectious diarrheas. A CBC, stool culture, and electrolytes are unlikely to be helpful in this mild case of acute diarrhea. You ask the nurse to limit sorbitol and lactose in the diet and hold the metformin for a few days while monitoring the blood glucose.

19–1, D. Learning objective: *Important points of a physical examination for diarrhea.* You visit the patient at the nursing home. She is now complaining of nausea and bloating along with the diarrhea. On rectal exam she has impacted stool caused by bed rest and narcotics. The diarrhea is due to liquid stool passing around the hard stool. Manual disimpaction results in a voluminous release of watery stool.

19–2, A. Learning objective: *Causes of acute infectious diarrhea.* The history suggests a common source outbreak (two children) and an invasive pathogen (bloody stool and fever). *Campylobacter* is the most commonly isolated bacterial cause of diarrhea in the United States. Salmonallosis, shigellosis, and enteroinvasive *Escherichia coli* are usually food-borne. Less common agents include *Vibrio parahaemolyticus, Aeromonas* species, and *Plesiomonas,* which are frequently related to freshwater or saltwater food products. *Yersinia enterocolitica* can also be food-borne. *Entameba histolytica* and *C. difficile* are less likely without a supporting history of foreign travel or recent antibiotic use, respectively. Other diagnoses to consider include *E. coli* 0157:H7 (although fever is unusual at the time of presentation), inflammatory bowel disease, intussusceptions, and appendicitis (unusual in both patients).

19–2, B. Learning objective: *Questions that will help in the diagnosis and management of infectious diarrheas.* The children live on a dairy farm and frequently drink raw milk that their father brings home. The parents don't drink milk (possible source of *Campylobactor, E. coli O157:H7*). They don't have a pet reptile (*Salmonella*) or kitten or puppy (*Yersinia*). Their mother is careful in food preparation and the rest of the family, including a 6-month-old breast-fed brother, is well. Neither girl has had a splenectomy, is HIV positive, has sickle cell anemia, liver disease, or other blood dyscrasia. They are at low risk for disseminated disease. Neither is pregnant or has taken antibiotics recently.

19–2, C. Learning objective: *Treatment of acute invasive diarrheas.* Many physicians would obtain a culture and start emperic antibiotic therapy. Observation would also be acceptable, with the provision that worsening symptoms should prompt a return for reevaluation. Quinolones are recommended for those at high risk for complications.

19–2, D. Learning objective: *Complications of infectious diarrheas.* *Campylobactor* bacteremia is rare in the immunocompetent host. It is associated as a trigger of Guillain-Barré syndrome, reactive arthritis, and mesenteric adenitis with appendicitis. *Campylobactor* infection is a reportable disease to the state health department.

▶ DIZZINESS

20–1, A. Learning objective: *Differential diagnosis of vertigo.* This patient most likely has benign positional vertigo. She describes a spinning sensation, which is the characteristic of vertigo—especially associated with head movement.

20–1, B. Learning objective: *Cost-effective testing for dizziness.* The Dix-Hallpike test will usually be positive with reproduction of symptoms and nystagmus.

20–2, A. Learning objective: *Differential diagnosis of dizziness.* Feeling of impending fainting, associated with erect posture, is the hallmark of orthostatic hypotension.

20–2, B. Learning objective: *Effective bedside testing for dizziness.* Doing orthostatic blood pressure and pulse reading will help make the diagnosis. A drop in systolic blood pressure of 20 mmHg or in diastolic blood pressure of 10 mmHg or more is considered to be diagnostic of orthostatic hypotension.

▶ DYSPEPSIA

21–1, A. Learning objective: ***Understand the differential diagnosis of upper abdominal pain.*** The most likely diagnosis is functional (non-ulcer) dyspepsia.

21–1, B. Learning objective: ***Understand the management of upper abdominal pain.*** Since he is over the age of 50, current recommendations suggest upper GI endoscopy to rule out cancer.

21–2, A. Learning objective: ***Understand treatment options for gastric ulcer.*** Sucralfate, H_2-blockers, and proton-pump inhibitors (PPIs) are all options. PPIs have the highest success rate but are also the most expensive.

21–2, B. Learning objective: ***Understand follow-up required for gastric ulcer.*** A post-treatment esophagogastroduodenoscopy is unlikely to be beneficial if the patient responds well to treatment. On the other hand, if symptoms persist, repeat endoscopy is indicated.

▶ DYSPNEA

22–1, A. Learning objective: ***Know the appropriate testing in patients with chest pain.*** ABGs would be the most appropriate choice because the patient has tachypnea, tachycardia, and chest pain and this would be the best way to evaluate her respiratory condition.

22–1, B. Learning objective: ***Know the differential diagnosis of chest pain.*** Pulmonary embolus needs to be ruled out, and a spiral CT of the chest is the current standard of care for diagnosing pulmonary embolus. Other tests to consider are ventilation perfusion scan and pulmonary arteriogram.

22–2, A. Learning objective: ***Know the evaluation of heart disease.*** An echocardiogram will assess left ventricular function and alcohol-related heart disease.

22–2, B. Learning objective: ***Know the differential diagnosis of heart disease.*** Alcoholic cardiomyopathy is most likely given this patient's history. Treatment should include alcohol cessation, diuretics, afterload reduction, and ionotropic agents.

▶ DYSURIA

23–1, A. Learning objective: ***Key historical findings in a female patient with dysuria.*** Key points from history include a sexual history, specifically new partners, description of discharge, duration of symptoms, past history, location of burning sensation, and other symptoms.

23–1, B. Learning objective: ***Recognize appropriate laboratory testing.*** Appropriate lab tests include urinalysis, urine culture, culture of urethral discharge, and possibly DNA testing of the discharge for chlamydia and gonorrhea.

23–1, C. Learning objective: ***Know the likely causes of dysuria in a sexually active female.*** The most likely causes include a urinary tract infection, *Chlamydia trachomatis* with watery mucoid discharge, *Neisseria gonorrhoeae* with yellow or gray thick discharge, or fungus with thick, curdlike, white, pruritic discharge.

23–2, A. Learning objective: ***Know key historical questions for a patient with dysuria and systemic symptoms.*** Key points from the history include the duration of symptoms, history of stones (herself and other family members), sexual history, costovertebral angle pain, nausea, and vomiting.

23–2, B. Learning objective: ***Know appropriate testing and systemic symptoms in a patient with dysuria.*** Appropriate testing would include a urinalysis, urine culture, ultrasound of the abdomen, and radiographic imaging of the kidneys, ureters, and bladder.

23–2, C. Learning objective: ***Know the causes of dysuria in a patient with systemic signs and symptoms.*** Potential causes for this patient's presentation include acute pyelonephritis, or a pyelonephritis secondary to obstruction from a stone. She could also have an acute abdomen from an appendicitis, ectopic pregnancy, or pelvic inflammatory disease.

▶ EARACHE

24–1, A. Learning objective: ***Differential diagnosis of earache in a child.*** This young boy may have either acute otitis media or otitis media with effusion.

24–1, B. Learning objective: ***Important historical data to obtain.*** Exposure to smoking and day care attendance are risk factors for otitis media. The fact that the patient is afebrile and happy makes OM less likely.

24–1, C. Learning objective: ***Physical findings in otitis media.*** The tympanic membrane should be examined for evidence of effusion and mobility.

24–1, D. Learning objective: ***Follow-up for otitis media.*** The child should be reexamined in two to four weeks to document resolution of the effusion.

24–2, A. Learning objective: ***Differential diagnosis for external pain and ear drainage.*** The child has either otitis externa or otitis media with pus draining from a perforated tympanic membrane.

24–2, B. Learning objective: ***Appropriate exam of a draining ear.*** With a history of pain and drainage, otoscopy is essential for visualization of the tympanic membrane.

24–2, C. Learning objective: ***Treatment of otitis externa.*** A topical fluoroquinolone/steroid drop would be a good treatment option.

▶ FATIGUE

25–1, A. Learning objective: ***Pharmacologic treatment of fibromyalgia.*** The selective serotonin re-uptake inhibitors (SSRIs) such as Zoloft are helpful with pain control as well as disturbed sleep patterns related to depression. They have also been useful with hot flashes. Additionally, they have a favorable side effect profile and are reasonably safe.

25–2, A. Learning objective: ***Recognition of sleep apnea.*** Daytime fatigue, memory loss, snoring, and weight gain are consistent with the diagnosis of sleep apnea.

25–2, B. Learning objective: ***Treatment of sleep apnea.*** Weight loss would be the initial treatment of choice. The patient may also benefit from continuous positive airway pressure (CPAP) or pharyngeal reduction surgery.

▶ GASTROINTESTINAL BLEEDING

26–1, A–B. Learning objective: ***Know the initial evaluation of GI bleeding.*** In acute settings such as this, airway, breathing, and circulation should be included in the first evaluation. A rapid clinical assessment should give an idea as to how much blood the patient has lost. Then the patient should be transferred immediately to the ER. The patient is vomiting blood and therefore has an upper GI bleed, and this should be confirmed by insertion of an NG tube.

26–1, C–D. Learning objective: ***Learn the basic evaluation techniques and associated treatment plans for upper and lower GI bleeds.*** Endoscopy is usually the initial evaluation in GI bleeds. This patient needed an esophagogastroduodenoscopy (EGD), which revealed a mucosal tear at the gastroesophageal junction—

a Mallory-Weiss tear. Although EGDs offer the therapeutic options of banding, embolization, and injection of vasopressin, Mallory-Weiss tears often heal with observation alone.

▶ HEADACHE

27–1, A. Learning objective: ***Know what studies are indicated for a tension-type headache.*** This patient is presenting with symptoms consistent with a tension-type headache. No radiologic or laboratory studies are indicated.

27–1, B. Learning objective: ***The differential diagnosis for tension-type headaches.*** The differential diagnosis should also include "rebound" or medication-overuse headaches given this patient's history of daily analgesic useage.

27–2, A. Learning objective: ***Know the "red-flag" findings of a headache.*** "Red-flag" findings on exam would include fever, neck stiffness, asymmetry on neurological exam, and abnormal fundal or papillary exam.

27–2, B. Learning objective: ***Recognition of migraine symptoms.*** The history and exam are consistent with migraine with aura. This patient has a unilateral, throbbing headache with associated phonophobia and vomiting.

27–2, C. Learning objective: ***Treatment options for a migraine-type headache.*** Treatment options would include migraine-specific agents, especially those such as sumatriptan that can be given either intranasally or subcutaneously because the patient is vomiting. The associated nausea and vomiting can be treated with antiemetics and intravenous fluids.

▶ HEARTBURN

28–1, A. Learning objective: ***Recognize red flags of heartburn.*** This history is quite consistent with heartburn. Other questions that might help exclude more worrisome conditions include questions about weight loss or night sweats and questions to rule out cardiac disease. No lab testing is indicated at this time.

28–1, B. Learning objective: ***Pharmacologic and nonpharmacologic treatments for gastroesophageal disease.*** Initial recommendations would include lifestyle modifications, especially dietary modifications. Avoiding greasy meals, alcohol, and lying prone within three hours of eating should improve his symptoms. Smoking cessation would certainly be recommended, and exercise would probably help. Elevating the head of the bed may help. It would be reasonable to prescribe H_2-blockers or a proton-pump inhibitor (PPI) if lifestyle modifications fail.

▶ HIGH CHOLESTEROL

29–1, A. Learning objective: *Assess cardiovascular risk factors.* Risk factors other than dyslipidemia include current cigarette smoking, hypertension (≥ 140/90 mmHg) or currently being treated, diabetes mellitus, HDL-C less than 40 mg/dL, family history of premature cardiovascular disease (father, brother, or son before age 55; mother, sister, or daughter before age 65), male age 45 or older, female age 55 or older, obesity, and physical inactivity.

29–1, B. Learning objective: *Classify patients into appropriate risk categories.* This patient would be low risk (10-year risk < 10%) with no risk factors.

29–1, C. Learning objective: *Determine treatment plan and goals based on risk category and LDL-C level.* Since his LDL-C goal is less than 160 mg/dL, no treatment is indicated. He should be encouraged to maintain a healthy lifestyle.

29–1, D. Learning objective: *Discuss lipid-screening principles.* He should be screened again in five years.

29–2, A. Learning objective: *Discuss the effect of a myocardial infarction on cholesterol levels.* LDL-C levels decrease within a matter of hours following a myocardial infarction and may stay low for up to three months. The first cholesterol level would be most indicative of her true, baseline level; a pre-MI value would be the best indicator.

29–2, B. Learning objective: *Determine treatment plan and goals based on risk category and LDL-C level.* Her LDL-C goal is less than 100 mg/dL since she has known coronary heart disease (CHD).

29–2, C. Learning objective: *Discuss lipid-screening principles.* Her son should be screened for dyslipidemia and have a risk assessment. He should modify any risky behaviors that he does have; if he does not currently have any modifiable risk factors, he should be encouraged to maintain his healthy lifestyle.

29–3, A. Learning objective: *Discuss lipid-screening principles.* His non–HDL-C is 236. Fasting lipids to determine LDL-C should be ordered since his TC and HDL-C are both abnormal.

29–3, B. Learning objective: *Determine treatment plan and goals based on risk category and LDL-C level.* Since his CHD risk is greater than 20% (CHD equivalent), his LDL-C goal is 100 mg/dL. If his 10-year risk is 19%, his LDL-C goal is 130 mg/dL.

29–3, C. Learning objective: ***Determine treatment plan based on risk category and LDL-C level.*** Since his risk category is CHD-equivalent, drug therapy would be initiated if the LDL-C is 130 mg/dL or higher.

29–3, D. Learning objective: ***Assess secondary causes of dyslipidemia.*** Secondary causes include diabetes mellitus, chronic renal failure, obstructive liver disease, and hypothyroidism. Drug causes should be ruled out by history (progestins, corticosteroids, anabolic steroids, and protease inhibitors).

29–4, A. Learning objective: ***Describe treatment for metabolic syndrome.*** Weight loss and increased physical activity are the two main goals of treatment.

29–4, B. Learning objective: ***Discuss metabolic syndrome.*** These individuals are high CHD risks regardless of LDL-C levels.

29–4, C. Learning objective: ***Describe treatment for metabolic syndrome.*** Drug therapy for the patient with metabolic syndrome includes treatment of hypertension, elevated TG, and decreased HDL-C, plus a daily aspirin to reduce the prothrombotic state.

▶ HYPERTENSION

30–1, A. Learning objective: ***The diagnosis of hypertension is made only after confirmed readings of elevated blood pressure (BP) on two separate occasions.*** The measurement should be repeated after the patient has been sitting quietly. Use a BP cuff appropriate for the size of the patient's arm. Take two readings in each arm and compare. Values that differ by more than 5 mmHg require additional BP readings that should then be averaged. Ideally the patient should have had nothing to eat, drink, or smoke for one hour. A BP 140/90 mmHg or higher is consistent with hypertension, but until this is confirmed with two additional readings on a separate occasion the diagnosis is provisional.

30–1, B. Learning objective: ***Recognize the presence of comorbid conditions, end-organ damage, or possible causes of secondary hypertension.*** Obtain a complete family and social history to identify risk factors for both hypertension and comorbid conditions such as diabetes and hyperlipidemia. In particular, exercise habits, alcohol use, and tobacco use should be quantified. Review of systems should focus on the central nervous, cardiovascular, and endocrine systems to identify presence of cerebrovascular disease, coronary disease, peripheral vascular disease, diabetes, or pheochrocytoma. The physical examination should pay particular attention to the presence of obesity, striea, retinopathy, carotid bruits, jugular venous distension, ventricular gallops, rales, abdominal bruits, peripheral pulses, pedal edema, and neurologic deficits.

30–1, C. Learning objective: ***The initial diagnostic evaluation should be limited to the tests most likely to identify comorbid conditions, end-organ damage, and the common secondary causes of hypertension.*** The initial diagnostic evaluation should include a CBC, electrolytes, BUN, creatinine, glucose, uric acid, lipid profile, urinalysis, and electrocardiogram. These tests will identify the majority of patients with comorbid conditions such as diabetes and hyperlipidemia as well as those with common end-organ disease such as nephropathy, coronary disease, and left ventricular enlargement. Additionally, secondary causes of hypertension such as renal disorders and hyperaldosteronism will be detected.

30–1, D. Learning objective: ***The initial treatment of hypertension is therapeutic lifestyle change (TLC).*** Even before the diagnosis of hypertension is confirmed, this patient should be instructed to undertake an aerobic activity such as walking, dancing, cycling, or swimming for 30 minutes four days out of the week. These activities involve large muscle groups and can be undertaken in a social or group context, which will increase the probability of it becoming a habitual activity. Food consumption should be balanced with caloric expenditure to maintain a BMI of 19.0–24.9. Salt intake should be restricted to 6 g daily (equal to of 2 g of sodium daily). Alcohol intake should not exceed two equivalents for men and one equivalent for women. (A 12-ounce beer, 4-ounce glass of wine, and 1 ounce of distilled spirits each constitute one alcohol equivalent.) Once the diagnosis is confirmed and after six months of TLC (being male constitutes having one risk factor), if the treatment goal BP of less than 140/90 mmHg is not met, medication should be initiated.

30–2, A. Learning objective: ***Investigate changes in adherence to prescribed treatment regimens when a treatment goal BP is not achieved.*** A thorough nonjudgmental line of questioning should be undertaken to identify any changes in this patient's lifestyle. This includes her level of activity, diet, and consumption of alcohol or use of tobacco. Additionally the use of any over-the-counter or herbal remedies should be explored. Finally it should be determined if the patient is able to adhere to the prescribed drug treatment plan. Some of the reasons patients are unable to achieve adherence include dosing schedules more frequent than once daily, expense, and undesirable effects of medication. These possibilities should be explored with the patient.

30–2, B. Learning objective: ***Secondary causes of hypertension should be considered when treatment goal BP is not achieved in a previously well-controlled patient.*** The leading cause of secondary hypertension is renal artery stenosis. Clues to this diagnosis include the presence of diffuse atherosclerosis and the presence of an abdominal bruit over the area of one or both renal arteries, particularly in a patient over 50. An acute rise in serum creatinine after administration of an angiotensin converting enzyme inhibitor or angiotensin II receptor blocker also suggests the diagnosis.

Other causes of secondary hypertension to be considered include primary renal disease, pheochromocytoma, primary aldosteronism, Cushing's syndrome, and coartation of the aorta.

30–2, C. Learning objective: ***The majority of hypertensive patients require multiple medications to achieve treatment-goal blood pressure.*** Even in the absence of secondary causes, more than one medication is usually required to control hypertension. The use of multiple medications in lower doses is likely to be better tolerated than a single medication at a higher dose. Possibilities for this patient include drugs from the other four classes: β-blockers, ACE inhibitors/angiotensin receptor blockers (ARBs), calcium channel blockers, and α-adrenergic blockers. The choice of drug selected for additional BP lowering might depend on the presence of other diagnoses. Hypertensive patients with diabetes or CHF would be expected to benefit from ACE inhibitors or ARBs; those with CAD would do well with β-blockers. However, β-blockers should be used cautiously in patients with severe obstructive pulmonary disease or severe peripheral vascular disease.

▶ LOWER EXTREMITY PAIN & SWELLING

31–1, A. Learning objective: ***Recognize deep venous thrombosis.*** This patient had an acute onset of unilateral pain and swelling with erythema and tenderness after prolonged travel. This presentation should always raise the possibility of a deep vein thrombosis (DVT). Other risk factors for this would include estrogen usage, smoking, and family history of DVT.

31–1, B. Learning objective: ***Know the appropriate test for diagnosing DVT.*** Venous Doppler studies are the noninvasive test of choice when there is clinical suspicion of a DVT. The test is readily available, reasonably inexpensive, and clinically reliable.

31–1, C. Learning objective: ***Know the initial management strategy for DVT.*** A patient with DVT needs to be anticoagulated. Typically, this is accomplished with IV heparin or subcutaneous low-molecular-weight heparin products. An oral warfarin product such as Coumadin is initiated after 24 hours and titrated to a therapeutic level; usually this would be an international normalization ratio (INR) of 2.0 to 2.5. Most patients are admitted to the hospital for initial treatment of DVT.

31–2, A. Learning objective: ***Recognition of cellulitis.*** The most likely diagnosis in this patient is cellulitis caused by the recent skin break. The diagnosis is further supported by his clinical exam of redness and warmth. In addition, diabetics will frequently have elevated blood sugars during an infectious process.

31–2, B. Learning objective: ***Know the treatment for acute cellulitis.*** Superficial skin infections are commonly caused by staphylococcal and streptococcal bacteria. Appropriate treatment would include antibiotics such as extended spectrum penicillins or cephalosporins. Diabetics are more likely to have *pseudomonas* as a causative agent, thus requiring an antibiotic such as a fluoroquinolone. Reliable patients can be managed on an outpatient basis but will require close follow-up.

▶ LYMPHADENOPATHY

32–1, A. Learning objective: ***Lymphadenopathy that lasts less than two weeks or more than a year with no progressive increase in size has a very low likelihood of being neoplastic.*** Most likely, this patient has bacterial pharyngitis.

32–1, B. Learning objective: ***Evaluation of exudative pharyngitis with cervical adenopathy.*** Perform a rapid streptococcus test; if negative, perform a throat culture. Begin empirical treatment with penicillin.

32–2, A. Learning objective: ***Evaluation of clavicle mass.*** Excisional biopsy is the diagnostic procedure of choice in this case. Fine-needle aspiration—even with the advent of new immunohistochemical analytical techniques—has lesser diagnostic yield because of the limited amount of tissue that undergoes evaluation. In this patient, red flags are raised because the patient is young, the size of the lymph node is larger than 1 cm, and the location is an extremely common one for cancer.

32–2, B. Learning objective: ***Left supraclavicular lymphadenopathy is often associated with carcinoma.*** One or two enlarged lymph nodes in a young person indicates Hodgkin's disease and Reed-Sternberg cells are pathognomonic of Hodgkin's disease.

▶ RASHES

33–1, A. Learning objective: ***Know the characteristic signs and symptoms of urticaria.*** Urticaria (hives) is the most likely diagnosis. Urticaria is an allergic process in which new wheals evolve as old ones resolve. As seen with this patient, itching is the hallmark symptom in urticaria. Acute urticaria often is caused by an allergic reaction to a medication. The sulfa in the trimethoprimsulfamethoxazole is the most likely offending agent. It is only life-threatening if the allergic reaction also involves the airway. Differential diagnosis includes erythema multiforme, which is also a common drug reaction to sulfa medications.

33–1, B. Learning objective: ***Learn how to manage urticaria.*** The best course of management is to make sure that the patient stops the current sulfa antibiotic. Simultaneously he should start taking an H_1 antihistamine to treat the allergic reaction. The first generation antihistamines such as diphenhydramine, chlorpheniramine, and hydroxyzine are very effective for acute urticaria. Diphenhydramine and chlorpheniramine are available over-the-counter and are relatively inexpensive. The second generation H_1 antihistamines such as astemizole, loratadine, desloratadine, and cetirizine cause less sedation and are better tolerated in the daytime for chronic use. More severe and resistant cases may require a course of oral prednisone.

33–2, A. Learning objective: *Learn the common causes of a widespread pruritic rash.* The differential diagnosis includes atopic dermatitis, contact dermatitis, drug eruption, and a viral exanthem. The absence of fever, lack of unusual topical exposures, and negative medication history along with the family history make atopic dermatitis (AD) the most likely diagnosis. Also this pruritic papular eruption with scale found in the popliteal fossa is classic for AD. These patients often have either a personal or family history of asthma, allergic rhinitis, or conjunctivitis. Most atopic dermatitis is not caused by specific allergens, but is set off by a number of trigger factors in patients with a strong genetic predisposition to develop eczematous eruptions.

33–2, B. Learning objective: *Learn the best course of management for atopic dermatitis.* The best course of management starts with reducing exposure to skin irritants and using emollients to moisten the skin. The allergic and inflammatory component is treated with a low potency topical steroid such as 1% hydrocortisone. A cream may be adequate, but an ointment is preferred if the skin is very dry or cracked. The absence of crusts or exudate makes a secondary bacterial infection less likely and avoids the need to use an antibiotic. The itching and sleep disturbance may be treated with a first-generation antihistamine as discussed in Case 33–1.

▶ SLEEP PROBLEMS

34–1, A. Learning objective: *Identify common causes of insomnia from history and physical exam information.* It is likely that both individuals have a sleep-related disorder. The husband apparently snores very loudly, has hypertension, is obese, and reports excessive daytime sleepiness. These are the hallmark findings for sleep apnea. However, it would also be useful to inquire into his prostate symptoms and whether he is waking up to urinate. Review his blood pressure medications. The wife likely suffers from periodic limb movements. The most relevant piece of history comes from the husband when he states she is active in bed. Her diabetes can also contribute to insomnia if her sugar is not well controlled, as can arthritis or any cause of chronic pain. Menopausal women often have difficulty sleeping secondary to vasomotor symptoms. Finally, inquire into the couple's social history and sleep routine to rule out contributions from alcohol or poor sleep hygiene.

34–1, B. Learning objective: ***Initiate an appropriate insomnia work-up for patients.*** The initial step is to complete a more thorough history and physical exam including reviewing all medications the couple is on. Completing a two-week sleep diary may help. Although perhaps not necessary to make the diagnosis, given the suspicion of sleep apnea for the husband and a movement disorder for the wife, a sleep study may yield confirmatory information.

34–1, C. Learning objective: ***Be able to articulate basic treatment options for movement-related sleep disorders and obstructive sleep apnea.*** Assuming the wife has periodic limb movements or restless leg syndrome, the most likely successful course of treatment involves dopaminergic medications (such as the Parkinson-type medications). First-line treatment for sleep apnea is losing weight; however, for many patients this proves too difficult. Continuous positive airway pressure masks keep the soft tissues from collapsing and blocking the airway. If this fails, there are several surgical options for removing or modifying the soft palate.

34–2, A. Learning objective: ***Identify elements placing patients at risk for insomnia.*** Although the exact nature of her insomnia is unclear, she has numerous risk factors—including age, being institutionalized, fairly recent loss coupled with change of environment, tobacco use, COPD medication that could be theophylline, and a diagnosis of GERD, which appears to be untreated. Additionally, the patient provides a good story for a diagnosis of depression (anhedonia, sleep, weight gain).

34–2, B. Learning objective: ***Develop a list of investigative studies in an elderly patient complaining of insomnia.*** The patient should be instructed on how to keep a sleep diary for two weeks. Given the description of her problem it is unlikely that a sleep study would offer much insight. B_{12}, folate, and TSH would be useful studies looking for possible causes of her symptoms, such as pseudodementia or depression.

34–2, C. Learning objective: ***Initiate a treatment plan for long-term-care patient who presents with insomnia.*** Instruct the patient on proper sleep hygiene. For example, encourage her to be out of bed during the day and only get in bed to sleep. Also, she should not smoke prior to bed. If the patient's GERD is contributing to her symptoms, it should be treated; likewise, if the patient is on theophylline for her COPD, this should be changed. Environmental disturbances also play a significant role in disrupting institutionalized patients' sleep. Moving her away from the nurse's station, less frequent vitals, and minimizing other light and sound may be helpful. Finally, if the patient turns out to have depression, treat the symptoms with an appropriate sedating antidepressant. Benzodiazepines and other sleep agents only mask the problem and thus should be avoided in this patient, who likely has correctable causes for her insomnia.

▶ SORE THROAT

35–1, A. Learning objective: ***Know the differential diagnosis for causes of pharyngitis.*** Viral and bacterial strep pharyngitis are likely candidates.

35–1, B. Learning objective: ***Know the criteria for diagnosis of strep pharyngitis.*** The patient has two criteria for strep and has unknown strep culture. A strep screen and culture should be performed.

35–1, C. Learning objective: ***Know the criteria for treatment of pharyngitis with antibiotics.*** Do not send this child home with antibiotics. He has no adenopathy and does not meet temperature criteria or known exposure. It is acceptable to wait until the culture results are back.

35–2, A. Learning objective: ***Know the history to take for patients with pharyngitis.*** Additional history of cough, fatigue, rash, and physical examination including throat and cervical area is appropriate.

35–2, B. Learning objective: ***Know the indications for laboratory testing for patients with pharyngitis.*** Ordering of laboratory tests depends on the clinical course. This is a classic presentation for mononucleosis. The diagnosis is usually made after 10 days of illness when conventional testing will be positive.

35–2, C. Learning objective: ***Know the important features of the clinical course of mononucleosis.*** If this is mononucleosis, the course is variable, but usually lasts about six weeks.

▶ SYNCOPE

36–1, A. Learning objective: ***Identify symptoms consistent with syncope versus other conditions.*** While this patient has dizzy spells, she may more likely be describing presyncope. She does not have actual loss of consciousness, which is part of the definition of syncope. Other likely explanations of her symptoms include panic attacks and anxiety. Hyperventilation can result in hypocarbia, which classically presents with these symptoms.

36–1, B. Learning objective: ***Describe appropriate evaluation and management of syncope.*** This patient's symptoms may be reproduced by having her hyperventilate. Therefore an appropriate intervention would be to have her rebreathe carbon dioxide using a paper bag. In the absence of cardiac risk factors or findings, an extensive workup may not be necessary, but an electrocardiogram (EKG) would be important to rule out arrhythmia or ischemia. Unusual causes in this patient might include thyrotoxicosis or adrenergic overactivity and more extensive blood work might be helpful if simple interventions do not help.

36–2, A. Learning objective: ***Identify high-risk patients presenting with syncopal episodes.*** This patient has comorbid heart disease and is describing probable cardiac arrhythmias with ischemia. In general, new onset or worsening pattern of symptoms are more worrisome for disease. Also, specific cardiac or neurologic symptoms require timely evaluation.

36–2, B. Learning objective: ***Describe appropriate evaluation and management of syncope.*** In addition to the EKG, cardiac testing including exercise treadmill is indicated. Exercise-limited symptoms may also require evaluation by echocardiogram to identify valvular disease or cardiomyopathy. If palpitations are a prominent symptom, ambulatory Holter monitoring or cardiac event monitoring is a reasonable test.

▶ VAGINAL BLEEDING

37–1, A. Learning objective: ***Know the signs and symptoms of polycystic ovary syndrome (PCOS).*** This is a classic case of PCOS. Anovulatory, irregular cycles occur due to multiple follicular cysts on the ovary. Hypothyroidism, another endocrine disorder, can affect menstrual cycles, but usually does not cause hirsutism.

37–1, B. Learning objective: ***Know the disorders related to PCOS.*** Patients with PCOS have a higher incidence of diabetes and other obesity-related diseases. In addition, the patient may have difficulty getting pregnant.

37–2, A. Learning objective: ***Know evaluation strategies for postmenopausal bleeding.*** Additional history should include hormonal therapy, previous abnormal bleeding, and other medical illnesses such as diabetes and hypertension.

37–2, B. Learning objective: ***Know management strategies for postmenopausal bleeding.*** This patient is at high risk of carcinoma, and so an endometrial biopsy and ultrasound should be performed.

► VAGINAL DISCHARGE

38–1, A. Learning objective: *List causes of vaginal discharge.* The clinical features are most consistent with a *Trichomonas* infection. Bacterial vaginosis can present with this history, but the cervix is usually not inflamed and the discharge is usually more gray and thin. The history of an unsuccessful trial of antifungal medication makes a *Candida* infection unlikely.

38–1, B. Learning objective: *Recognize a common presentation for* Trichomonas *infection.* On saline wet mount exam, you should find motile protozoa along with many white blood cells. Coinfection with bacterial vaginosis is possible, so clue cells may also be present.

38–1, C. Learning objective: *Appropriately counsel a patient with a sexually transmitted infection.* *Trichomonas* vaginitis is a sexually transmitted disease. She should use a barrier method such as condoms to prevent future infection. The patient should be advised to inform all recent sexual partners that they need to be treated. She should not resume sexual relations with any partner until both have completed a course of medication to prevent reinfection. The name of the infection needing treatment should be written down and given to the patient to give to her partners for their doctor to read.

38–2, A. Learning objective: *Recognize a common presentation for yeast vaginitis.* *Candida* yeast infection is common after a course of oral antibiotics. You expect to see hyphae or budding yeast on potassium hydroxide (KOH) exam.

38–2, B. Learning objective: *Recognize advantages and disadvantages of oral versus topical treatment.* Topical antifungals are less expensive and do not cause systemic side effects. Oral fluconazole is given as a single dose and does not require local application.

► VOMITING

39–1, A. Learning objective: *Know the differential diagnosis for vomiting in a woman of reproductive age.* The differential diagnosis should include viral illnesses, hepatitis, food poisoning, gallbladder disease, medication side effects, appendicitis, and pregnancy. Your list of potential diagnoses must include morning sickness owing to early pregnancy.

39–1, B. Learning objective: *Know the additional history to obtain from a woman of reproductive age with vomiting.* Additional history should include last menstrual period, contraception, and unprotected intercourse.

39–1, C. Learning objective: ***Know which tests should be ordered for a woman of reproductive age with vomiting.*** A urinalysis will screen for dehydration and ketones in the urine, signs of dehydration. A urine or serum pregnancy test also would help differentiate the causes of the symptoms.

39–2, A. Learning objective: ***Know the differential diagnosis for a child with vomiting.*** Your differential diagnosis should include viral illnesses, medication side effects, food poisoning, foreign substance ingestion, hepatitis, and appendicitis. In a younger child (less than 1 year of age) also consider congenital abnormalities of the gastrointestinal tract in your differential diagnosis.

39–2, B. Learning objective: ***Know the lab and imaging studies that may need to be performed for a child with vomiting.*** CBC and radiographic studies will help confirm the diagnosis of appendicitis. Some institutions prefer ultrasound examination, while others prefer CT or MRI for further definition of the problem.

39–3, A. Learning objective: ***Know the differential diagnosis for common causes of food poisoning.*** *Staphylococcus aureus* is a common cause of food poisoning mediated by a heat-stable enterotoxin that causes rapid onset of symptoms lasting one to two days. Foods that are frequently associated with staphylococcal food poisoning include meat products; salads such as egg, tuna, chicken, potato, and macaroni; and bakery products such as cream-filled pastries. *Escherichia coli* takes about one week for symptoms to occur and rarely causes vomiting. *Giardia lamblia* causes diarrhea without vomiting and is associated with drinking water from contaminated rivers or streams. *Bacillus cereus* causes watery diarrhea and abdominal cramping within six hours of ingestion and is often associated with rice products.

▶ FAMILY VIOLENCE

40–1, A. Learning objective: ***Know the signs and symptoms of child abuse.*** The timing of the injury, the remoteness of the dryer from the sofa, and the nature of the injury all raise the level of suspicion.

40–1, B. Learning objective: ***Know how to evaluate for child abuse.*** Obtain information about other injuries and assess family risk factors.

40–2, A. Learning objective: ***Know what to look for on physical exam when evaluating for possible elder abuse.*** Look for bruises, poor hygiene, healed lacerations, occult fractures, and pressure ulcers.

40–2, B. Learning objective: ***Know how to obtain a history and conduct an interview in a situation of possible elder abuse.*** The assessment would continue with obtaining additional history in a nonthreatening way. This would involve talking in private and looking for signs of social isolation, coercion, and signs of depression.

40–2, C. Learning objective: ***Know the management strategy for elder abuse.*** If all lab and physical findings are negative, then close follow-up should be attempted to establish the continuum of care.

▶ ASTHMA/COPD

41–1, A. Learning objective: ***Know the major cause of acute exacerbation in patients with COPD.*** The major causes are infections. The organisms include *Streptococcus pneumoniae, Haemophilus influenzae, Moraxella catarrhalis, Chlamydia pneumoniae, Mycoplasma pneumoniae,* viruses, and *pseudomonas* (most severe).

41–1, B. Learning objective: ***Know which lab tests should be ordered in COPD patients.*** A chest x-ray will show an increase in the volume of the lung fields with flattening of the diaphragm. There will be a decrease in vascular markings and a hyperlucency over the lung fields. Pulmonary function tests would show a FEV_1/FRC ratio below 0.75, which is not reversible after β_2-agonist treatment. A pulse oximetry reading would be below the mid-90s percent range. Finally, an ABG would show a higher than normal CO_2 value with compensatory metabolic alkalosis.

41–1, C. Learning objective: ***How to treat an acute exacerbation of COPD.*** There are five things to do when treating an acute exacerbation of COPD: This patient needs O_2 via nasal cannula or CPAP, a beta$_2$-agonist, oral corticosteroids, IV fluid resuscitation, and broad-spectrum antibiotic coverage until the organism and sensitivities are known.

41–1, D. Learning objective: ***How to treat chronic COPD.*** Albuterol is just for rescue therapy. A chronic COPD patient needs long-term preventive medication. First of all, smoking cessation should be encouraged. Secondly, if the PaO_2 is below 55 mmHg, he should be on home oxygen therapy. Finally, a combined inhaled corticosteroid and long acting β_2-agonist would be beneficial. He should also get a yearly flu shot and a pneumococcal shot.

41–2, A. Learning objective: ***Recognize concerning signs for a worsening asthma attack.*** There are several signs of an asthma attack. The most concerning is the presence of pulsus paradoxis of greater than or equal to 25 mmHg. That is a fall of systolic blood pressure of 25 mmHg or greater on inspiration. Secondly, look for the following signs of fatigue: Children will present with two- to three-word sentence dyspnea, accessory muscle use, retractions, and diaphoresis. Finally, if an arterial blood gas is drawn and the CO_2 is normal or increasing, this is a sign of fatigue and impending respiratory failure.

41–2, B. Learning objective: ***How to treat an asthma attack.*** Oxygen will never hurt a child during an asthma attack. You need to immediately start systemic corticosteroid therapy. The systemic steroids may take some time to start working so, in the meantime, give nebulized racemic epinephrine treatment to maintain airway patency. Finally, be ready for intubation if the child shows signs of fatigue.

41–2, C. Learning objective: ***Know which lab tests and other diagnostic studies to order for asthma.*** An arterial blood gas can be obtained to examine the acuity of the attack. Special attention is placed on the CO_2 and pH. A chest x-ray may show some hyperinflation, but it could be normal. Pulmonary function tests will show obstructive disease (FEV_1/FRC ratio ≤ 0.75) that improves after β_2-agonist treatment. There should be an increase in the FEV_1 of greater than 12%. Other tests that can be done are skin testing or RAST testing; these are IgE sensitization testing techniques.

41–2, D. Learning objective: ***Understand current recommended long-term therapy for asthma.*** His symptoms are consistent with severe persistent asthma. The current recommendations for treatment include the maintenance therapy of high-dose inhaled corticosteroids and a long-acting β_2-agonist. There are combination inhalers, such as Advair. He can continue to use his short acting β_2-agonist as needed for rescue therapy. The addition of leukotriene inhibitors can be added for synergistic effects. If adequate control is still not obtained, use oral steroid treatment as a last resort.

▶ ANGINA & CORONARY ARTERY DISEASE

42–1, A. Learning objective: ***Recognize acute coronary syndrome and the importance of prompt EKG.*** This patient has a classic acute coronary syndrome (ACS) presentation, and the goal is to have an EKG within 5 minutes so that thrombolysis can be started within 30 minutes if ST elevations are seen on the EKG and if the patient has no contraindications to thrombolysis.

42–1, B. Learning objective: ***Identify the vital information needed in an initial ACS work-up.*** Assess character, intensity, location, timing, and radiation of the pain and if the patient has had any similar pain in the past. Ask about any accompanying symptoms and what brought the symptoms on. Assess for all the main risk factors including age, smoking, hypertension, high cholesterol, obesity, physical inactivity, family history, diabetes, and history of heart disease. Define the patient's past medical and surgery history as well as allergies and medications.

42–1, C. Learning objective: ***Be able to order the appropriate initial therapies and labs for an ACS without EKG changes.*** Order chewed aspirin, sublingual nitro, supplemental oxygen, a β-blocker, heparin, IV access, and morphine for pain. Also order chest x-ray, serial cardiac enzymes, serial EKGs, CBC, basic metabolic panel, PT/PTT, and a urinalysis. GP IIb/IIIa receptor antagonists should be added with positive enzymes.

42–2, A. Learning objective: ***Know how to recognize and assess someone at high risk for coronary artery disease (CAD).*** This patient already has many serious risk factors including family history, age, sex, hypertension, smoking, physical inactivity, and obesity. Even though this patient is asymptomatic it is important to do a thorough assessment. Evaluation should include CBC, BUN and creatinine, fasting lipid profile, and blood sugar. A baseline EKG and chest x-ray would also be wise.

42–2, B. Learning objective: ***Know how to address risk factors in an asymptomatic patient at high risk for CAD.*** This patient needs appropriate counseling on weight loss, exercising, and quitting smoking. He should also be on 81 mg of aspirin a day and a β-blocker to control his blood pressure.

42–2, C. Learning objective: ***Know how to use noninvasive testing in a high-risk patient without symptoms.*** It would be very reasonable to address this patient's concerns as well as gain useful prognostic information by having him perform an exercise EKG. It would be beneficial for the patient's confidence, and it may uncover significant CAD.

▶ BREAST DISEASE

43–1, A. Learning objective: ***Know the history to take when evaluating a breast mass in a post-menopausal woman.*** Historical information regarding the persistence of the mass, any changes over time, and the evaluation of this patient's risk factors for breast cancer are all important.

43–1, B. Learning objective: ***Know the key findings of the physical examination of the breasts in a postmenopausal woman.*** The clinical exam can give many clues. The "classic" description of a malignancy is a single, hard, immobile lesion greater than 2 cm. The presence of axillary or superclavicular lymphadenopathy is also concerning. The presence of a smooth, well-demarcated mobile mass consistent with a cyst can be treated with aspiration at the time of initial exam. If it resolves completely, the patient and physician can be reassured.

43–1, C. Learning objective: ***Know the indications for breast biopsy in a postmenopausal woman.*** It is essential to remember that a palpable breast mass, even with normal radiological studies, must be further evaluated to include a tissue diagnosis.

43–2, A. Learning objective: ***Know the history to take when evaluating a breast mass in a premenopausal woman.*** It is important to identify the color, site, and spontaneity of the discharge as well as any masses noted, nipple stimulation, trauma, or medications. A review of symptoms related to hypothyroidism such as fatigue, weight gain, dry hair and skin, as well as amenorrhea, should also be done.

43–2, B. Learning objective: ***Know the key findings of the physical examination of the breasts in a premenopausal woman.*** A unilateral, uniductal discharge requires evaluation by mammogram and galactogram if performed in your area as well as surgical consultation. A bilateral milky discharge is most likely endocrinologic. A discharge associated with a mass is very concerning for malignancy. A woman who is appropriate for screening mammography should have a mammogram regardless of your findings on exam.

43–3, A. Learning objective: ***Know the history to take when dealing with breast pain.*** Cystic mastalgia in a young woman is most likely caused by fibrocystic changes. Her history is consistent with the peaking before menses and the lumpy feel to her breasts.

43–3, B. Learning objective: ***Know the treatment options for mild to moderate breast pain.*** Treatment recommendations are reassurance, lifestyle changes (low-fat high-carbohydrate diet, avoidance of caffeine, vitamin E or evening primrose oil) as well as topical nonsteroidal anti-inflammatory medications and changing her oral contraceptive to one with a higher progestin activity.

43–3, C. Learning objective: ***Know the treatment options for severe breast pain.*** If pain is restricting lifestyle, and lifestyle changes do not resolve her symptoms, further changes in her oral contraceptive may help. Danazol in doses of 100 to 200 mg daily may also help. Remember to counsel the patient regarding the significant side effects of weight gain, acne, amenorrhea, and hirsutism.

▶ CANCER PREVENTION & SCREENING

44–1, A. Learning objective: ***Try to include some routine prevention at every visit.*** Any of the listed options is reasonable. Whatever you do should be in the context of overall routine health maintenance, which includes other noncancer-related screens and preventive actions. Prioritization is important. If the visit was in the late fall, for example, spending time assuring she obtained the flu shot is probably more worthwhile than advising about cancer.

44–1, B. Learning objective: ***Optimize the medical record and office as an aid in getting prevention done.*** All of the listed options can assist you. Prevention information should be easily visible and accessible (e.g., electronic medical record or flow-sheet prompts about items due or when last done per lists in chapter tables; education materials and test requisition forms readily available). The problem list and progress note entries can also be helpful.

44–2, A. Learning objective: ***Be proactive in addressing cancer-related issues.*** The depression screen is the best idea in this scenario. Examples of brief actions include the following: stress the importance of frequent visits to you even if he is feeling well; check the chart about documentation of advanced directives; schedule a follow-up visit solely to talk about living with cancer; perform a depression screen; clarify the patient's understanding of the extent and severity of the cancer. The other answers in the case list are either counterproductive or of minimal or no merit in this patient (although the baseball talk certainly could build rapport for future, more personal discussions).

44–2, B. Learning objective: ***Use the medical record as a "memory-card" for important cancer care issues.*** Family history is unlikely to be relevant to the present management. The problem list should document cancer specifics (e.g., "small cell lung cancer, lung mets, s/p radiation") and other cancer-related issues (e.g., depression, anorexia); information about advances directives and consultants and significant others should be easily found.

▶ HEART FAILURE

45–1, A. Learning objective: ***Create a differential diagnosis for heart failure based on history and physical exam.*** There are many causes of fatigue in the older patient. Include in your differential: heart failure, chronic lung disease, anemia, diabetes mellitus, hypothyroidism, renal failure, etc.

45–1, B. Learning objective: ***Name the signs and symptoms of heart failure.*** Exertional dyspnea, cough, fatigue, edema, S3, rales, JVD.

45–2, A. Learning objective: ***Order appropriate diagnostic tests for hematamesis and chest pain.*** You should order an EKG, chest x-ray, CBC, BUN, and creatinine.

45–2, B. Learning objective: ***Discuss the etiology of heart failure.*** Hypertension (most common) and coronary artery disease are the two most common causes of left-sided heart failure. In this case, we know that she is a diabetic, which places her at risk for atherosclerosis and coronary artery disease.

▶ DEMENTIA

46–1, A. Learning objective: ***Know the most common causes of dementia.*** The most likely etiology is dementia of the Alzheimer's type (60–70% of dementias are caused by Alzheimer's disease). The next most likely cause is vascular dementia.

46–1, B. Learning objective: ***Understand the key parts of the dementia history.*** Ask about specific examples where the patient had trouble with finances. It is important to ask the patient if he notices memory lapses. Make sure to ask how this problem has impacted the family as a whole. Ask questions pertaining to the patient's home life. Get a timeline of symptom onset and progression. Also, ask about agnosia, apraxia, and aphasia.

46–2, A. Learning objective: ***Understand a typical clinical vignette of vascular dementia.*** Given this scenario, the most likely cause is vascular dementia. The patient has many risk factors for stroke. Also, vascular dementia tends to proceed in a stepwise fashion rather than a continuous one (the patient's cognitive problems stay the same until there is a relatively acute worsening followed by a plateau at that level—like a ladder).

46–2, B. Learning objective: ***Understand appropriate diagnostic tests to order for vascular dementia.*** The next step would be to obtain an MRI. A CT scan may be helpful, but an MRI would best show vascular insults to the brain.

▶ DEPRESSION & ANXIETY

47–1, A. Learning objective: ***Create a differential diagnosis of mood disorders.*** First, the woman presents information that suggests both manic and depressive episodes. In order to confirm this, you must assess to ensure she meets the criteria for both episodes. For depression, first ask if she has days when she has a depressed or hopeless mood. During those days does she overeat or lose her appetite? Does she have trouble falling or staying asleep? Does she have interest in things she usually finds pleasurable? Does she have a lack of energy? Is she able to concentrate? Does she feel guilty or worthless? Does she ever want to harm herself? If she answers yes to five or more of these questions, and this *impairs her social or occupational functioning,* then she is having depressive episodes. To assess for a manic episode, questions should include:

When you feel like you do today, do you need very much sleep? Do you feel like you need to talk a lot? Are you having difficulty getting things accomplished either at work or around the house? Are you participating in pleasurable activities that may also be risky, such as shopping and spending a lot of money or having multiple sexual partners? Again, if she has three of these symptoms (many of which are observable in session, such as increased self-esteem or grandiosity—"I am God's gift to man"), and it *impairs her social or occupational functioning,* then she may be diagnosed as bipolar I. If she describes her mania in such a way to suggest it is hypomanic (does not impair functioning), a bipolar II diagnosis is more appropriate.

47–1, B. Learning objective: *Recognize comorbid conditions associated with mood disorders.* This patient has already told you that she participates in risky sexual behavior. This indicates she is at an increased risk to participate in other risky behaviors that are often comorbid with mood disorders (drug and alcohol use). You should also assess for her safety and the safety of others. Use the four question areas to determine if she is at suicide risk or at risk of harming others. Also assess for the type of environment she lives in. If she is a potential harm to society, does she live in a controlled environment or is she on her own? Does she have economic, familial, or community support? Is she in a safe environment or is she enduring abuse?

47–1, C. Learning objective: *Design a treatment plan for bipolar I disorder.* Appropriate treatment for bipolar I disorder requires a combination of pharmacotherapy and psychotherapy. A mood stabilizer would be the appropriate first-line agent. The addition of an antipsychotic would be appropriate adjunctive treatment until the mood stabilizer has reached appropriate levels. Coordinated treatment with the primary care physician, psychiatrist, and therapist (team approach) would be ideal.

47–2, A. Learning objective: *Recognize the symptoms of post-traumatic stress disorder.* The most appropriate diagnosis is post-traumatic stress disorder. The common symptoms are reexperiencing of an extremely traumatic experience (e.g., rape, murder, motor vehicle accident), followed by hyperarousal and subsequent attempts to avoid these reexperiences.

47–2, B. Learning objective: *Distinguish between acute stress disorder (ASD) and post-traumatic stress disorder (PTSD).* The difference between ASD and PTSD is the amount of time since the event. In PTSD the symptoms must last more than four weeks.

47–2, C. Learning objective: *Create a management plan for post-traumatic stress disorder.* The most appropriate treatment for PTSD is management of symptoms and helping the patient process the traumatic event. Psychological treatment early on is important so that symptoms do not continue to worsen. Pharmacotherapy aimed at reducing the anxiety reaction may also be warranted. Short-term benzodiazepines and the use of an SSRI could be helpful for this patient.

▶ DIABETES MELLITUS

48–1, A. Learning objective: ***State the diagnostic criteria, as outlined by the American Diabetic Association (ADA), for the diagnosis of diabetes.*** Diabetes can be diagnosed by the following: a fasting plasma glucose (FPG) of 126 mg/dL or greater, a 75-gram oral glucose tolerance test (OGTT) tested at two hours that is 200 mg/dL or greater, or a random blood glucose that is 200 mg/dL or greater. In order to be diagnostic of diabetes, each of these tests must be repeated on a separate day, unless accompanied by the unequivocal sign of diabetes—polyuria, polydipsia, and unexplained weight loss. The FPG is the preferred method and the method that should be used in this patient.

48–1, B. Learning objective: ***Identify key areas of the history that are important in a newly diagnosed diabetic.*** During the initial evaluation, the patient should be classified as a type 1 or type 2 diabetic and should be questioned about the presence or absence of diabetic complications or the presence of additional risk factors. Information to be gathered includes the following: symptoms of diabetes; results of diagnostic testing; history of hypertension or dyslipidemia; medications that may affect blood glucose levels; history of exercise; eating patterns; presence of any factors that might interfere with management—lifestyle, economic, cultural, education; use of tobacco, alcohol, or controlled substances; family history of diabetes or atherosclerosis; prior or current infections of skin, foot, dental, and genitourinary system; symptoms of end-organ disease associated with diabetes including eye, cardiovascular, nerve, kidney, genitourinary, cerebrovascular, and foot complications; and reproductive and sexual history.

48–1, C. Learning objective: ***Identify key areas of the physical exam that are important to focus on in a newly diagnosed type 2 diabetic.*** The physical examination should focus on the following: height and weight; blood pressure, including orthostatic measurements; the eye (for cataracts and retinopathy); mouth; thyroid; heart; abdomen (for hepatomegaly); peripheral pulses; feet (for ulceration, infection, or sensory loss, as measured with a monofilament); skin; and neurologic system (dulling of vibration, pain, temperature, and possible loss of ankle jerks). In this patient, a vaginal exam is also needed because of her presenting complaint. Signs of diseases that can cause secondary diabetes (hemochromatosis, Cushing's, and pancreatic disease, for example) should be sought.

48–1, D. Learning objective: ***Identify what labs are needed to establish a baseline, to identify any end-organ disease, and to identify comorbid risk factors.*** Initial testing should include a HbA_{1C}, fasting lipid profile (total cholesterol, HDL cholesterol, LDL cholesterol, and triglycerides), urine screen for microalbuminuria, serum BUN and creatinine, and a urinalysis for ketones, protein, sediment, or signs of infection. A TSH and EKG should be ordered if clinically indicated.

48–1, E. Learning objective: ***Outline an appropriate management strategy for the control of diabetes.*** Diabetes management should include a team that consists of the patient, the patient's family, the physician, and other healthcare professionals. In her case, she should see an ophthalmologist for a baseline dilated eye exam and a diabetic educator who can teach her about the self-management of her disease and the potential complications of non-control. Calorie restriction and exercise prescription would be the initial steps in managing this overweight, adult diabetic. As long as her baseline labs are all stable, she should be followed-up in three months. If diet and exercise do not result in a significant drop in the HbA_{1C}, then medication therapy should be considered.

48–2, A. Learning objective: ***Understand the importance of identifying lifestyle issues that might interfere with a patient's control of diabetes.*** This patient experienced a significant loss and needs to be evaluated for depression. Depression may interfere with a person's motivation to control his or her diabetes, ability to make wise choices about diet, or interest in exercise. If this gentleman was found to be clinically depressed, and a decision was made to treat him with medication, then a medication would have to be selected that would not interfere with his diabetes. In addition, he would benefit from a consultation with the diabetic educator, to help him find a diabetic diet that works within his lifestyle and capabilities.

48–2, B. Learning objective: ***List what labs and interventions are needed to monitor a diabetic for glycemic control, end-organ disease, and comorbid risk factor control.*** HbA_{1C} reflects the state of glycemia over the proceeding 8 to 12 weeks and should be monitored at least every 3 to 4 months for those with HbA_{1C} more than 2% above the upper limits of normal, and every 6 months for those with greater control. Lipids should be measured every 3 to 4 months until the goal is met, and then annually. Urine should be screened for microalbumin annually and then, once positive, at each visit. Dilated eye exams should be performed annually. Pneumococcal vaccine should be given as recommended and influenza vaccine should be provided annually. Aspirin therapy should be considered on an individual basis.

48–2, C. Learning objective: ***Understand which antihypertensive medications are recommended in a type 2 diabetic and how this recommendation changes once microalbuminuria***

becomes apparent. Calcium channel blockers, ACE inhibitors, β-blockers, and diuretics can all be used in type 2 diabetics and can be selected according to individual patient profiles; for example, a β-blocker would be used in a diabetic who has a history of a myocardial infarction. However, in patients with diabetes and microalbuminuria, ACE inhibitors can slow the progression of diabetic nephropathy, while none of the other medications have been shown to do this.

48–2, D. Learning objective: ***Identify what parameters are used in making the decision to switch to insulin therapy. Briefly outline how this transition is made.*** Insulin therapy is used in all type 2 diabetics who have failed treatment with diet, exercise, and oral hypoglycemic medications (HbA_{1C} remains ≥ 8%). Diabetics on insulin should monitor their blood sugars daily; the frequency is usually determined by the types of insulins used and the frequency of injections. For type 2 diabetics, the longer-acting insulins, such as NPH insulin (0.1 to 0.2 U/kg) and insulin glargine (10 U), are most often started as a single evening or prebedtime dose. If the initial nighttime dose does not bring the blood sugars within the expected range, the longer-acting insulin dose may be increased or the shorter-acting insulins, regular or insulin lispro, may be administered along with meals. Some insulins come as a combination of a short-acting and a longer-acting insulin, for example 70% NPH and 30% regular. While these combinations may make insulin administration easier, individually titrating each component becomes more difficult. Blood glucose measurements obtained by self-monitoring are used to further adjust the insulin dosage and to help prevent hypoglycemia. Type 2 diabetics are often continued on their oral hypoglycemic medication(s) after insulin is started.

▶ FAMILY DISCORD/DYSFUNCTION

49–1, A. Learning objective: ***Know the consequences of family dysfunction.*** This patient's fatigue is most likely owing to the family dysfunction caused by the stress arising from care of the elderly parent. With the parent requiring constant care, household routines and sleep patterns have very likely been significantly disrupted.

49–1, B. Learning objective: ***Learn about interventions that may be helpful to dysfunctional families.*** A referral to a community agency to secure temporary "respite" for caregivers of the elderly parent may significantly improve this family's function and decrease your patient's fatigue. Often, a family conference, during which plans can be made to relieve the caregiver of stress and most effectively use available community resources, can be helpful to the family. Family discord causes a substantial illness burden for a number of people, can often be treated, and may not be disclosed by many patients.

49–2, A. Learning objective: ***Describe the family life cycle and discuss developmental tasks for each stage.*** When working with this couple it is important to ensure that they have successfully accomplished the tasks of the "new couple" family life cycle stage (see Table 49–1). You will also need to begin introducing the tasks for the "childbearing/preschool family" stage, educating them about the nature of those tasks and resources in the community that can help them accomplish them.

49–2, B: Learning objective: ***Describe characteristics and behaviors associated with healthy families and with families who are at risk for dysfunction.*** Both husband and wife were raised in dysfunctional family systems. The husband is distant from his father and appears to have an overly close relationship with his mother. His mother and father are also emotionally distant from each other. Any relationship within a family that crosses subsystem boundaries (e.g., in this case where mother may be closer to her son than she is to her husband) is a "red flag" for family dysfunction. In this case it may lead to possessiveness and overinvolvement on the part of the husband's mother, creating potential conflict between her and his wife, and subsequently between husband and wife.

The wife is closer to her father, but distant from her mother, a relationship similar to that of her husband (i.e., closer relationship with the opposite gender parent). She also comes from a dysfunctional family system, although the issues may be somewhat different.

Over the course of the pregnancy, supportive family counseling would benefit this couple to help them understand the family systems in which they were raised so that they can establish a more functional relationship that doesn't replicate their dysfunctional nuclear family experience.

49–3, A. Learning objective: ***List those activities that describe a physician who practices family systems medicine.*** Everyone who is part of the family and who could help influence the decision making should be there. That would include all the siblings, with their spouses, and may include any friends or other relatives (e.g., cousins, aunts, uncles) who function "like family," and any influential third party who is respected by the family and who may influence them (e.g., a clergyman or another health professional). The final list should be agreed upon by the siblings, who are most involved with the final decision making.

49–3, B. Learning objective: ***List those activities that describe a physician who practices family systems medicine.*** Prepare for the conference following the plan suggested under the "Preliminary Work" section in Table 49–2.

49–3, C. Learning objective: ***List six functions of a family and five functional axioms that apply to family systems.*** A number of questions could be raised prior to the conference, including the following:

- What facts do I need to share with this family about their father and his disease?
- What roles do the siblings play in their relationships with one another?
- Who among the family members seems to have the most influence, or is it shared?
- How rigid or flexible is this system in its ability to change attitudes and behaviors?
- Has the family faced any similar issues in the past (like with their mother) and how did they resolve that problem?
- What is the mood or atmosphere in this family? How much affection do they seem to share with each other?
- What is this family's communication style? Will it facilitate or hinder resolution of the problem?
- What community resources might help this family manage this problem?
- Will I be able to help this family reach a resolution, or will I need to refer them to a family therapist to resolve the problem?

49–3, D. Learning objective: ***List those activities that describe a physician who practices family systems medicine.*** Plan to run the conference following the outline suggested in Table 49–2 in the section "Agenda for Leading a Family Conference."

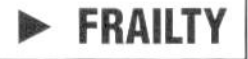

▶ FRAILTY

50–1, A. Learning objective: ***List the prehospitalization signs of frailty.*** This patient's prehospitalization signs of frailty were age, recent changes, perhaps depression, chronic disease, congestive heart failure, and osteoarthritis.

50–1, B. Learning objective: ***Identify the precipitants of acute frailty.*** The precipitants of acute frailty included preexisting conditions, falls, and pain medications.

50–2, A. Learning objective: ***Identify at least two physical markers of frailty in this patient.*** This patient's weight loss, cognitive impairment, and chronic disease are all physical markers of frailty.

50–2, B. Learning objective: ***Identify at least one adverse outcome of this patient's frailty.*** The adverse outcomes of this patient's frailty include sarcopenia, falls, and inability to arise from the chair.

▶ HEALTHCARE MAINTENANCE

51–1, A. Learning objective: ***Describe age-appropriate and gender-appropriate cancer risks and screening protocols.*** For women under the age of 50 the most significant cancer risks are related to cervical dysplasia and breast disease. In addition, a review of the family history may reveal additional cancer concerns for specific individuals. In this case the family history is unremarkable; therefore, the cancer risks are cervical and breast disease. Screening for cervical cancer is via Pap smear beginning within three years of first intercourse or by age 21, whichever is first. Screening should be every year for at least three years. Thereafter the interval may be increased to every three years in women with no abnormal results and no significant risk factors. Breast cancer screening may include education concerning breast self-examination, physician-performed manual breast examination, and mammography every one to two years.

51–1, B. Learning objective: ***Describe age-appropriate and gender-appropriate cancer risks and screening protocols.*** For males over the age of 50 the major cancer concerns are lung, colon, and prostate. Family history or past history may reveal other cancer concerns as well (e.g., occupational exposure to known carcinogens or high levels of unprotected exposure to sunlight). In this case, the patient has no significant historical risks but does have a family history of colon cancer in a first-degree relative. For this patient, recommendations for screening would include colon cancer screening, probably via colonoscopy, and a discussion of the risks, benefits, and limitations of screening for prostate cancer. Screening for prostate cancer, if elected, would include a digital rectal examination and prostate specific antigen.

51–2, A. Learning objective: ***Describe age-appropriate developmental milestones.*** A 5-year-old child with normal development should be able to demonstrate most or all of the following: dresses independently, grooms independently including washing hands and brushing teeth, eats independently including simple preparation, draws a stick figure person with multiple body parts, copies drawings, counts objects easily. Language includes nouns, verbs, adjectives, and prepositions, and speech is fully understandable. Can run with facility, balance on one foot for a prolonged period of time, and jump, hop, and skip.

51–2, B. Learning objective: ***Describe age-appropriate vaccination schedules.*** If all vaccinations were completed at the age of 2 as recommended under current guidelines and the child is not a member of a high-risk group, he will need the final preschool vaccinations, which include the DtaP #5, IPV #4, and MMR #2. The history should be carefully reviewed to ensure that the entire hepatitis B series was completed and that the child either received the varicella vaccine or has documentation of the natural disease.

▶ LIVER & BILIARY TRACT

52–1, A. Learning objective: ***Know the most appropriate laboratory tests to order for a patient with suspected liver disease.*** The most appropriate laboratory tests to order for this patient include a liver function panel, hepatitis profile, and complete blood count. The symptoms this patient exhibits are consistent with an episode of acute hepatitis.

52–1, B. Learning objective: ***Know that with chronic hepatitis C, therapy is beneficial and based on certain factors of the hepatitis C virus present.*** After an initial acute episode of hepatitis C, 85% to 90% of people remain chronically infected with the virus. Untreated, this chronic infection can lead to multiple symptoms of chronic disease, liver failure, and hepatocellular carcinoma. Therapy is based on the viral load and the genotype present. In this instance a quantitative hepatitis C virus RNA and hepatitis C virus genotype should be ordered.

52–2, A. Learning objective: ***Know the most appropriate imaging study to order in a patient with suspected gallbladder disease.*** An ultrasound of the liver and gallbladder will yield the most information. This patient's symptoms are consistent with gallbladder disease, most likely cholecysitis, which is often associated with cholelithiasis.

52–2, B. Learning objective: ***Know the most appropriate therapy for an elderly patient with acute cholecystitis, coexisting cholelithiasis, and type 2 diabetes mellitus.*** The treatment of acute cholecystitis in this setting requires antibiotic therapy directed at the most common pathogens *Enterbacteriaceae,* enterococci, bacteroides, and *Clostridium* species. In addition, an urgent surgical consultation is necessary to appropriately time cholecystectomy. Elderly patients with coexisting diabetes mellitus are at risk to develop gangrene of the gallbladder.

52–3, A. Learning objective: ***Know how to interpret liver function tests and apply those results to clinical practice.*** The most likely cause of the elevation of this patient's liver enzyme elevation is simvastatin. Since long-term use of simvastatin can cause significant liver damage, and since there are alternatives to simvastatin use, it would be most prudent to stop this medication and monitor liver function tests to see if they return to baseline.

52–3, B. Learning objective: ***Know how to approach the work-up of elevation of liver enzymes in the absence of any obvious potential causative factor such as medication side effect.*** If a medication as the cause of elevated liver enzymes has been eliminated, this patient must be investigated for other causes of hepatocellular damage. Elicitation of a more in-depth history regarding alcohol use, possible exposure to viral hepatitis, or familial disorders affecting the liver must be accomplished. If excess alcohol has been eliminated as a causative factor, then blood for hepatitis profile, serum ferritin, serum ceruloplasmin, and antimitochondrial antibodies should be drawn. Depending on the results, it may be necessary to do further testing such as a liver biopsy or imaging studies to determine the cause.

► MENOPAUSE

53–1, A. Learning objective: ***Understand the differential diagnosis of the symptomatic late menopausal female.*** Your differential diagnosis includes depression, osteoporosis, testosterone deficiency, and estrogen deficiency.

53–1, B. Learning objective: ***Develop a rational approach to the investigation of the symptomatic late menopausal female.*** Mammogram, Pap smear, and DXA scan will be most appropriate for a late menopausal patient presenting with these symptoms.

53–1, C. Learning objective: ***Describe appropriate recognition and treatment of an osteoporotic female—especially to differentiate late initiation of hormone replacement therapy (HRT) from symptomatic care.*** The patient is likely to benefit from the following treatments: calcium, vitamin D, bisphosphonates, estrogen vaginal cream/ring, and testosterone.

► NUTRITION & OBESITY

54–1, A: Learning objective: ***List the causes of sudden unexplained weight loss.*** The most likely underlying causes of weight loss are malignancy, gastrointestinal disorder, or depression/dementia.

54–1, B: Learning objective: ***Describe a plan to evaluate a patient's unexplained weight loss.*** Evaluation should include complete history and physical examination, mental status examination, basic laboratory studies such as CBC, blood chemistries, serologies for celiac disease, and screening for cancers common to his age group, such as colorectal cancer and prostate cancer.

54–2, A: Learning objective: ***Set realistic weight loss goals for overweight/obese individuals.*** A weight loss of no more than 10% of current weight, at an average rate of not more than 1 to 2 lb per week is reasonable, and may in fact be aggressive. This would amount to a 17-lb weight loss over 9 to 18 weeks maximum. Encourage the patient that a weight loss of even 10 lb would be helpful to her overall health, and that not gaining any more weight is a priority.

54–2, B: Learning objective: *Counsel patients in safe and effective methods to lose weight.* In order to lose 1 to 2 pounds per week, the patient must have a caloric deficit of 3500 to 7000 kcal per week, or 500 to 1000 kcal per day. She should use a combination of reduction of intake with increased activity to meet that goal. She should focus on lifestyle changes that will be relatively easy to maintain in the long run, rather than drastic changes in diet and/or exercise that would probably result over the long term in her regaining any weight lost.

▶ PREGNANCY

55–1, A. Learning objective: *List the steps in the management of a pregnant patient.* It is important to determine the location of the patient's pregnancy and her estimated gestational age (EGA), as well as to determine if rhogam is indicated for isoimmunization prevention.

55–1, B. Learning objective: *Create a differential diagnosis for pregnancy.* Differential diagnosis would include ectopic pregnancy, intrauterine pregnancy, possible miscarriage, or dysplastic or neoplastic disease of the genital system.

55–1, C. Learning objective: *Order tests appropriate for determining pregnancy.* A quantitative HCG test along with antibody screening and ABO and Rh typing should be done. This should be followed by an ultrasound of the internal genitals. Further testing or procedures can be planned depending on the results of the above tests and a more specific physical exam.

55–2, A. Learning objective: *Know the benefits of folic acid.* The patient should be on folic acid (400 micrograms) to help prevent the development of neural tube defects (from spina bifida occulta to anencephaly) that might occur should she conceive.

55–2, B. Learning objective: *Discuss relevant and important issues with patients during preconception visits.* You should take a good family history looking for any congenital or familial risk factors and arrange the appropriate counseling for them.

▶ PERIOPERATIVE CARE

56–1, A. Learning objective: *Performing a history and physical exam provides two thirds of diagnoses associated with increased perioperative risk.* This patient has a high probability of underlying coronary artery disease. He is sedentary, smokes cigarettes, has a strong family history of coronary artery disease, is overweight, and is hypertensive. Therefore, he is at risk for a perioperative MI, arrhythmia, and death. He also is at risk for pulmonary complications from cigarette smoking and thromboembolic phenomena secondary to obesity.

56–1, B. Learning objective: *The history and physical exam guides perioperative laboratory testing and studies.* Your patient should have a baseline EKG, as well as an exercise treadmill test (ETT). The ETT will allow you to unmask coronary artery disease (CAD) by provoking ischemic changes and will also give you valuable information about his functional capacity, i.e., an exact measurement of the number of metabolic equivalents (METS). (If he were having major vascular surgery, he would need stress imaging instead of an ETT.)

56–1, C. Learning objective: *Cigarettes should be stopped eight weeks or longer before surgery.* Because the patient is scheduled for surgery in two weeks, you would not tell this patient to quit smoking before his surgery. It is hypothesized that quitting smoking less than eight weeks before surgery can lead to pulmonary complications from increased mucous production.

56–1, D. Learning objective: *β-blockers reduce perioperative morbidity and mortality in patients who have CAD or are at risk for CAD.* His ETT (before β-blockade) showed reasonable functional capacity and no ischemia, but his risk factors render him as possibly having undiagnosed CAD (false-negative ETT). Thus, he should be started on a β-blocker and continue on it in the postoperative period to reduce the chance of him dying from an MI or arrhythmia. Giving him a β-blocker has the added advantage of treating his hypertension, although it is not at a level thought to cause perioperative risk.

56–2, A. Learning objective: *Your patient's ausculatory findings are a better predictor of pulmonary complications than are pulmonary function tests or a chest radiograph.* You should talk with the orthopedic surgeon and anesthesiologist, who will most likely decide to delay surgery until after treatment and resolution of her lung findings. The wheezes should clear after a couple doses of an albuterol MDI inhaler using a spacer.

56–2, B. Learning objective: *COPD is a major risk factor for postoperative pulmonary complications, especially in symptomatic patients.* This risk can be reduced by at least optimizing their pulmonary status if time permits. This patient is also at risk for a thromboembolic event because of her fracture and obesity, and reduced mobility postoperatively.

56–2, C. Learning objective: *Exposure to exogenous corticosteroids at any time over a six-month period (some say a year) may cause suppression of the hypothalamic-pituitary axis.* Your patient has two indications for systemic steroids. The first is to help control her COPD. The second is to provide stress doses of corticosteroids because she received prednisone three months ago and is at risk for suppression of the hypothalamic-pituitary axis. This can cause hypotensive shock because the normal increase in ACTH and cortisol production in response to stress (surgery) is compromised. Other medications would include oxygen (reduction of postoperative wound infections) and inhaled albuterol (as noted in Part A).

56–2, D. Learning objective: *Corticosteroids should be continued through the postoperative period to reduce the risk of pulmonary complications.* Steroids do not increase surgical wound infections. Oxygen would be maintained for the first two hours postoperatively. Also, because of her increased chance of clot formation, prophylactic low-molecular-weight heparin should be started 12 to 24 hours after her surgery.

▶ SCHOOL/BEHAVIORAL PROBLEMS—ADD/ADHD

57–1, A. Learning objective: *Know the differential diagnosis of ADHD-like behavior problems.* A common pitfall for physicians is to close their minds about diagnoses prematurely. A child with this presentation is almost textbook ADHD; however, a physician doesn't want to miss a treatable diagnosis. When thinking about the differential diagnosis, think in terms of four categories: (1) general medical problems such as hearing or vision problems, hypothyroid, asthma, medications, lead toxicity, enuresis/encopresis, and malnutrition; (2) neurologic causes such as learning disability, tic disorder, seizures, developmental delays, brain injury, and sleep disorders; (3) psychiatric problems such as oppositional defiant disorder, conduct disorder, anxiety, depression, obsessive-compulsive disorder, and substance abuse; (4) environmental conditions such as parental psychopathology, child neglect/abuse, family dysfunction, poor parenting, and improper learning environment.

57–1, B. Learning objective: *Diagnostic criteria for ADHD.* The child must be under the age of 7 and been having symptoms for longer than six months in two different settings. You need to ask questions to rule out organic diseases that could cause behavior problems. The child must meet the DSM-IV criteria for ADHD. Finally, an organic cause of the behavior must be ruled out.

57–1, C. Learning objective: *Know that lab tests are not needed to make the diagnosis of ADHD.* No, your history and physical exam revealed nothing, thus leading away from an organic cause to this disease. There is no laboratory test for the diagnosis of ADHD. It may be pertinent to do intellectual testing and ADHD behavior screening questionnaires at both home and school to assist with your diagnosis of ADHD.

57–1, D. Learning objective: *Treatment options for ADHD.* There are four treatment options. *Psychosocial interventions* encourage the children to participate in sports or other recreational activities to promote self-esteem and improve positive peer relationships. *Behavioral interventions* provide positive rewards to encourage appropriate behaviors. *Educational interventions* are aimed at teaching the child and parents to develop areas of strengths, adapt to areas of special needs, and remediate skill deficiencies. *Pharmacologic options* are the most preferred and have proven to be efficacious. Medication options include Ritalin, Adderall, Concerta, and Stratera.

57–1, E. Learning objective: *Side effects of the methylphenidate drugs.* The side effects include insomnia, appetite suppression, stomach pain, headache, decreased growth velocity, hypertension, and the worsening of tics (involuntary muscular movements).

57–2, A. Learning objective: *Causes of oppositional defiant disorder (ODD).* In a child with these symptoms you need to make sure there are no organic causes to the disease. By ruling out vision, hearing, thyroid, and toxic ingestion problems you can move on to other psychiatric evaluations of this child. First, assess the child's surroundings, looking for environment or parental stressors that could cause this behavior. Assess to see if the child is always like this, or just at school. In addition, make sure to screen for other comorbid psychiatric illnesses, especially ADHD.

57–2, B. Learning objective: *Diagnostic criteria for ODD.* The diagnostic criteria are the observation of a pattern of negativistic, hostile, and defiant behavior in a child under 8 for the last six months. He must have four of the eight traits described in the DSM-IV criteria for ODD.

57–2, C. Learning objective: *Lab work or exam findings needed to diagnose ODD.* ODD is a clinical diagnosis. However, it is important to do a good history and physical to rule out any organic cause for the behavior problem.

57–2, D. Learning objective: *Treatment of ODD.* The treatment of ODD is difficult and time consuming. Children with other comorbid psychiatric illnesses are much more difficult to treat. Treatment usually is focused around cognitive behavioral therapy. It may be best handled by a specialist in the field (child and adolescent psychiatrist).

57–2, E. Learning objective: *Prognosis for a child with ODD.* The prognosis for ODD is variable. The majority of the prognosis depends on the timing and intensity of intervention for the child.

▶ SEIZURES

58–1, A. Learning objective: *List the possible diagnoses of seizure disorders in a young man.* Most likely this patient had a complex partial seizure that did alter the consciousness. Nausea and light-headedness may be warning symptoms preceding the seizure. These episodes may include staring and unresponsiveness, lip smacking, picking at the clothes, and hand wringing. During a typical complex partial seizure, the patient will appear "out of touch" for 30 to 90 seconds, and will display automatisms (e.g., lip smacking, picking at clothing).

58–1, B. Learning objective: *List the predisposing factors for seizures.* Risk factors for seizures include a history of febrile seizures, possible earlier auras or brief seizures not recognized as seizures, and a family history of seizures. Possible predisposing events include prior head trauma, stroke, tumor, or vascular malformation. Possible precipitating events include sleep deprivation, electrolyte or metabolic abnormalities, systemic disease, acute infection, alcohol, and use of either legal or illegal drugs.

58–1, C. Learning objective: *Consider appropriate tests for this patient.* Complete blood count (with differential and platelet count) and standard chemistry battery (e.g., electrolytes, magnesium, calcium, glucose, creatinine, liver enzymes) are indicated in a patient presenting with an unexplained seizure. Careful history, neurologic examination, EEG, and, if necessary, neuroimaging usually clarify the diagnosis. Because the differentiation between seizures and disorders that may mimic seizures is often based primarily on history, the importance of obtaining an eyewitness account cannot be overemphasized.

58–2, A. Learning objective: *Consider the differential diagnosis of the patient.* The patient had a generalized seizure. But if the initial evaluation would not suggest a cause of the episode, or a nonseizure cause is suspected, conditions like syncope, transient ischemic attacks and stroke, migraine, vertigo, sleep disorders, and pseudoseizures should be considered.

58–2, B. Learning objective: *Recognize that history and physical examination of a generalized seizure disorder.* A typical generalized tonic-clonic seizure begins with a loss of consciousness and a tonic phase, which consists of generalized stiffening of the body and extremities. The tonic phase then gradually merges with the clonic phase, which evolves from high-frequency, low-amplitude to low-frequency, high amplitude rhythmic clonic jerks. Motor movements more prominently affecting one side of the body suggest a secondary generalized seizure. The postictal state following generalized tonic-clonic seizures is characterized by transient stupor, confusion, and sleepiness that lasts minutes to hours. Perform a complete general physical examination to look for signs of systemic disease, infection, and trauma. Perform a thorough neurologic examination focused on finding deficits suggesting a cerebral lesion.

58–2, C. Learning objective: *Select a medical treatment strategy for the patient with seizures.* In a patient presenting acutely with an unexplained seizure, first determine whether there is an acute medically or surgically amenable cause of the seizure. Expect most patients to respond well to one or more antiepileptic drugs (AEDs). Start treatment with a low dose of a single AED; increase the dose gradually. The drug of choice for most generalized epilepsy syndromes is valproate. The most responsive of the generalized seizures are absence seizures, which respond well to valproate or ethosuximide.

► SUBSTANCE ABUSE

59–1, A. Learning objective: *Be able to recognize the symptoms and time frame of alcohol-related complications.* This person is suffering from acute alcohol withdrawal.

59–1, B. Learning objective: *Know the treatment modalities that should be considered for a patient in alcohol withdrawal.* While some individuals do fine without any medical management, this person will require sedation (e.g., a benzodiazepine such as ativan) to manage withdrawal symptoms. He will also require nutritional fortification.

59–1, C. Learning objective: *Be able to formulate a long-term treatment guideline for a patient with an addiction.* Once the patient is lucid, it is important to assess his stage of readiness to change. If the person is interested in overcoming his alcohol addiction, and with his long-standing history, this individual would do best with an intensive inpatient program, followed by an intensive outpatient program and participation in a support group (such as Alcoholics Anonymous). It is also important to assess the patient for any comorbid conditions (with this person it is probably grieving). If there is a significant psychological condition, both psychotherapy and pharmacotherapy will be helpful.

59–2, A. Learning objective: *Be able to recognize the signs and symptoms of stimulant use/overdose.* This patient has probably overdosed on a stimulant (e.g., cocaine, amphetamine, methamphetamine).

59–2, B. Learning objective: *Know the medical complications of stimulant overdose and how they are treated.* There are many medical issues that could arise with this patient; they include treating the patient for any of the following conditions:

Seizure: IV benzodiazepines, barbiturates
Hypotensive episode: IV 0.9% NaCl, dopamine, norepinephrine
Hypertensive episode: benzodiazepine sedation, nitroprusside 0.1 mcg/kg/min, titrate to effect if severe/end-organ damage
Conduction disorder of the heart: lidocaine, amiodarone, phenytoin
Body temperature above normal: control agitation, evaporative cooling
Feeling anxious: IV benzodiazepines, large doses may be needed
Monitoring of patient: vital signs, EKG, electrolytes; renal/hepatic function, PT/PTT or INR, ABGs if severe.

59–2, C. Learning objective: ***The most appropriate treatment plan for a patient who has overdosed on an abused substance.*** For this individual, you should recommend that the patient go to an intensive inpatient treatment center that specializes in substance addiction.

▶ SEXUALLY TRANSMITTED DISEASES

60–1, A. Learning objective: ***Identify the more common infective organisms in urethritis.*** *N. gonorrhoeae* and *C. trachomatis* are the two most common causes of classic urethritis. Occasionally, patients can present with *E. coli* and mycoplasmal infections as well. In rare instances in males, candidal infections can manifest as urethritis.

60–1, B. Learning objective: ***Know the significance of associated symptoms in a urethritis patient.*** This patient also has strong evidence for epididymitis infection (testicular pain and inguinal lymphadenopathy). The causative organisms for this condition in a young male are the same as for urethritis and would include a similar treatment plan.

60–1, C. Learning objective: ***Be aware of special consideration that should always be given to cases of urethritis in sexually active patients.*** Because of high prevalence of both *N. gonorrhoeae* and *C. trachomatis*, these patients should always be treated for both organisms. A sample treatment plan could include ceftriaxone 125 mg IM once and azithromycin 1 gram by mouth once.

60–2, A. Learning objective: ***Recognize a classic presentation of PID.*** This patient exhibits both adnexal tenderness and cervical motion tenderness. The instance of the patient jumping off the table during the exam is known as the chandelier sign and is considered almost diagnostic for PID.

60–2, B. Learning objective: ***Know the work-up that should be performed in a PID patient.*** In this particular instance, a wet mount and KOH prep should be done to rule out *Gardnerella vaginalis* and candidal infection. Because they are the most likely organisms, a culture for gonorrhea and chlamydia should also be performed. A CRP and sedimentation rate can give some insight to the degree of infection but, in this particular case with pronounced exam findings, they are probably unnecessary.

60–2, C. Learning objective: *List other tests that should be performed based on the social history.* Given the past instances of multiple sex partners and IV drug use, it would be wise to counsel the patient about being screened for HIV and hepatitis B and C. These are conditions common in certain high-risk populations and should be addressed in this patient. Additionally, a pregnancy screen should be performed to rule out an ectopic pregnancy.

▶ THYROID DISEASE

61–1, A. Learning objective: *Recognize that thyroid disease is in the differential of many disease processes.* This patient could easily be diagnosed with generalized anxiety or depression with anxious features.

61–1, B. Learning objective: *Know the appropriate tests to order for patients with symptoms consistent with hyperthyroidism.* Blood tests always start with a free T4 and a thyroid stimulating hormone (TSH). In a patient with hyperthyroid symptoms, a high free T4 and low TSH are consistent with primary thyroid disease. If the high free T4 is associated with a normal or high TSH, consider an MRI scan of the pituitary looking for an adenoma. A thyroid scan is indicated when laboratory is consistent with hyperthyroidism to differentiate the multiple primary causes.

61–1, C. Learning objective: *Learn how to interpret TSH results.* The TSH has an inverse relationship to the level of circulating thyroid hormone levels. If the TSH is low, the levels of T3 and T4 will likely be elevated. If the TSH is low, total and free T3 and T4 levels should be drawn. If the TSH is high, the patient is hypothyroid and can be managed by following TSH levels until they are normal, although some clinicians will also follow T4 levels along with TSH levels.

61–1, D. Learning objective: *Know the dysrhythmias associated with thyroid disease.* Since elevated thyroid hormone levels can predispose patients to cardiac dysrhythmias, including sinus tachycardia and atrial fibrillation, an irregular pulse in a patient with a thyroid disorder should be followed up with an EKG and further evaluation if the dysrhythmia does not clear after treatment of the thyroid disorder.

61–2, A. Learning objective: *Remember the importance of history and physical findings when a thyroid nodule is palpated.*

A 65-year-old male has an increased likelihood of thyroid cancer because of his age. Is there a family history of thyroid cancer? Does the patient smoke (other head and neck cancers)? Are there any problems with swallowing or hoarseness? On physical exam is there any cervical lymphadenopathy? History of head or neck radiation is important.

61–2, B. Learning objective: ***Be comfortable with the initial lab and imaging evaluation of a thyroid nodule.*** Again start with the free T4 and TSH. If patient is euthyroid, a fine-needle aspiration (FNA) is in order. A high TSH would make Hashimoto's thyroiditis more likely, but thyroid cancer may coexist. Ultrasonography may help to further define the problem.

61–2, C. Learning objective: ***Know the treatment for a malignant thyroid nodule.*** The treatment of choice for a malignant thyroid nodule is surgical removal, with appropriate consultation with oncologists or endocrinologists experienced in treating thyroid malignancies.

61–2, D. Learning objective: ***Be aware of complications that may arise from thyroid surgery.*** Complications of thyroid surgery include hypothyroidism, hypoparathyroidism and subsequent hypocalcemia, and damage to the recurrent laryngeal nerve.

► TRANSIENT ISCHEMIC ATTACK AND STROKE

62–1, A. Learning objective: ***Know the risk factors that predispose one to strokes.*** This woman has many risk factors for atherosclerosis, and therefore atherothrombotic disease. For the history of present illness, it would be important to know the time course of this patient's aphasia. We need to elicit from the patient and/or bystanders (family, friends, neighbors) how long the patient has been suffering from her current condition. If the patient is presenting within three hours of the onset of symptoms, and there is no evidence of intracranial hemorrhage on a noncontrast CT, the administration of a thrombolytic agent (t-PA), should be considered. If the patient presents within six hours, intra-arterial thrombolysis may be considered. It would also be important to ask if the symptoms have worsened, remained the same, or improved over time. It is also paramount that we ask about any other symptoms that may be overshadowed by the aphasia, such as numbness, weakness, or loss of vision. Additionally, we would want to know about any history of prior cerebrovascular accidents, coronary artery disease, congestive heart failure, myocardial infarction, and atrial fibrillation. We should also ask if there is any family history of stroke or hypercoagulable states.

62–1, B. Learning objective: ***Know the specific imaging modalities for brain ischemia.*** There are several imaging studies that would be appropriate to order. First, a noncontrast CT scan of the head is indicated. Although areas of infarction may not be visible on CT for up to 48 hours, a CT scan should rule out hemorrhage and alternative causes for the neurologic deficit such as a tumor. In order to consider thrombolysis, the noncontrast CT scan must show no evidence of a hemorrhage or cerebral ischemia involving more than one third of the territory of the middle cerebral artery. To better identify the areas of ischemia, we can order an MRI of the brain, which is able to show areas of tissue undergoing ischemic changes within just a few hours of the onset of the stroke. Magnetic resonance angiography (MRA) can be done at the same time and has the ability to demonstrate large artery occlusive disease in the internal carotid or middle cerebral artery. Carotid duplex studies are a noninvasive alternative to determine any disease within the carotids. If the patient has a transient ischemic attack (TIA) or recovers well from a stroke, and has stenosis greater than 70% within the carotids, then a carotid endarterectomy may be warranted. Conventional angiography is the gold standard method of determining vascular anatomy. An angiogram may be performed prior to a carotid endarterectomy to precisely determine the degree of stenosis and may also look at the degree of intracranial stenosis to more carefully target therapy. Finally, a transesophageal echo may be ordered to get detailed information about the cardiac structures and the aorta; on it you should look for defects such as a patent foramen ovale or wall motion abnormalities that may predispose a patient to a cerebrovascular accident. Additionally, in a patient with several risk factors for atherothrombosis, as in this case, severe aortic arch disease may be present, putting the patient at risk for emboli from the arch to travel to the cerebral circulation.

62–1, C. Learning objective: ***Know common lesions that may present in a stroke patient.*** In Broca's aphasia, a patient's ability to comprehend written and spoken language is relatively preserved, but a patient's speech output is slow, poorly articulated, and dysmelodic. Patients with Wernicke's aphasia have difficulty comprehending spoken or written language, yet are able to speak with great fluency. The speech is often incomprehensible and contains neologisms. Broca's area is in the dominant frontal lobe and Wernicke's is in the dominant temporal lobe; the middle cerebral artery supplies both areas.

62–2, A. Learning objective: ***Know the common presentations of a TIA.*** This patient is describing the phenomenon of amaurosis fugax, which is a transient monocular blindness. It is a form of TIA caused by retinal ischemia.

62–2, B. Learning objective: ***Know the parameters of a TIA.*** The most likely diagnosis of this man's disorder is a transient ischemic attack (TIA). TIAs are rapidly resolving ischemic neurologic deficits that generally last 5 to 15 minutes, but by definition may last up to 24 hours.

62–2, C. Learning objective: ***Know the risks posed by a TIA.*** Approximately one third of patients with a TIA will subsequently suffer a major stroke.

▶ TRAUMA

63–1, A. Learning objective: ***Understand what structures are injured from a lateral blow to the knee.*** In this type of injury, the most common structures to be injured are the ACL, MCL, and medial meniscus, also called the "terrible triad" of knee injuries.

63–1, B. Learning objective: ***Know what important structure, in addition to the "terrible triad," can be damaged from a lateral blow to the knee.*** The popliteal artery can be severely damaged and severed in an ACL injury or knee dislocation. The faint pulses and pale skin tone are clues to this injury.

63–1, C. Learning objective: ***Recognize the need for urgent hospital-based evaluation and treatment for neurovascular damage.*** In this instance, the patient should be transported to a hospital with an immediate vascular surgery consult.

63–1, D. Learning objective: ***Recognize the need to forgo in-office testing.*** As stated above, this patient requires immediate surgical consult. If there was any doubt about his possible injury (legs were not pale, pulse stronger, etc.), a Doppler ultrasound could be performed to assess for distal blood flow.

63–2, A. Learning objective: ***Recognize common signs of head trauma.*** The bruising about the eyes and apparent disruption of smell indicate a nasal fracture with probable fracture of the cribriform plate. The bruising at the base of the skull indicates a fracture there as well. Fluid in the ears is another sign that can indicate a basilar skull fracture.

63–2, B. Learning objective: ***Recognize the signs of less apparent head injuries.*** While the previous injuries require evaluation, so does the symptom of wanting to go to sleep following a period of being awake (called the lucid interval). This loss of consciousness could indicate progressing damage to the brain through tissue swelling or a hematoma.

63–2, C. Learning objective: ***Understand the evaluation that should be performed for head injuries.*** In this case, the strongly suspected skull fractures could be imaged with x-ray. However, a better picture could be obtained with a CT scan, which would show both the fractures and a possible hematoma causing the new onset of drowsiness in this patient.

63–2, D. Learning objective: ***Know the most emergent con-***

cern with a head injury patient. In all cases of closed skull injuries, the most immediate concern is swelling of the brain or of a hematoma putting pressure on the brain. This can be assessed by a CT scan and requires immediate neurosurgical evaluation and treatment.

PRACTICE TEST

1. What is the most common diagnosis of patients presenting with abdominal pain in the primary care setting?
   A. Peptic ulcer disease
   B. Irritable bowel syndrome
   C. Appendicitis
   D. No clear diagnosis
   E. Cholelithiasus

2. In evaluating patients with abdominal pain, it is important to do all of the following *except:*
   A. Take an appropriate history that explores all issues relevant to the abdominal pain
   B. Perform a careful physical examination
   C. Order a standard battery of laboratory and diagnostic tests for all patients
   D. Determine the acuity and severity of the condition
   E. Hospitalize patients who are seriously ill or in need of an urgent diagnosis

3. Disorders of which of the following organ systems may result in abdominal pain?
   A. Gynecologic
   B. Genitourinary
   C. Gastrointestinal
   D. Cardiovascular
   E. All of the above

4. A 24-year-old woman has an Hb of 10.3 ng/dL and MCV of 80 when she is 28 weeks pregnant. What is the next step in management?
   A. Check serum ferritin, TIBC, and iron levels
   B. Check folate level
   C. Check TSH
   D. Check reticulocyte count and peripheral smear
   E. Start ferrous sulfate 325 mg/day

5. A 54-year-old Native American man presents to your office complaining of increased fatigue over the past few weeks. His wife of 20 years died one month ago. He denies any alterations in sleep, but his appetite has decreased significantly. Past medical history includes hypertension and asthma. He has never had surgery and has not been taking his daily diuretic since his wife's death. The patient does not smoke. He has a history of alcohol and drug abuse. Physical exam is remarkable for dry oral mucosa, pale conjunctivae, and tachycardia. What is the likely cause of this patient's weakness?
   A. Iron deficiency
   B. Vitamin B_{12} deficiency
   C. Folate deficiency
   D. Both vitamin B_{12} and folate deficiency

6. What is the most common cause of anemia?
   A. Alcohol abuse
   B. Poor nutrition
   C. Iron deficiency
   D. Advanced age
   E. Leukemia

7. An 85-year-old woman is brought into the office by her daughter, who complains that her mother's hygiene has declined. The patient states that she has "old-age" joint pain and she has other things to worry about besides "making myself pretty." Further history reveals that the patient has difficulty combing her hair and getting out of a chair. Review of systems is unremarkable. On physical exam, there are mild changes of her DIPs of the bilateral fingers and marked proximal muscle weakness. What is the diagnosis?
   A. Temporal arteritis
   B. Rheumatoid arthritis
   C. Polymyalgia rheumatica
   D. Fibromyalgia
   E. Osteoarthritis

8. In the previous case (Question 7), how would you treat this patient?
   A. High-dose steroids
   B. Low-dose steroids
   C. SSRIs

D. Methotrexate
E. Acetaminophen

9. A 42-year-old man presents to the acute care clinic with "arm and hand pain" after falling. He states that he slipped on the ice and fell onto his outstretched hand. Inspection reveals moderate soft tissue swelling. What is the most likely fracture?
   A. Boxer's fracture
   B. Colles' fracture
   C. Scaphoid fracture
   D. Monteggia's fracture
   E. Galeazzi's fracture

10. In the previous case (Question 9), the patient fractured the distal radius.
    A. True
    B. False

11. A 55-year-old man with a prosthetic right hip presents with pain, swelling, and limited movement of the joint. Physical exam reveals warmth, edema, and erythema over the joint. You prepare for arthrocentesis. The likely pathogen is:
    A. *Streptococcus pneumoniae*
    B. *Escherichia coli*
    C. *Staphylococcus aureus*
    D. *Pseudomonas aeruginosa*

12. A 45-year-old man reports intense low back and leg pain after a fall last night. He has decreased muscle strength in both lower extremities, and hyperreflexia. He is in otherwise good health. What history is critical to this assessment?
    A. Range of motion of his lumbar spine
    B. History of intravenous drug use
    C. Past history of low back pain
    D. Incontinence or urinary retention symptoms

13. A 50-year-old man reports two weeks of persistent low back pain symptoms aggravated by activity. He has been staying in bed most of the time to get pain relief. He denies fever, cancer history, or bowel or bladder symptoms. He has been using ibuprofen with only minimal effect. There are no leg symptoms. He has no abnormal neurologic findings on exam. What would you recommend?

A. X-rays of the lumbar spine
B. Increase ibuprofen to prescription-level dose and offer physical therapy
C. Blood work to include CBC and ESR
D. MRI of the lumbar spine

14. A 65-year-old man presents with worsening back pain symptoms over the past six weeks that were initially present only with activity but now present all the time. He gets minimal symptom relief with NSAIDs. His past medical history is significant for prostate cancer five years ago that was treated with surgery. What laboratory test would be most helpful at this time to further evaluate his symptoms?
    A. Prostate-specific antigen testing
    B. CBC
    C. ESR
    D. Urinalysis

15. The mother of a 5-year-old boy states that she is concerned about his refusal to sleep in his own bed. This problem behavior began within the last month, subsequent to their move to an apartment. They lost their home to foreclosure because his father has been out of work for six months. What is the appropriate next step?
    A. Refer the family to a pediatric psychologist for an evaluation of an underlying mood or anxiety disorder.
    B. Suggest the parents consult with a family therapist in order to address undetected family structure problems contributing to his difficulty.
    C. Reassure the mother that the behavior is normal for a 5-year-old and that he will grow out of it in time.
    D. Suggest that the behavior is likely a reaction to the loss of a familiar environment and that they talk with their son about how to help make his new bedroom a safe place for him to sleep.

16. A 12-year-old boy, in the company of his custodial grandmother, relates that he is on the verge of flunking the second semester in sixth grade. He was evaluated in the third grade and diagnosed with attention deficit hyperactivity disorder (ADHD) based on his inability to pay attention and keep still and an evaluation by his teachers and the school psychologist. What is the best next step?

A. Prescribe an appropriate stimulant medication and schedule a two-week follow-up appointment.
B. Refer to a child psychiatrist for neuropsychological testing.
C. Perform an MRI of the brain.
D. Call the Department of Social Services to request a home visit and evaluation of the grandmother's suitability as a parent.

17. All of the following conditions may result in sudden death *except:*
    A. Myocardial infarction
    B. Tension pneumothorax
    C. Pericarditis
    D. Pulmonary embolus
    E. Aortic dissection

18. The most common cause of chest pain in the outpatient setting is:
    A. Cardiac
    B. Gastrointestinal
    C. Pulmonary
    D. Musculoskeletal
    E. Psychological

19. Treatment of myocardial infarction includes all of the following *except:*
    A. Heparin
    B. Aspirin
    C. Thrombolytic if less than six hours since onset of pain
    D. β-blocker
    E. Oxygen

20. A 23-year-old patient presents with a five-day history of runny nose, cough, fever (maximum temperature of 37.8°C), and myalgia. She is not a smoker. There is no history of sputum production, shortness of breath, or chest tightness. Vital signs are blood pressure 125/80, pulse 85, respirations 18, temperature 37.7°C. There is no cyanosis or respiratory distress. Exam reveals a clear nasal discharge, slightly erythematous pharynx, and clear lungs. Which of the following is the next step in the evaluation and treatment of this patient?

A. Measure peak flow.
B. Obtain a chest x-ray.
C. Recommend rest and use of a vaporizer.
D. Treat with a broad-spectrum antibiotic.
E. Treat with a β-agonist inhaler.

21. A patient presents with URI symptoms. Which of the following is a finding that would necessitate further evaluation?
    A. Cough
    B. Fever
    C. Headache
    D. Rales
    E. Yellow-green nasal discharge

22. A 53-year-old woman presents with a 10-week history of cough and increased sputum production. She has smoked one pack of cigarettes per day for the past 20 years. She has no fever, nasal congestion, headache, or shortness of breath. Her vital signs are normal. Lung exam reveals an increased AP diameter and a distant wheeze. The rest of the exam is normal. Which of the following is the next step in evaluating and treating this patient's cough?
    A. Chest x-ray
    B. CT scan of the chest
    C. Empiric antibiotic and reexamination
    D. Sinus x-ray
    E. Sputum Gram stain and culture

23. A middle-aged couple is planning a sea cruise to Alaska. After reading about recent outbreaks of viral gastroenteritis on cruise ships, they are concerned enough to see you prior to their departure. Both are in good health and not on any medications. What would you advise?
    A. Antibiotic prophylaxis against diarrhea using metronidazole
    B. Loperamide tablets to be used if necessary
    C. Typhoid immunization
    D. Wearing a mask when at shipboard events to avoid respiratory droplets

24. A 50-year-old man complains of one week of loose stools, four to six per day, without blood or mucus. He has felt

great; in fact, he quit his two-pack-per-day smoking habit the day before his diarrhea began. Physical exam is normal. You suspect:

A. Food poisoning due to *Staphylococcus aureus*
B. Irritable bowel syndrome
C. He is chewing sugarless gum or breath mints to help him quit smoking.
D. Proctitis due to inflammatory bowel disease

25. Acute diarrhea is usually caused by:

A. Infectious agents
B. Dietary changes
C. Inflammatory bowel diseases such as ulcerative colitis and Crohn's disease
D. Hyperthyroidism

26. Central vertigo is often associated with:

A. A severe form of subjective spinning sensation
B. Diplopia
C. Rapid compensation
D. Severe nausea or vomiting

27. Disequilibrium is classified as:

A. A rotational sensation; whirling or spinning
B. Loss of balance
C. A vague sensation of giddiness
D. The perception of impending faint

28. The Dix-Hallpike maneuver is used in the diagnosis of:

A. Presyncope
B. Migraine
C. Benign positional vertigo
D. Psychogenic dizziness

29. Which of the following is a "red-flag" symptom for patients with dyspepsia?

A. Nausea
B. Black stool
C. New-onset diarrhea or constipation
D. Heartburn

30. Which of the following tests is not used for *Helicobacter pylori* testing?
    - **A.** Stool antigen
    - **B.** Blood culture
    - **C.** Mucosal biopsy
    - **D.** Urea breath test

31. Which of the following modalities is best for diagnosing functional dyspepsia?
    - **A.** EGD
    - **B.** Serum *H. pylori* antibody
    - **C.** Medical history
    - **D.** Physical exam

32. Which of the following is suggestive of a pulmonary embolus?
    - **A.** Low D-dimer
    - **B.** Normal respiratory rate
    - **C.** Jugular venous distension
    - **D.** Abnormal ventilation-perfusion scan

33. Signs of respiratory failure include all of the following *except:*
    - **A.** Cyanosis
    - **B.** Quiet chest
    - **C.** Low CO_2
    - **D.** Rising CO_2 on repeat ABGs

34. A true statement about wheezing is:
    - **A.** Wheezing is diagnostic for asthma.
    - **B.** Wheezing associated with pulsus paradoxus is suggestive of a good prognosis.
    - **C.** Wheezing associated with paradoxical chest movement is a sign of respiratory failure.
    - **D.** The severity of asthma is associated with the intensity of wheezing.

35. After presenting with fevers, chills, and painful urination, a 27-year-old woman gasps and nearly jumps off the exam table when you percuss her costovertebral angle. What is the most likely cause of her pain?

A. Pelvic inflammatory disease
B. Acute pyelonephritis
C. Urethritis caused by an aggressive fungal infection
D. *Neisseria* infection of the upper urinary tract

36. A 21-year-old man is suspected of having a *Neisseria gonorrhoeae* infection. What would his discharge most likely resemble?

A. White and curdlike
B. Clear and watery
C. Yellow and thick
D. Blood-tinged mucus

37. A 55-year-old woman who has smoked two packs of cigarettes per day for 30 years presents for the first time with painful urination of five months duration. Her physical exam is negative for any findings. After obtaining urinalysis, you learn she has 7 RBCs per high-powered field and no WBCs were seen at all. What should you do next?

A. Treat with an appropriate antibiotic
B. Order an intravenous pyelogram
C. Ask her to drink plenty of water and return when the stone passes
D. Refer her to a urologist for cystoscopy

38. An 11-month-old boy is brought in by his father in January. He has been sniffling for a week and is now pulling at his right ear. He is eating normally. Today, he has a temperature of 37.2°C. He is happy in the exam room until you attempt otoscopy, at which point he starts crying. Both tympanic membranes are very red, have normal movement, and are translucent. You recommend to the father that:

A. He fill a prescription of amoxicillin
B. He give his child Tylenol and Benadryl
C. Not worry unless his child develops a fever
D. He take his child to be evaluated by audiology

39. Three months after being diagnosed with acute left otitis media, an 18-month-old girl returns for follow-up. Her parents say she is healthy, and she is happy in the exam room. Her left tympanic membrane has reduced mobility and is pearly and translucent with air-fluid levels. You recommend that:

A. She should have tympanostomy tubes placed by ENT.

B. She should be evaluated by audiology and a speech therapist.

C. She should start a course of amoxicillin.

D. She should have no further follow-up.

40. A 9-year-old girl presents with ear pain of one-week duration and decreased hearing on the right. Her mother has been trying to Q-tip™ the right ear daily. On physical exam, she is afebrile. The right tympanic membrane cannot be visualized because of impacted cerumen. Your next step is to:

    A. Force water into the ear to dislodge the cerumen.

    B. Add a few drops of docusate sodium (Colace) and attempt suction in 30 minutes.

    C. Send her home with a prescription for ciprofloxacin/ dexamethasone drops.

    D. Reassure the mother and give her a coupon for more Q-tips.

41. Which of the following statements is true about fatigue?

    A. It is not important to treat concurrent pain.

    B. Fatigue that lasts more than six months is owing to a psychological disorder.

    C. A patient can have physical and psychological causes of fatigue simultaneously.

    D. It is necessary to order extensive lab work to diagnose fibromyalgia.

42. A 40-year-old woman complains: "I'm tired all the time." History reveals that she is working 60 hours per week between two jobs because her husband is disabled from a back injury. Also, her 17-year-old son recently was arrested for shoplifting. In the past six months her menses have become very heavy and now last ten days instead of six. Which of the following should be done first?

    A. Check CBC

    B. Check TSH

    C. Refer to a psychiatrist

    D. Start an antidepressant

43. A 17-year-old boy presents for vomiting bright red blood this morning. He has had nausea and decreased energy for the past month, but no fever, diarrhea, or vomiting. He has had

decreased interest in activities with his friends, and his grades in school have been dropping. Findings on physical exam indicate dry mucous membranes and pallor. Laboratory findings indicate a slightly decreased hemoglobin and mild increase of gamma-glutamyl transpeptidase activity. What is the most likely cause of the hematesis?

A. Peptic ulcer disease

B. Infectious mononucleosis

C. HIV

D. Schizophrenia

E. Alcohol-induced gastritis

44. An 82-year-old man with severe atherosclerosis presents with chest pain. He takes one baby aspirin a day. Cardiac catherization is successful, but later in the day severe abdominal pain develops. The patient passes a large amount of bloody stool. What is the most likely cause of the hematochezia?

A. Colon cancer

B. Mesenteric ischemia

C. NSAID gastritis

D. Diverticulosis

E. Diverticulitis

45. A 68-year-old woman presents with new, throbbing temple pain on the left side, decreased vision in the left eye, and pain with chewing. What is your working diagnosis?

A. No further evaluation, tension-type headache

B. No further evaluation, typical new migraine presentation

C. Red-flag symptoms warrant further evaluation, consider arteritis

D. Immediate noncontrasted CT of the head

46. Which of the following is not a characteristic of cluster headaches?

A. More common in women than men

B. Often associated with autonomic signs/symptoms

C. Usually unilateral in distribution

D. Primarily retro-orbital in location

47. Which of the following is true of migraine preventive therapy?
    A. Should only be used if having more than five headaches per week
    B. The same regimen should be used for every patient.
    C. Sumatriptan is a migraine preventive therapy.
    D. Many medications are used for migraine prophylaxis and should be tailored to the patient's history and needs.

48. Which of the following symptoms suggests a need for more thorough work-up of heartburn?
    A. Substernal burning at night
    B. Acid taste in the mouth
    C. Weight loss
    D. Recurrent sore throat

49. Which of the following medications is *not* a common cause of heartburn?
    A. Fosamax (Aledronate)
    B. Potassium
    C. Prednisone
    D. Calcium supplements

50. All of the following are recommended as lifestyle modifications for preventing heartburn *except:*
    A. Weight loss
    B. Smoking cessation
    C. Elevate the head of the bed
    D. Increasing dietary fat

51. A 50-year-old man presents for a fasting lipid profile. He does not smoke and his family history is negative for cardiovascular disease. He weighs 155 lb and his height is 68 inches. Blood pressure is 118/72 and fasting blood glucose is 92 mg/dL. The patient jogs a couple of miles every other day. His 10-year risk for coronary heart disease is assumed to be:
    A. <10%
    B. 10–19%
    C. 20–29%
    D. 30–39%

52. For the patient in the preceding question, his LDL-C goal is:
    A. <100 mg/dL
    B. <130 mg/dL
    C. <160 mg/dL
    D. <190 mg/dL

53. A 54-year-old woman presents for cardiovascular risk assessment. Her sister had a stroke at age 66. She takes no medications. In evaluating her for dyslipidemia, you find that her HDL-C is 45 mg/dL and her LDL-C is 120 mg/dL. Her fasting glucose is 200, and a follow-up glycosylated hemoglobin is 10. Her blood pressure is 136/84. What is this patient's LDL-C goal?
    A. 100 mg/dL
    B. 130 mg/dL
    C. 160 mg/dL
    D. 190 mg/dL

54. For the patient in the preceding question, at what level of LDL-C would you consider initiating drug therapy?
    A. 100 mg/dL
    B. 130 mg/dL
    C. 160 mg/dL
    D. 190 mg/dL

55. A 65-year-old woman with confirmed hypertension has undertaken 12 months of therapeutic lifestyle changes (TLC). She is taking no medications. Her physical examination reveals a healthy woman with no evidence of end-organ damage. Urinalysis, CBC, electrolytes, BUN, creatinine, uric acid, fasting glucose, and fasting lipids are normal. EKG is normal. Her blood pressure in the office has consistently been 142/90 mmHg. What is the most appropriate recommendation at this time?
    A. Emphasize adherence with TLC for an additional three months.
    B. Start HCTZ 25 mg daily.
    C. Start combination antihypertensive therapy with two drugs at lower dose.
    D. Evaluate for secondary causes of hypertension.

56. A 55-year-old man with type 2 diabetes and hypertension is being seen every three months for chronic disease manage-

ment. His diabetes is acceptably controlled on a single oral hypoglycemic agent. His blood pressure continues to run 150/95 on HCTZ 25 mg daily. He feels well, and physical examination reveals no evidence of end-organ damage. However, his urine albumin excretion is greater than 300 mg/day, BUN is 35 mg/dL, and serum creatinine is 1.8 mg/dL. What medication change would be most appropriate to consider at this time?

A. Increase the dose of thiazide diuretic.

B. Add a β-blocker.

C. Add an angiotensin converting enzyme inhibitor.

D. Add a calcium channel blocker.

57. A 60-year-old man who is a new patient comes to the office with a chief complaint of a headache. He has a history of hypertension and has been treated previously but has not taken medication consistently. His blood pressure is 200/110 confirmed in both arms. He looks uncomfortable, but well. What should your approach to the patient be?

A. Admission to the hospital for stabilization of a hypertensive emergency.

B. Attempt to normalize blood pressure in the office immediately.

C. Evaluate for the presence of acute end-organ damage and if none is present, recommend therapeutic life style changes (TLC) with close follow-up.

D. Evaluate for the presence of acute end-organ damage and if none is present, review TLC and start BP-lowering medication with close follow-up.

58. A 55-year-old woman presents to the office with a history of pain in her left calf for two days. She underwent arthroscopic surgery on her left knee three weeks ago. She went off hormone replacement therapy one year ago. The patient smokes a half pack of cigarettes per day. What is the most likely diagnosis?

A. Acute phlebitis

B. Shin splints

C. Osteoarthritis in the left hip

D. Septic arthritis in the left knee

59. The woman in the previous question returned to work five days ago (after the knee arthroscopy), and she has used up her "paid time off." Her telemarketing job involves sitting at a desk for the eight-hour shift except for two 5-minute breaks

and 30 minutes for lunch. A venous ultrasound indicates that she does not have deep vein thrombosis. How would you manage this situation?

A. Hospitalize her on intravenous heparin until she is therapeutic on Coumadin.

B. Start her on acetaminophen 500 mg every four hours (while awake) for pain control.

C. Instruct her supervisor to allow her to walk around for five minutes each hour.

D. Instruct the patient to avoid climbing stairs until the pain in her calf resolves.

60. A 70-year-old diabetic man presents to the emergency department one day after he slipped on ice and fell, twisting his left ankle. Physical exam is significant for moderate swelling over the lateral malleolus and trace dorsalis pedis pulse bilaterally. Appropriate initial management includes all of the following *except*:

A. MRI of the left ankle

B. X-ray of the left ankle

C. Acetaminophen 650 mg every four hours as needed for pain

D. Ice for 15 minutes at a time up to four times per day for the next two days

61. A 50-year-old man, previously healthy, presents to his primary care physician with chest pain, fatigue, night sweats, and weight loss over the past four months. He states he has been under stress recently. He also complains of lumps in his neck. On exam, temperature is 36.7°C, pulse 80, respirations 20, blood pressure 108/70. He has enlarged cervical lymph nodes and bilateral epitrochlear lymph nodes varying in diameter between 1 and 2 cm. He has hepatomegaly (liver edge is palpated approximately 3–4 cm below the left costal edge). His spleen is just palpable. Excisional lymph node biopsy reveals diffuse small cleaved cells (diffuse poorly differentiated lymphocytic) histology. What is the most likely diagnosis?

A. Hodgkin's disease

B. Non-Hodgkin's disease

C. AIDS

D. Infectious mononucleosis

62. An 18-year-old college student presents to the local health center with a three- to four-week history of fatigue, malaise, fever, chills, and sore throat. She is on the college basketball and track team. She has no energy, has difficulty waking up in the mornings, and is experiencing generalized aches and pain all over. On exam, temperature is 38.4°C, pulse 100, respirations 20, blood pressure 100/70. Examination of her throat reveals pharyngeal hyperemia with exudates in both tonsillar areas. She has significant cervical lymphadenopathy. On abdominal examination, the tip of the spleen is felt. Bacterial throat culture was negative, and monospot test was positive. What is the most likely diagnosis?

A. Hodgkin's lymphoma

B. Infectious mononucleosis

C. Streptococcal pharyngitis

D. Fibromyalgia

63. A 28-year-old man has had a rash on his face intermittently for the last three years. It gets worse with stress and itches around his moustache. He is otherwise in good health and does not have any other symptoms. On physical exam there is erythema and scale across his eyebrows, cheeks, and near his moustache. With close-up inspection, the scale is visible under his moustache and eyebrows. What is the most likely diagnosis?

A. Psoriasis

B. Seborrhea

C. Atopic dermatitis

D. Acne rosacea

E. Contact dermatitis

64. A 34-year-old woman has had a new rash on her arms and legs for two days. She just got back from a weeklong backpacking trip in the mountains. The rash is very pruritic and is driving her crazy. She has multiple vesicles on her extremities and there is one area on the leg where the vesicles seem to be arranged in a line. There are some excoriations and one area of crusting. What is the most likely cause of this rash?

A. A contact dermatitis to the bug repellant that she applied daily to her arms and legs

B. An allergic reaction to the SPF 30 sunscreen she was using to avoid sunburns

C. An allergic response to the oleoresin found in the poison ivy or poison oak plant

D. Bug bites from chiggers or the vicious mosquitoes that plagued them during her trip

E. Neurodermatitis caused by the anxiety of returning to the world of work and responsibilities

65. A 68-year-old African-American man is in the clinic for a routine follow-up for his well-controlled hypertension and on further questioning reports that he is finally going to retire. He has been under a lot of stress at work and they are refusing to give him the time off that he needs to help care for his ill wife. All of this worry has caused him to toss and turn for the last two weeks and now he feels exhausted but remains unable to sleep. Assuming he is otherwise healthy, what is the appropriate treatment at this visit?

A. Reassure him and schedule a follow-up visit in two weeks.

B. Prescribe a benzodiazepine.

C. Prescribe a sedating antidepressant.

D. Prescribe a dopaminergic agent.

66. A 55-year-old man is brought in by his wife because she is tired of him falling asleep as soon as he sits down in his chair after work, where he often remains all night. He states that although he sleeps eight hours a night he does not feel rested during the day. On physical exam you note that his weight has remained stable at 250 lb, his blood pressure remains elevated despite your addition of a second agent, and there is 2+ edema in the ankles. What is the most appropriate intervention at this point?

A. Zolpidem (Ambien)

B. Melatonin

C. Change hypertension medication

D. Sleep study

67. A 30-year-old woman presents for an initial visit to obtain her annual exam. Under review of systems she complains of not being able to sleep. She wakes up often and especially has a hard time falling asleep as she pours over everything that happened at work and what needs to be done tomorrow.

Even her partner's sleep is disrupted because she grinds her teeth. Her past medical history is remarkable for "stomach problems" and cocaine abuse but the patient states she successfully completed rehabilitation. During the exam she is fidgety and wrings her hands. What is the most likely underlying diagnosis for the patient's insomnia?

A. Anxiety disorder
B. Restless leg syndrome
C. Substance-induced sleep disorder
D. Circadian rhythm disturbance

68. Worried parents bring in their 9-month-old son because he has become very sick in the last 12 hours. The child's voice is changed and he is very irritable, warm, and drooling. In your clinic, he has a temperature of 39.8°C, is lethargic, and is foaming at the mouth. What is your next step in management?

A. Reassure the parents that this is a self-limiting disease and discharge home.
B. Complete your physical exam, including assessing tonsil size.
C. Obtain lateral neck x-rays and keep the child as calm as possible.
D. Give the child a shot of penicillin and discharge home.

69. A 5-year-old girl presents to your clinic with two days of sore throat. She attends day care, and several of her classmates have been diagnosed with strep throat. She has a temperature of 38.3°C, enlarged, pus-covered tonsils, and cervical lymphadenopathy. If she is untreated, the most likely complication is:

A. Nothing. She will have no sequelae even without an antibiotic.
B. Rheumatic fever
C. Peritonsillar abscess
D. Scarlet fever

70. The reflex compensatory mechanisms for syncope include all of the following *except:*

A. Baroreceptor reflex
B. Renin-angiotensin release
C. Dopamine release
D. Peripheral vasoconstriction
E. Carotid sinus response

71. The initial test of choice for evaluating syncope includes:
    A. Complete blood count (CBC)
    B. Chemistry profile
    C. Electrocardiogram (EKG)
    D. Noncontrast computed tomography of head
    E. Urine drug screen

72. Vasovagal syncope can be caused by which of the following?
    A. Micturition
    B. Eating
    C. Prolonged standing
    D. All of the above

73. The appropriate action in postmenopausal bleeding is:
    A. Reassure the patient
    B. Provide progestins
    C. Ask for menstrual calendar charting from the patient
    D. Hysterectomy
    E. Endometrial biopsy and/or endometrial stripe evaluation with ultrasound

74. Endometrial biopsy demonstrates hyperplasia. Treatment should be:
    A. Cyclic estrogen therapy
    B. Hysterectomy
    C. Endometrial ablation
    D. Progestins and rebiopsy in three to six months
    E. Observation

75. A 27-year-old woman presents with a one-week history of vaginal discharge. The discharge is thin and gray. On wet prep exam, you observe epithelial cells with bacteria adherent to the cell membranes. There is a slight amine odor when you add a drop of KOH. The most likely diagnosis for this patient is:
    A. Allergic vaginitis
    B. Bacterial vaginosis
    C. *Candida* vaginitis
    D. *Trichomonas* vaginitis
    E. Atrophic vaginitis

76. The treatment of choice for *Trichomonas* vaginitis is:
   A. Clindamycin topical
   B. Fluconazole oral
   C. Terconazole topical
   D. Metronidazole oral
   E. Ceftriaxone intramuscular

77. Which of the following is least likely to be seen in *Candida* vaginitis?
   A. Thick, white, "cottage cheese–like" discharge
   B. pH 4.0
   C. Amine odor
   D. Budding yeast and hyphae
   E. Vulvar and vaginal erythema

78. An 8-month-old girl is brought in after vomiting a small amount of greenish-brown fluid. For several days, she has been crying uncontrollably and drawing her legs up to her chest. She has been "colicky" in the past, but her cries are louder and more urgent. Her last bowel movement was mixed with blood and mucus. What is the diagnostic modality of choice in this patient?
   A. CT scan of the abdomen
   B. Barium or air enema
   C. Exploratory laparotomy
   D. Abdominal ultrasound

79. A 57-year-old woman is brought into the emergency department by police after she was found driving recklessly. Family members state she has "not been herself lately" and is increasingly inappropriate and belligerent with others. History reveals a 40-year history of smoking two packs a day, hypertension, and chronic bronchitis. The patient states that she wakes up with a terrible headache and is extremely nauseated with episodes of emesis every day to every other day. Vital signs are temperature 36.9°C, blood pressure 167/97, respirations 20, pulse 96. Physical exam reveals papilledema and right-sided weakness, along with wheezing and dullness to percussion in the right upper lung field. What is the most likely cause of her symptoms?

A. Glioma
B. Primary brain tumor with metastases to lung
C. Primary lung carcinoma with brain metastases
D. Mental status changes secondary to pneumococcal pneumonia

80. Which of the following items is *not* a common type of elder abuse?
A. Financial abuse
B. Sexual abuse
C. Neglect
D. Physical abuse

81. Which of the following is a sign of sexual abuse in a child?
A. Malnutrition
B. Inadequate clothing
C. Delays in physical development
D. Recurrent urinary tract infections

82. A 34-year-old waiter with a known history of asthma presents to the emergency room with complaints of severe shortness of breath, cough, and wheezing. His vitals are temperature 37°C, blood pressure 154/84 mmHg, respirations 32, pulse 104. With inspiration, his blood pressure falls to 112/70 mmHg. On lung examination, there are loud, high-pitched wheezes and a prolonged expiratory phase. Which of the following physical examination findings is of most significance in evaluating this patient?
A. Hypertension
B. Loud wheezing
C. Prolonged expiratory phase
D. Pulsus paradoxus
E. Tachycardia

83. A 76-year-old man with long-standing COPD presents to the clinic for his semiannual examination. The patient is a long-time smoker (2 packs per day for 50 years). He had a right upper wedge resection two years ago for adenocarcinoma, and at that time had severe obstructive disease. A recent chest CT showed apical bullae and severe emphysematous changes. The patient has moderate dyspnea on exertion and often has shortness of breath with minimal activity. On this visit, the patient relates that he is even more short of

breath at rest and is almost unable to perform any physical activity as a result. Which of the following would most strongly suggest the need to initiate home oxygen therapy?

A. Exercise-induced oxygen desaturations <92%

B. Resting arterial PaO_2 showing an alveolar arterial gradient >12 mmHg

C. Resting arterial PaO_2 < 55 mmHg

D. Resting PaO_2 > 40 mmHg

E. Room air oxygen saturation <92%

84. A 61-year-old man with a smoking history of 2 packs per day for 40 years presents with increasing dyspnea on exertion. He also has developed a productive cough, which has persisted over most of the past two years. He denies any other medical problems and has never been hospitalized for evaluation of his symptoms. On physical examination, his vitals are blood pressure 132/74 mmHg, pulse 70, and respirations 30. On lung examination, there are crackles throughout, with a prolonged expiratory phase in both lung fields. There is an increased anteroposterior chest diameter. Heart sounds are regular but distant. A chest x-ray film reveals hyperinflation of both lung fields and a normal-sized heart. Which of the following would most likely be expected on pulmonary function tests?

A. Decreased forced expiratory volume in 1 second (FEV_1) to forced vital capacity (FVC) ratio

B. Decreased total lung capacity

C. Decreased residual volume

D. Increased FEV_1

E. Increased FVC

85. A 65-year-old man with a well-documented history of stable angina is in for an office visit. He is otherwise healthy. He is on aspirin, β-blockers, long-acting nitrates, and he also uses sublingual nitroglycerin frequently. He cannot climb a flight of stairs without severe angina. His most recent episode was four days ago. An EKG today is normal. What is the next step?

A. Dipyridamole perfusion study

B. Coronary angiography

C. Draw cardiac enzymes

D. Addition of a calcium channel blocker

86. A 69-year-old diabetic woman who you know well comes in to the clinic with a chief complaint of profound fatigue. She denies chest pain at any time. You review her insulin regimen and her sugar diary with her, which seems to show good control. Her other medications include an ACE inhibitor for hypertension, a statin for high cholesterol, and 81 mg of aspirin. A physical exam is unremarkable and her vitals are blood pressure 110/70, pulse 88, temperature 37.5°C, and respirations 16. An EKG shows Q waves with no ST elevation, troponins elevated, and CKMB normal. An EKG from one year ago is normal. What is the most likely diagnosis?

A. Patient is having a non–ST-elevation MI

B. Patient had an ST-elevation MI 24 hours ago

C. Patient had a non–ST-elevation MI 24 hours ago

D. Patient had an ST-elevation MI 4 days ago

87. A 72-year-old man with no history of angina presents with moderate chest pressure that radiates to his left shoulder. It started 20 minutes ago when he was scooping the snow on his sidewalk. Based on this information, what is the most appropriate classification of the patient at this time?

A. Unstable angina

B. Acute coronary syndrome

C. Myocardial infarction

D. Stable angina

88. What should you recommend for a 28-year-old woman with cyclic breast pain, worst prior to menses, with a normal physical exam?

A. The Atkins diet

B. Evening primrose oil and topical NSAIDs

C. Danazol

D. Mammogram

89. Bilateral, milky nipple discharge is most likely caused by:

A. Nipple stimulation

B. Hyperthyroidism

C. Ductal ectasia

D. Malignancy

90. A 65-year-old woman presents with a palpable hard lesion in the breast. Her mammogram is normal. Your next step is:

A. Reassurance and follow-up mammogram annually
B. Ultrasound evaluation
C. Repeat exam five days after her next menses
D. Surgical consultation

91. According to the United States Preventive Service Task Force, how often should women at risk for HPV infection have Pap smears?
A. Every six months
B. Every two to three years
C. Every six months, starting two years after the onset of sexual activity
D. Every year

92. The first step in screening a patient for cancer is:
A. Taking a personal and family history
B. Ordering lab tests
C. Ordering genetic studies
D. Performing a focused physical exam

93. A 67-year-old man with a history of coronary artery disease presents with three-word dyspnea and bilateral 2+ pitting edema. Acute management includes:
A. β-blocker
B. Calcium channel blocker
C. HCTZ
D. Furosemide

94. A 69-year-old woman being treated for congestive heart failure (CHF) has an ejection fraction of 55%. What type of CHF does she have?
A. Left-sided
B. Right-sided
C. Systolic
D. Diastolic
E. Low output

95. Use of digoxin in symptomatic systolic heart failure increases life expectancy.
A. True
B. False

96. A 77-year-old woman complains of loss of memory for the last few months. She relays several specific examples of her memory problems. Upon cognitive testing she frequently says "I don't know" to your questions. Physical exam and lab tests are normal. What is the next step in diagnosing this condition?

    A. CT scan of head

    B. Ask more history questions pertaining to her mood/spirits

    C. Put her on an acetylcholinesterase inhibitor prophylactically

    D. Refer her for neuropsychological testing

97. An 80-year-old woman is brought into your clinic by her son. He relates that she has been acting oddly and saying things that do not make sense for the past couple of days. These symptoms tend to worsen in the early evening. Her medical history is significant for hypertension, diabetes mellitus type 2, acute myocardial infarction, congestive heart failure, and a recent (last week) bout of pneumonia for which she was hospitalized. Given this information, what is the most likely diagnosis?

    A. Alzheimer's dementia

    B. Vascular dementia

    C. Mixed (vascular/AD) dementia

    D. Delirium

98. A 76-year-old man is brought to your office by his adult daughter. She tells you that he has had difficulty keeping track of his finances recently. She thinks this is odd because he is a retired accountant and has had no trouble with this before. She states that he is able to feed and clothe himself. Physical exam is normal. MMSE is 23. A CBC, CMP, TSH, and vitamin B_{12} are all within normal limits. A CT of the head is also normal. What is the next step in management for this patient?

    A. Referral to an assisted living community

    B. Intensive cognitive-behavioral therapy

    C. Put the patient on an acetycholinesterase inhibitor

    D. Put the patient on an SSRI

99. A 35-year-old woman tells you that she is tired of riding an emotional roller coaster. She has periods of depressed mood countered with days of feeling really good. She is not experiencing social or occupational difficulties but the mood

swings bother her. Which diagnosis is the most appropriate for this woman?

A. Dysthymic disorder

B. Major depressive disorder

C. Bipolar I disorder

D. Cyclothymic disorder

E. Bipolar II disorder

100. A 45-year-old man complains of difficulty sleeping. He states that he can never relax and is always worried about something. His wife is both concerned and irritated with him because he is "worrying himself sick." He isn't sure what is wrong with him. What is the most appropriate diagnosis?

A. Major depressive disorder

B. Panic disorder

C. Obsessive compulsive disorder

D. Generalized anxiety disorder

E. Agoraphobia

101. The most appropriate first-line, pharmacological agent for an elderly woman with major depressive disorder who has multiple medical problems (coronary artery disease, diabetes, ulcerative colitis, and gastroesophageal reflux disease) is:

A. Sertraline

B. Buproprion

C. Nafazodone

D. Venlafaxene

E. Amitriptyline

102. During the last six months, a 45-year-old obese African-American woman with a history of type 2 diabetes has been attempting to control her diabetes with diet modification and exercise. She has lost 5 lb during this time. Her most recent HbA_{1C} was 8.2. You have decided to start her on a medication for her diabetes. What is the best initial therapy for this patient?

A. NPH insulin

B. Acarbose

C. Metformin

D. Sulfonlyurea and troglitazone

103. A 52-year-old Latino man comes to your office for his "yearly" exam. He considers himself in good health but he does not exercise. He is obese and has a body mass index (BMI) of above 25 kg/m^2. His mother was diabetic. You decide to screen him for diabetes. A fasting glucose level is 135 mg/dL. When repeated four days later it is 127 mg/dL. The next step in this patient's management would be to:

A. Diagnose impaired fasting glucose (IFG) and screen him again in one year.

B. Measure a two-hour postprandial glucose after a 75-g glucose load.

C. Tell the patient he has type 2 diabetes and begin diet and exercise therapy.

D. Begin an oral hypoglycemic agent.

104. A 35-year-old woman with type 2 diabetes comes in for a routine visit. She is a nonsmoker. Her blood pressure is 136/85. Her physical exam shows no evidence of end-organ damage. Her preprandial blood sugars have been less than 110 mg/dL. Laboratory test results are as follows: her HbA_{1C} is 6%, total cholesterol is 196 mg/dL, LDL is 92 mg/dL, HDL is 52 mg/dL, and triglycerides are 143 mg/dL. Her urine screen is negative for microalbumin. Which of the above physical exam findings or labs is greater than that which is recommended as a goal for treatment in a type 2 diabetic?

A. BP of 136/85

B. Preprandial blood sugars of <110 mg/dL

C. Total cholesterol of 196 mg/dL

D. HbA_{1C} of 6%

105. In a patient with diabetes mellitus and hypertension who has just screened positive for mild microalbuminuria, which of the following antihypertensive medications would be the best choice for treatment?

A. A calcium channel blocker

B. An angiotensin converting enzyme inhibitor

C. β-blocker

D. A diuretic

106. Which one of the following demonstrates a troublesome family rule?

A. It's okay to interrupt one another's conversation at any time in order to be heard.

B. Every family member needs his or her own space at home.

C. Parents ask what the children think before making family decisions.

D. Everyone speaks for himself or herself.

107. When working with troubled families, physicians should do which one of the following?

A. Reinforce the members who are doing things right.

B. Determine who the troublemaker(s) is (are) in the family.

C. Reinforce the family's basic structure and behavior patterns.

D. Assume that a family member's symptoms may serve a function within the family.

108. A family that is emotionally separated with little family loyalty, involvement among family members, sharing of feelings, parent-child closeness, or time spent together describes a family that is:

A. Enmeshed

B. Chaotic

C. Disengaged

D. Rigid

109. An 85-year-old man presents to the office after a fall from which he was unable to get up. His daughter found him and brought him to your office for a checkup. In the office he appears cachectic. The physical exam is remarkable for muscle wasting and osteoarthritis in the hands. He is unable to arise from the chair or transfer from supine to sit without assistance. Which of the following will be least helpful in the work-up of this patient?

A. Height and weight

B. Diet and medication history

C. Routine lab work

D. Hip x-ray

E. Hospitalization

110. A 96-year-old man with chronic renal insufficiency, hypertension, slow walking gait, and a history of frequent falls presents to the office for a routine checkup. His weight is down 20 lb, blood pressure is 140/86, BUN 88, creatinine 4.3,

hemoglobin 9, HCT 30. The patient lives independently with his wife and is cognitively intact. Which of the following would you ascertain first?

A. His wishes regarding dialysis and other life-extending therapies

B. His overall nutritional and hydration status

C. His wife's continued ability to care for him

D. His willingness to participate in a rehab program

E. His current functional capacity and satisfaction with life

111. An 89-year-old woman has seen you in the office frequently over the last three months complaining of weakness and shakiness. She experiences early morning awakening with marked anxiety, recent weight loss, and a generalized slowing down. Her appetite is poor. Past medical history is positive for chronic obstructive pulmonary disease and anxiety. She is widowed and lives alone. The patient weighs 112 lb, height is 5 feet 6 inches, and essential tremor is present. Blood pressure is 130/76; heart rate is 98. Chest is clear to auscultation with diminished breath sounds. Which of the following best explains her increasing frailty?

A. Advanced age

B. Weight loss

C. Depression

D. Weakness and slowed gait

E. All of the above

112. In the case in the previous question, which tests are least likely to rule out a specific medical cause(s) for her symptoms?

A. CBC, complete chemistry profile

B. Morning cortisol level

C. Chest x-ray

D. Thyroid profile

E. EKG

113. The leading cause of death in patients over the age of 55 is:

A. Cancer

B. Endocrine disorders

C. Heart disease

D. Pneumonia

E. Renal disorders

114. Each of the following requires a total of two vaccines *except:*

A. Varicella after age 13

B. Measles, mumps, rubella

C. Catch-up for hepatitis B for a 2-year-old child who received the first in the newborn nursery but has received none since

D. Catch-up for a 5-year-old child who never received polio vaccine

115. A 9-month-old child should be able to demonstrate which of the following developmental tasks?

A. Sitting without assistance

B. Two or more words

C. Walking up stairs

D. Peddling a bicycle

116. In adults, jaundice is usually seen at bilirubin levels of:

A. Less than 2 mg/dL

B. Between 1 and 2 mg/dL

C. Greater than 0.2 mg/dL but less than 2 mg/dL

D. Greater than 2.5 mg/dL

117. The most appropriate treatment for patients with asymptomatic chronic cholelithiasis is:

A. Observation

B. ERCP for stone removal

C. Intravenous antibiotics

D. Antacids

118. Perimenopause begins with which of the following?

A. The onset of the first hot flash

B. The first break in regular cyclicity in women of the appropriate age

C. Usually around 40 years of age

D. After the cessation of menses for more than 12 months

119. The usual treatment for the symptomatic perimenopausal patient, with frequent hot flashes, sleep disturbance, and irritability, would be which of the following?

A. Low-dose fixed ratio oral contraceptives
B. Oral testosterone
C. High-dose oral estrogen alone
D. High-dose oral progesterone alone

120. Which of the following physical findings is *not* present in untreated menopause?
A. Pale vaginal mucosa
B. Small vaginal introitus
C. Loss of vaginal rugal folds
D. Enlarged cervix and uterus

121. A 65-year-old woman, not on hormone replacement, presents with vaginal bleeding. The next step in management should be?
A. Reassurance
B. Hysterectomy
C. High-dose hormone replacement therapy
D. Endometrial biopsy

122. A 54-year-old man with a long history of alcohol abuse develops chronic pancreatitis. He is able to stop drinking, but continues to complain of loose stools, especially after fatty meals, indicative of steatorrhea. This symptom indicates that he is at risk for which of the following nutrient deficiencies?
A. Vitamin A
B. Vitamin B_6
C. Vitamin C
D. Folate

123. A mother brings her 15-year-old daughter to the office because she is concerned that the daughter is too thin. Which of the following would make you concerned that the girl has an eating disorder?
A. The daughter is also concerned that she is too thin.
B. The daughter participates on the school basketball team.
C. The daughter seems preoccupied with food and food magazines.
D. The mother is thin and the father is overweight.

124. A patient asks you how quickly he will lose 1 pound when he wants to lose weight gradually and decreases his food intake by 100 kilocalories per day. What would you tell him with your understanding of how many kilocalories it takes to lose 1 pound?

A. 25 days
B. 30 days
C. 35 days
D. 40 days
E. 45 days

125. A patient relates a history of a lifetime of dieting. He asks your advice on which current diet program would work best for him. You would advise him to:

A. Exercise at least 15 minutes per day.
B. Eliminate all soda pop from his diet.
C. Decrease fat in his diet.
D. Determine what he is doing that causes his energy imbalance.
E. Follow the high-protein, high-fat plans that offer immediate weight loss results.

126. Appropriate screening tests in an early uncomplicated pregnancy include all of the following *except:*

A. Hemoglobin
B. Rubella
C. Repeat HCG levels
D. Pap smear

127. The last menstrual period (LMP) begins on the:

A. First day of the last normal period
B. Last day of the last normal period
C. First day of the last bleeding episode
D. Last day of the last bleeding episode

128. The appropriate dose of folic acid supplementation in the diet of a woman hoping to conceive is:

A. 40 milligrams
B. 400 micrograms
C. 4 grams
D. 100 milligrams

129. You are called to evaluate a 62-year-old man who has recently (24 hours post-op) undergone abdominal surgery in a veteran's hospital to release adhesions that were secondary to an appendix rupture several decades ago. Currently, he has newly elevated blood pressure, mild tachypnea, a low-grade fever, and appears to have a slightly depressed mood. He is being given 800-mg ibuprofen TID, a PPI, low-molecular-weight heparin, and TED hose, and he has a 25-mg fentanyl patch. A CBC and BMP drawn that day are normal. His wound appears clean, dry, and intact with no sign of infection. He has been ambulating over the last 12 hours. What parameters of his postoperative care need to be reassessed?

   A. Infection prophylaxis
   B. DVT/PE prophylaxis
   C. Pain control
   D. Review of sterile surgical technique

130. A 46-year-old man presents for a preoperative evaluation two weeks prior to surgery to repair a torn rotator cuff suffered during a league softball game. The patient's history is significant for diabetes, which is well controlled, and a half-pack-per-day smoking habit. He currently does not have any angina, chest tightness, or shortness of breath. What cardiac work-up is necessary in this patient?

   A. EKG and an exercise stress test
   B. EKG
   C. EKG and a stress echo
   D. Cardiac catheterization

131. A 7-year-old boy is referred by his school for psychiatric evaluation. The teachers have noticed that, in the past year, he has been unable to sustain attention in class and has been fidgeting and talking to his peers during class. He seems unable to wait for others to finish speaking and keeps interrupting and blurting out answers before questions are completed. At home, his parents state that he is forgetful and loses things easily. Which of the following is the most likely diagnosis?

   A. Attention deficit/hyperactivity disorder (ADHD)
   B. Bipolar disorder
   C. Conduct disorder
   D. Post-traumatic stress disorder
   E. Rett syndrome

132. A 14-year-old girl comes into the clinic for follow-up of her ADHD. She is currently on methylphenidate and doing well in school. All of the following are common side effects of methylphenidate drugs *except:*

   A. Insomnia
   B. Precocious puberty
   C. Appetite suppression
   D. Hypertension
   E. Cardiac arrthymia

133. A 12-year-old is brought into the clinic by his mother. He has been having trouble with math in school for the past two and a half years. He does well in all other subjects and has not received any additional help in school. His IQ is 95. He is well behaved in school and doesn't have any attention or behavior problems. What is the diagnosis and why?

   A. Mental retardation because of failing grades in school
   B. Learning disability because of normal behavior yet difficulty in school
   C. Mental retardation because of IQ below 95
   D. Learning disability because of IQ below 95
   E. Learning disability because of trouble in math but acceptable skills in other subjects

134. The parents of a 7-year-old boy, who has had continuing problems with daydreaming and "staying focused" in school, are told by the boy's second-grade teacher that he often becomes inattentive and nonresponsive (although still appears awake) during class. Assuming this is seizure related, what medication would be most appropriate?

   A. Benzodiazapine
   B. Phenobarbitol
   C. Ethosuximide
   D. Ritalin
   E. Lithium

135. In the example in the previous question, in what category of seizures would this be classified?

   A. Generalized seizure
   B. Simple partial seizure
   C. Grand mal seizure
   D. Complex partial seizure
   E. Tonic-clonic seizure

136. A 45-year-old man was admitted to the hospital for alcohol detoxification. You have successfully treated him with no adverse events. He is currently stable and is ready for discharge. When you talk to him about staying away from alcohol he states that he really wants to stop but does not currently have a plan and says that he can just stay away from alcohol. What stage of readiness for change is this person?

A. Precontemplation
B. Contemplation
C. Preparation
D. Action
E. Maintenance

137. A 28-year-old woman presents to your clinic today for a routine physical. During the physical you ask her about her use of substances. She states that she does not use any illegal drugs but likes to go to parties. When asked specifically about alcohol consumption she states that she drinks to intoxication three to six times a month (five to seven beers). She denies any problems with the law. She denies increasing tolerance. Which category best describes her use of alcohol?

A. Alcohol abuse
B. Alcohol misuse
C. Alcohol dependence
D. Normal drinking pattern for her age
E. High risk for alcoholism

138. A 50-year-old man presents to your clinic for right upper quadrant pain. He reports that he has been drinking for 25 years with multiple driving-while-under-the-influence (DUI) offenses. He is alienated from his family and has been fired from more than 15 jobs because of his drinking. He reports that he is scared and wants to stop drinking. What is the most appropriate treatment plan for this person?

A. Inpatient detox, outpatient therapy
B. Inpatient detox, intensive outpatient therapy
C. Inpatient detox, intensive inpatient therapy and a prescription for an SSRI
D. Inpatient detox, intensive inpatient therapy
E. A prescription for naltrexone

139. A 21-year-old man presents with a complaint of a sore on his penis. Which of the following historical factors will assist you most in making your diagnosis?

A. The patient's sexual partner has a similar lesion.

B. The ulcer is painless.

C. The patient has felt feverish.

D. The lesion has been present for five days.

140. A 22-year-old man presents with a complaint of discharge from the penis for the past three days. You make a diagnosis of chlamydial infection. The patient denies any allergies to medications. Which of the following is an appropriate treatment regimen?

A. Ceftriaxone 125 mg IM one time plus doxycycline 100 mg twice a day for seven days

B. Azithromycin 1 g one time plus doxycycline 100 mg twice a day for seven days

C. Ciprofloxacin 500 mg twice a day for seven days

D. Metronidazole 2 g one time plus erythromycin base 500 mg four times a day for seven days

141. A 24-year-old woman presents with a complaint of vaginal discharge. She also complains of lower abdominal pain, dyspareunia, and fever. She states she has recently changed sexual partners but has not been using condoms. Her last menstrual period was two weeks ago, and it was normal. Which of the following physical exam findings would help you make a diagnosis of pelvic inflammatory disease?

A. A shallow ulcer on the labia majora, draining a yellow exudate

B. Genital warts located on the cervix on speculum exam

C. Thick white vaginal discharge, showing budding hyphae under the microscope

D. Cervical motion tenderness on bimanual exam

142. The most frequent cause of hyperthyroidism is:

A. Grave's disease

B. Hashimoto's thyroiditis

C. Adenoma

D. Toxic nodular goiter

143. If the levothyroxine dose is changed today, when should the TSH be rechecked?

A. One day
B. One week
C. Two weeks
D. Four weeks
E. Four months

144. A 33-year-old woman presents with her hair coarsening, skin drying, and fatigue. In the initial evaluation of her thyroid, which tests should be ordered?

A. TSH, total T4
B. Total T4, free T4
C. TSH, antithyroid antibodies
D. Free T4, TSH

145. The most common cause of ischemic stroke is:

A. Vasospasm
B. Cerebral embolism
C. Severe hypotension
D. Arterial dissection
E. Cerebral hemorrhage

146. A 68-year-old man presents to the emergency department with weakness and numbness in his left hand and the left side of his face for the last half hour. As he is wheeled back to a bed, he notes that his symptoms have spontaneously resolved. Treatment of this man's disorder may include:

A. Antiarrhythmic drugs
B. β-blockers
C. Antiseizure drugs
D. Thrombolytic therapy
E. Antiplatelet drugs

147. A 28-year-old woman comes to your office two hours after being in a motor vehicle accident. She states she struck the upper portion of her nose on the steering wheel during the collision. She currently has nasal swelling, bruising about the eyes, and marked tenderness in the upper cheeks and bridge of her nose. Bleeding from the nose has been minimal. She has coughed up clots of blood every few

minutes since the accident and has felt nauseous since then as well. Should this patient be referred to ENT specialists?

A. No, she obviously has a simple broken nose.

B. No, the blood she is coughing up is clotted so it should stop soon.

C. Yes, this could represent a cribriform plate fracture.

D. Yes, she could have a basilar skull fracture that requires ENT/neuro evaluation.

E. Yes, the clotted blood represents ongoing bleeding of a posterior nasal artery.

148. A parent brings her 11-year-old son to the clinic for evaluation of a dog bite. She tells you the family cocker spaniel bit her son on his hand when he tried to take a chew toy away from the dog. The skin on the hand has several puncture wounds that are not currently bleeding and one 2-cm laceration that is bleeding. Both the dog and patient are up-to-date with their immunizations. What is your treatment strategy?

A. Suture all the wounds.

B. Suture all the wounds and prescribe antibiotics.

C. Loosely cover wounds with a sterile bandage and prescribe a broad-spectrum antibiotic.

D. Tell the patient's mother to get rid of the dog.

E. Suture the laceration but not the puncture wounds.

PRACTICE TEST ANSWERS

1. D
2. C
3. E
4. E
5. D
6. C
7. C
8. B
9. B
10. A
11. C
12. D
13. B
14. A
15. D
16. A
17. C
18. D
19. C
20. C
21. D
22. A
23. B
24. C
25. A
26. B
27. B
28. C
29. B
30. B
31. C
32. D
33. C
34. C
35. B
36. C
37. D
38. C
39. B
40. B
41. C
42. A
43. E
44. B
45. C
46. A
47. D
48. C
49. D
50. D
51. A
52. C
53. A
54. B
55. B
56. C
57. D
58. A
59. C
60. A
61. B
62. B
63. B
64. C
65. B
66. D
67. A
68. C
69. A
70. C
71. C
72. D

73. E
74. D
75. B
76. D
77. C
78. B
79. C
80. B
81. D
82. D
83. C
84. A
85. B
86. D
87. B
88. B
89. B
90. D
91. D
92. A
93. D
94. D
95. B
96. B
97. D
98. C
99. D
100. D
101. A
102. C
103. C
104. A
105. B
106. A
107. D
108. C
109. E
110. A
111. E
112. B
113. C
114. D
115. A
116. D
117. A
118. B
119. A
120. D
121. D
122. A
123. C
124. C
125. D
126. C
127. A
128. B
129. C
130. B
131. A
132. B
133. E
134. C
135. D
136. C
137. A
138. D
139. B
140. A
141. D
142. A
143. D
144. D
145. B
146. E
147. E
148. C

Appendix I: Medical Abbreviations

Abbreviations for common medical terms are used extensively in medical records. When time is of the essence, and brevity is valued, members of medical teams can often communicate well using such abbreviations. There are several disadvantages to their use, however, particularly in light of the frequency of medical errors. Not all specialties use the same abbreviations, even for the same condition. If a consulting team uses an abbreviation that the primary team is not familiar with, then confusion may result. In addition, abbreviations can be harder to read than if the whole word is spelled out. There are some abbreviations (such as mcg and mg) that look very similar and can cause dangerous errors. These abbreviations occur particularly in medication orders. Drug names should not be abbreviated in orders because this is the most common place where misreading occurs, often leading to severe consequences. The 2004 Joint Commission on Accreditation of Healthcare Organizations National Patient Safety Goals state that every hospital must have a list of Unacceptable Medical Abbreviations. It is important that every student, resident, physician, and staff member be aware of this list and not use these abbreviations.

Below is a brief list of abbreviations that should not be used because they have been the source of frequent medication errors. (See Cohen MR [ed]: Medication Errors. Washington, DC: American Pharmacists Association, 1999, for more information.) Next is a list of commonly used abbreviations that are consistent for most hospitals and specialties across the country.

Avoid These Abbreviations

Unacceptable Abbreviation	Intended Meaning	Misinterpretation
MSO_4, $MgSO_4$, MS	Morphine sulfate, magnesium sulfate	Drugs may be confused
cc	Cubic centimeters	Misread as "U" (units)
QD, QID, QOD	Once daily, four times a day, every other day	Mistaken for each other
Zero after a decimal (1.0)	1 mg	Misread as 10 mg

Common Medical Abbreviations	
AAA	Abdominal aortic aneurysm
a–a gradient	Alveolar to arterial gradient
Abd	Abdominal
ABG	Arterial blood gas
AC	Acromioclavicular
ACL	Anterior cruciate ligament
ADH	Antidiuretic hormone
AI	Aortic insufficiency
AFB	Acid fast bacilli
AKA	Above knee amputation
ALL	Acute lymphocytic leukemia
AML	Acute myelogenous leukemia
ANA	Antinuclear antibody
AOM	Acute otitis media
AP	Anteroposterior
ARDS	Acute respiratory distress syndrome
ARF	Acute renal failure
AS	Aortic stenosis
ASCVD	Atherosclerotic cardiovascular disease
ASD	Atrial septal defect
ASHD	Atherosclerotic heart disease
AV	Atrioventricular
A-V	Arteriovenous
BBB	Bundle branch block
BE	Barium enema
BID	Twice a day
BKA	Below the knee amputation
BM	Bone marrow or bowel movement
BMR	Basal metabolic rate
BOM	Bilateral otitis media
BP	Blood pressure
BPH	Benign prostatic hypertrophy
BPM	Beats per minute
BRBPR	Bright red blood per rectum
BRP	Bathroom privileges
BS	Bowel or breath sounds or blood sugar
BUN	Blood urea nitrogen
Bx	Biopsy

continued

Common Medical Abbreviations *continued*	
C&S	Culture and sensitivity
CA	Cancer
Ca	Calcium
CABG	Coronary artery bypass graft
CAD	Coronary artery disease
CAT	Computerized axial tomography
CBC	Complete blood count
CC	Chief complaint
CF	Cystic fibrosis
CHF	Congestive heart failure
CHO	Carbohydrate
CML	Chronic myelogenous leukemia
CMV	Cytomegalovirus
CN	Cranial nerves
CNS	Central nervous system
CO	Cardiac output
c/o	Complaining of
COPD	Chronic obstructive pulmonary disease
CP	Chest pain or cerebral palsy
CRF	Chronic renal failure
CRP	C-reactive protein
CSF	Cerebrospinal fluid
CVA	Cerebrovascular accident or costovertebral angle
CVAT	CVA tenderness
CVP	Central venous pressure
CXR	Chest x-ray
DAW	Dispense as written
DC	Discontinue or discharge
DDx	Differential diagnosis
D5W	5% dextrose in water
DIC	Disseminated intravascular coagulopathy
DIP	Distal interphalangeal joint
DJD	Degenerative joint disease
DKA	Diabetic ketoacidosis
DM	Diabetes mellitus
DNR	Do not resuscitate
DOA	Dead on arrival
DOE	Dyspnea on exertion

continued

Common Medical Abbreviations *continued*

DPT	Diphtheria, pertussis, tetanus
DTR	Deep tendon reflexes
DVT	Deep venous thrombosis
Dx	Diagnosis
EBL	Estimated blood loss
EKG	Electrocardiogram
ECT	Electroconvulsive therapy
EMG	Electromyogram
ENT	Ears, nose, and throat
EOM	Extraocular muscles
ESR	Erythrocyte sedimentation rate
ET	Endotracheal
ERCP	Endoscopic retrograde cholangio-pancreatography
ETOH	Ethanol (used for alcohol)
EUA	Examination under anesthesia
FBS	Fasting blood sugar
FEV	Forced expiratory capacity
Fx	Fracture
GC	Gonorrhea
GI	Gastrointestinal
GSW	Gunshot wound
GTT	Glucose tolerance test
GU	Genitourinary
HA	Headache
HBP	High blood pressure
HCG	Human chorionic gonadotropin
HCT	Hematocrit
HDL	High density lipoprotein
HEENT	Head, eyes, ears, nose, and throat
Hgb	Hemoglobin
HIV	Human immunodeficiency virus
HLA	Histocompatibility locus antigen
HOB	Head of bed
HPF	High power field
HPI	History of present illness
HR	Heart rate
HS	At bedtime

continued

Common Medical Abbreviations *continued*	
HSV	Herpes simplex virus
HTN	Hypertension
Hx	History
I & D	Incision and drainage
I & O	Intake and output
ICU	Intensive care unit
ID	Infectious disease or identification
IDDM	Insulin dependent diabetes mellitus
IM	Intramuscular
INF	Intravenous nutritional fluid
IPPB	Intermittent positive pressure breathing
ITP	Idiopathic thrombocytopenic purpura
IV	Intravenous
IVC	Intravenous cholangiogram or inferior vena cava
IVP	Intravenous pyelogram
JVD	Jugular venous distention
KUB	Kidneys, ureters, bladder (x-ray)
KVO	Keep vein open
LAD	Left axis deviation or left anterior descending
LAE	Left atrial enlargement
LBBB	Left bundle branch block
LDH	Lactate dehydrogenase
LDL	Low density lipoprotein
LE	Lupus erythematosus or lower extremity
LLL	Left lower lobe
LMP	Last menstrual period
LOC	Loss of consciousness or level of consciousness
LP	Lumbar puncture
LUL	Left upper lobe
LV	Left ventricle
LVH	Left ventricular hypertrophy
MAO	Monoamine oxidase
MAP	Mean arterial pressure
MAST	Medical antishock trousers
MCH	Mean cell hemoglobin
MCL	Medial collateral ligament
MCP	Metacarpal phalangeal
MCV	Mean cell volume

continued

Common Medical Abbreviations *continued*

MDD	Major depressive disorder
MI	Myocardial infarction or mitral insufficiency
ml	Milliliter
MMR	Mumps, measles, and rubella
MRI	Magnetic resonance imaging
MRSA	Methicillin resistant *Staphylococcus aureus*
MS	Multiple sclerosis, mitral stenosis
MVA	Motor vehicle accident
MVI	Multivitamin injection
NAD	No active disease, no apparent distress
NAS	No added salt
NG	Nasogastric
NIDDM	Non–insulin-dependent diabetes mellitus
NKA	No known allergies
NPO	Nothing by mouth
NSAID	Nonsteroidal anti-inflammatory drug
NSR	Normal sinus rhythm
OB	Obstetrics
OCG	Oral cholecystogram
OD	Overdose or right eye
OM	Otitis media
OOB	Out of bed
OPV	Oral polio vaccine
OS	Left eye
OU	Both eyes
PA	Posteroanterior
PAC	Premature atrial contraction
PAP	Pulmonary artery pressure
PAT	Paroxysmal atrial tachycardia
PC	After eating
PDA	Patent ductus arteriosus
PE	Pulmonary embolus, physical exam
PEEP	Positive end expiratory pressure
PFT	Pulmonary function tests
PI	Primary investigator
PIP	Proximal interphalangeal joint
PKU	Phenylketonuria
PMH	Previous medical history

continued

Common Medical Abbreviations *continued*

PMI	Point of maximal impulse
PMN	Polymorphonuclear leukocyte
PND	Paroxysmal nocturnal dyspnea or postnasal drip
PO	By mouth
POD	Post-op day
PP	Postprandial, pulsus paradoxus
PPD	Purified protein derivative
PR	By rectum
PRBC	Packed red blood cells
PRN	As needed
PT	Prothrombin time or physical therapy
PTCA	Percutaneous transluminal coronary angioplasty
PTH	Parathyroid hormone
PTSD	Post-traumatic stress disorder
PTT	Partial thromboplastin time
PUD	Peptic ulcer disease
PVC	Premature ventricular contraction
PVD	Peripheral vascular disease
Q 4h	Every four hours, etc.
QNS	Quantity not sufficient
RA	Right atrium, rheumatoid arthritis
RAD	Right axis deviation
RAE	Right atrial enlargement
RDA	Recommended daily allowance
RIA	Radioimmunoassay
RLL	Right lower lobe
RML	Right middle lobe
R/O	Rule out
ROM	Range of motion
ROS	Review of systems
RRR	Regular rate and rhythm
RTA	Renal tubular acidosis
RTC	Return to clinic
RUQ	Right upper quadrant
RV	Residual volume
Rx	Treatment
SA	Sinoatrial
SBE	Subacute bacterial endocarditis

continued

Common Medical Abbreviations *continued*

SBFT	Small bowel follow through
SEM	Systolic ejection murmur
SGA	Small for gestational age
SIADH	Syndrome of inappropriate antidiuretic hormone
Sig	Write on label
SL	Sublingual
SLE	Systemic lupus erythematosus
SOAP	Subjective, objective, assessment, plan
SOB	Shortness of breath
SOM	Serous otitis media
SQ	Subcutaneous
STD(I)	Sexually transmitted disease (infection)
SVD	Spontaneous vaginal delivery
Sx	Symptoms
T & C	Type and cross
TAH	Total abdominal hysterectomy
TB	Tuberculosis
TIA	Transient ischemic attack
TIBC	Total iron binding capacity
TID	Three times a day
TLC	Total lung capacity
TMJ	Temporomandibular joint
TNTC	Too numerous to count
TPN	Total parenteral nutrition
TSH	Thyroid stimulating hormone
TURP	Transurethral resection of prostate
Tx	Treatment, transplant
UA	Urinalysis
UGI	Upper gastrointestinal
URI	Upper respiratory infection
V/Q	Ventilation-perfusion
VSS	Vital signs stable
WBC	White blood cell or count
WD	Well developed
WNL	Within normal limits
WPW	Wolff-Parkinson-White
ZE	Zollinger-Ellison

Appendix II: Formulary

This formulary includes medications that are commonly used in family medicine. Only the most common indications or uses are listed for each drug or drug category. Doses listed are for the adult population unless otherwise noted. Keep in mind that many patients require individualized dosing. Consult your pharmacy for detailed drug information.

Cost Key	
$	<$20
$$	$20–$40
$$$	$40–$60
$$$$	>$60

A. Allergy Products

Nasal Steroids—Fluticasone, Mometasone	
Common trade name(s):	Flonase (fluticasone), Nasonex (mometasone)
Therapeutic class:	Topical anti-inflammatory
Indications:	Allergic rhinitis
Dose:	2 sprays per nostril qd
Pediatric dose:	1 spray per nostril qd (Nasonex ≥2 yo, Flonase ≥4 yo)
Adverse effects:	Nosebleed, headache
Cost:	$$$–$$$$
Notes:	Considered gold standard in treatment of allergic rhinitis. It targets all the symptoms of allergic rhinitis. Onset effect ≥1 wk. Also useful in nonallergic rhinitis.

Non-Sedating Antihistamines—Fexofenadine, Desloratadine, Loratadine, Cetirizine	
Common trade name(s):	Allegra (fexofenadine), Clarinex (desloratadine), Claritin (loratadine), Zyrtec (cetirizine)
Therapeutic class:	Non-sedating H1 histamine blockers
Indications:	Allergic rhinitis, chronic idiopathic urticaria
Dose:	Allegra 60 mg po bid or 180 mg po qd
	Clarinex 5 mg po qd
	Claritin OTC 10 mg po qd
	Zyrtec 10 mg po qd
Pediatric dose:	Start at ¼ to ½ of adult dose
	Allegra (≥6 yo), Claritin (≥2 yo), Zyrtec (≥6 mo)
Adverse effects:	Dizziness, drowsiness
Cost:	$$ (Claritin-OTC and generic available)
	$$$$ (Allegra, Clarinex, Zyrtec)
Notes:	Effective in majority of symptoms associated with allergic rhinitis except nasal congestion. These agents are also commonly combined with decongestants (e.g., Allegra-D, Claritin-D, Zyrtec-D).

B. Analgesics

NSAIDs—Ibuprofen, Naproxen	
Common trade name(s):	Motrin (Ibuprofen), Anaprox DS, or Naprosyn
Therapeutic class:	NSAIDs, anti-inflammatory
Indications:	Pain, arthritis, acute gout, primary dysmenorrhea
Dose:	Motrin 600–800 mg tid or prn
	Anaprox DS 550 mg bid or prn
	Naprosyn 500 mg bid or prn
Dose adjustments:	Avoid in renal and hepatic impairment or reduce dose
Adverse effects:	Abdominal pain, dyspepsia, heartburn, nausea, dizziness, edema, blood pressure elevation, rash
	Serious: ulcer, GI bleeding, renal failure, hepatitis
Monitoring:	Blood pressure, renal function, GI bleeding, CBC
Cost:	$ (generics available)
Notes:	Elderly (age >65), history of PUD, concurrent corticosteroids or warfarin therapy are at high risk of NSAIDs-induced ulcers. Recommend COX-II inhibitors for these patients. Contraindicated in patients with aspirin allergy, nasal polyps, or asthma/bronchospasm.

COX-II Inhibitors—Celecoxib, Rofecoxib

Common trade name(s):	Celebrex (celecoxib)
Therapeutic class:	COX-II inhibitors, anti-inflammatory
Indications:	Acute pain, osteoarthritis, primary dysmenorrhea, rheumatoid arthritis
Dose:	Celebrex 100–200 mg po qd–bid Use higher dose for acute pain
Dose adjustments:	Celebrex—liver disease reduce dose by 50% Avoid in renal impairment patients
Adverse effects:	Abdominal pain, dyspepsia, fluid retention, peripheral edema, blood pressure elevation, rash Serious and rare: GI bleeding, renal and liver impairment
Monitoring:	Blood pressure, long-term use—monitoring for GI bleeding
Cost:	$$$$
Notes:	Celebrex contraindicated in patients with sulfa allergy (namely sulfonamides). Also not recommended if patient has aspirin allergy, asthma, or nasal polyps. COX-II inhibitors do have less ulcergenic effects than traditional NSAIDs. Candidates for COX-II inhibitors are >60 yo, concurrent corticosteroids or anticoagulants, history peptic ulcer disease. No antiplatelet activity.

Opioids—Acetaminophen w/ Codeine, Hydrocodone w/Acetaminophen

Common trade name(s):	Tylenol #3 (acetaminophen w/codeine) Lortab or Vicodin (hydrocodone w/acetaminophen)
Therapeutic class:	Opioid analgesic
Indications:	Moderate to severe pain
Dose:	Tylenol #3 1–2 po q4 prn Lortab or Vicodin 1–2 tabs q 4–6 hrs prn, max 8 tablets/24 hrs (4 gm of acetaminophen)
Adverse effects:	Constipation, nausea, vomiting, initial sedation, respiratory depression, urinary retention
Cost:	$–$$ (generics available)
Notes:	The maximum dose is based on the total dose of acetaminophen per day, 4 g per day. Multiple dosage strengths are available. Avoid in severe COPD. Risk of physical dependence, tolerance, and addiction with long-term use. Recommend short-term usage, PRN usage for acute pain or breakthrough pain. Long-acting opioids are preferred for chronic pain management. Controlled substance III (phone prescriptions are accepted).

C. Antihypertensives

- All antihypertensives are effective in treatment of hypertension. Selection of agent should be based on compelling evidence (outcome data that shows decreased morbidity or mortality in cardiovascular disease or other target organ damage), comorbid conditions, avoidance of unfavorable effects, easy dosing, cost, etc.
- Per JNC-VII, ACE inhibitors, ARBs (angiotensin II receptor blockers), β-blockers (BB), calcium channel blockers (CCB), and thiazide diuretics are all good initial choices, with diuretic being the preferred agent.
- Thiazides should also be included in any combination of above antihypertensives.
- Doses included here are for hypertension only.

Compelling Indications	Initial Therapy Options
Heart failure	Diuretic, BB, ACEI, ARB, aldosterone antagonist
Post MI	BB, ACEI, aldosterone antagonist
High CVD risk	Thiazides, BB, ACEI, CCB
DM	Thiazides, BB, ACEI, ARB, CCB
Chronic kidney disease	ACEI, ARB
Recurrent stroke prevention	Thiazides, ACEI

Angiotensin Converting Enzyme Inhibitors (ACEIs)—Lisinopril, Enalapril

Common trade name(s):	Zestril or Prinivil (lisinopril), Vasotec (enalapril)
Therapeutic class:	Angiotensin converting enzyme inhibitor
Indications:	HTN, CHF, AMI, CAD, microalbuminuria, DM nephropathy, recurrent stroke
Dose:	Zestril or Prinivil 10–40 mg po qd
	Vasotec 5–40 mg po per day as qd or bid
Dose adjustments:	Reduce dose or dosing interval in renal impairment
Adverse effects:	Cough, dizziness, headache, hyperkalemia, hypotension
	Serious: angioedema, renal dysfunction
Monitoring:	Renal function and serum potassium
Cost:	$ (generics available)
Notes:	Contraindicated in pregnancy and bilateral renal artery stenosis. In patients on diuretics or with hyponatremia, start on the lower end of initial dose to avoid hypotension and acute renal dysfunction. Although less effective in hypertensive African Americans than non–African Americans, ACEIs should still be used in patients with compelling evidence (CHF, DM, CAD, AMI). Addition of diuretic provides additive effects (Zestoretic, Vaseretic). Caution with ACEIs and potassium-sparing diuretic/potassium supplement.

Angiotensin II Receptor Blockers (ARBs)—Losartan, Valsartan

Common trade name(s):	Cozaar (losartan), Diovan (valsartan)
Therapeutic class:	Angiotensin II receptor blockers
Indications:	HTN, CHF, DM nephropathy
Dose:	Cozaar 50–100 mg po qd
	80–320 mg po qd
Adverse effects:	Dizziness, headache
	Serious: angioedema (less than ACEIs)
Monitoring:	Renal function and potassium
Cost:	$$–$$$
Notes:	Contraindicated in pregnancy and bilateral renal artery stenosis. Useful in patients intolerant to ACEIs due to cough. Commonly used with HCTZ (Diovan-HCT, Hyzaar).

β-Blockers—Atenolol, Metoprolol

Common trade name(s):	Tenormin (atenolol), Toprol or Toprol XL (metoprolol)
Therapeutic class:	Cardioselective β-blocker
Indications:	HTN, angina pectoris, CAD, AMI, CHF, arrhythmias, migraine prophylaxis, prophylaxis prior to surgery
Dose:	Tenromin 25–100 mg po qd for hypertension
	Toprol 12.5–100 mg bid
	Toprol XL 25–200 mg qd
Dose adjustments:	Tenromin—dose reduction in renal impairment
	Toprol or Toprol XL—dose reduction in hepatic impairment
Adverse effects:	Dizziness, tiredness, bradycardia, depression, bronchospasm, glucose intolerance, mask hypoglycemic reactions, lipid abnormality
Cost:	$ (generic available)
	$$$ (Toprol XL only)
Notes:	Do no abruptly discontinue β-blockers. Cardioselectivity is lost at higher dose. Do not avoid in diabetes unless risk outweighs benefit. Caution in asthma, COPD, and peripheral vascular disease. Metoprolol has FDA indication for CHF. Atenolol has fewer CNS side effects than metoprolol.

Calcium Channel Blockers—Amlodipine

Common trade name(s):	Norvasc
Therapeutic class:	Calcium channel blocker, dihydropyridine
Indications:	HTN, angina
Dose:	5–10 mg po qd
Dose adjustments:	Hepatic impairment—start at 2.5 mg po qd
Adverse effects:	Dizziness, flushing, headache, palpitation, peripheral edema
Cost:	$$$–$$$$

Diuretics—Hydrocholorthiazide (HCTZ) or Triamterene/Hydrocholorthiazide

Common trade name(s):	Hydrodiuril or Dyazide, Maxzide-25
Therapeutic class:	Thiazide diuretic
Indications:	HTN, edema
Dose:	12.5–25 mg po qd
Dose adjustments:	Not recommend with CrCl <25 mL/min
Adverse effects:	Dizziness, electrolyte abnormalities, hyperglycemia, hyperlipidemia, hyperuricemia, impotence, photosensitivity
Monitoring:	Serum potassium, sodium. Renal function
Cost:	$
Notes:	Considered first-line for uncomplicated HTN. Should be part of any combination antihypertensive regimen. Keeping the HCTZ dose at <25 mg per day minimizes most of the adverse effects. Triamterene does not offer any significant blood pressure effect, but is mainly used to counteract hypokalemia. Although indicated for edema, loop diuretics (e.g., furosemide) are more effective for this purpose. Should *not* avoid in patients with diabetes or hyperlipidemia. Avoid in patients with gout or on lithium therapy.

Diuretics—Furosemide

Common trade name(s):	Lasix
Therapeutic class:	Loop diuretic
Indications:	HTN, edema from CHF, cirrhosis, renal disease
Dose:	20–40 mg po qd–bid
Adverse effects:	Dizziness, hypotension, electrolyte depletion, rash
Cost:	$
Notes:	Fast onset but short duration of action; therefore, not first-line choice for HTN. Mainly for edema or HCTZ nonresponder (CrCl <25 mL/min)

D. Anti-infective Agents

Azithromycin

Common trade name(s):	Zithromax
Therapeutic class:	Macrolide antibiotics
Indications:	URI, mild community-acquired pneumonia, otitis media, STDs (chlamydia and gonorrhea)
Dose:	URI and mild pneumonia—500 mg po day 1 then 250 mg po days 2–5
	Chlamydia—1 g po × 1
	Gonorrhea—2 g po × 1
Pediatric dose:	URI and pneumonia—10 mg/kg/d day 1 then 5 mg/kg/d days 2–5. For pharyngitis use 12 mg/kg/d × 5d
	Otitis media—30 mg/kg/d × 1d or 10 mg/kg qd × 3d or 10 mg/kg/d day 1 then 5 mg/kg qd
Adverse effects:	Abdominal pain, diarrhea, nausea
Cost:	$$$
Notes:	Although indicated for otitis media, current guidelines recommend Zithromax as an alternative therapy when patient has type 1 penicillin allergy. For non–type 1 penicillin allergy, guidelines recommend cephalosporins (Ceftin, Omnicef, or Vantin) for otitis media. Amoxicillin is considered drug of choice for otitis media. Safe in pregnancy.

Amoxicillin

Common trade name(s):	Amoxil
Therapeutic class:	Penicillin antibiotics
Indications:	URI, otitis media
Dose:	URI—500 mg tid or 875 mg to 1 gm bid
Pediatric dose:	Otitis media (drug-resistant *S. pneumoniae*)—80–90 mg/kg/day po divided every 8–12 hr
Dose adjustments:	Renal impairment—give usual dose and extend interval to every 12–24 hr
Adverse effects:	Diarrhea, nausea, rash
Cost:	$ (generics available)
	$$–$$$ (brand only; 500 mg, 875 mg)
Notes:	Considered drug of choice for otitis media. In adults, recommend 1 gm (500 mg × 2, generic available) bid instead of 875 mg bid (brand only) for cost savings. Safe in pregnancy.

Amoxicillin/Clavulanate

Common trade name(s):	Augmentin, Augmentin XR
Therapeutic class:	Penicillin with β-lactamase inhibitor, broad spectrum
Indications:	Lower respiratory infections, otitis media, sinusitis, skin infections, urinary tract infection
Dose:	Augmentin 500 mg bid to 875 mg bid Augmentin XR 2000 mg (2 tabs) bid for community-acquired pneumonia or sinusitis
Pediatric dose:	Dose amoxicillin part 40 mg/kg/d divided into bid Dose amoxicillin part 80–90 mg/kg/d divided into bid for drug resistant otitis media
Dose adjustments:	Reduce dose in severe renal impairment
Adverse effects:	Diarrhea (most common), nausea, rash
Cost:	$$$$
Notes:	Clavulanate causes the higher diarrhea incidence. Use higher strength as bid instead of lower strength tid to minimize this side effect. In otitis media, augmentin is considered when patient failed amoxicillin for otitis media or suspecting β-lactamase–producing organisms. Need to use 80–90 mg/kg of amoxicillin component for otitis media. Safe in pregnancy.

Cephalexin

Common trade name(s):	Keflex
Therapeutic class:	First-generation cephalosporin
Indications:	Mainly use for infections caused by Staphylococcus in skin infections Other uses include urinary tract infections, respiratory tract infections
Dose:	500 mg po bid–qid
Dose adjustments:	CrCl <50 mL/min give usual dose every 12 hr
Adverse effects:	Abdominal pain, diarrhea
Cost:	$
Notes:	Use with caution in patients with penicillin allergy (cross sensitivity 2%). Safe in pregnancy.

Fluoroquinolones—Ciprofloxacin, Levofloxacin

Common trade name(s):	Cipro (ciprofloxacin), Levaquin (levofloxacin)
Therapeutic class:	Fluoroquinolones, broad spectrum
Indications:	Lower respiratory infection, pneumonia, prostatitis, skin infections, sinusitis, urinary tract infections, gonorrhea, infectious diarrhea
Dose:	Cipro 250–750 mg po bid
	Cipro 250 mg po × 1 for gonorrhea
	Levaquin 250–750 mg po qd
Dose adjustments:	Reduce dose for both Cipro and Levaquin in renal impairment
Adverse effects:	Dizziness, headache, diarrhea, nausea
Cost:	$$$$
Notes:	Not recommended in children under 18 yo and in pregnancy. Avoid coadministering with antacids, calcium, dairy products, iron. Cipro is used more for genitourinary infections. Levaquin (better susceptibility with *S. pneumoniae* and Streptococcus than Cipro) is used more for upper or lower respiratory infections.

Metronidazole

Common trade name(s):	Flagyl
Therapeutic class:	Antibacterial, antiparasitic
Indications:	Bacterial vaginosis, Trichomoniasis
Dose:	Bacterial vaginosis—500 mg po bid × 7d
	Trichomoniasis—2 g po × 1
Adverse effects:	Dizziness, headache, GI discomfort, nausea, symptomatic candida cervicitis/vaginitis, vaginal discharge
	Serious: peripheral neuropathy, disulfiram-like reaction
Cost:	$
Notes:	Avoid alcohol consumption.

Fluconazole	
Common trade name(s):	Diflucan
Therapeutic class:	Antifungal, azoles
Indications:	Vaginal candidiasis, oropharyngeal/esophageal candidiasis
Dose:	Vaginal candidiasis—150 mg po × 1 Oropharyngeal—200 mg po × 1 then 100 mg po qd × 2 wks
Dose adjustments:	Reduce dose by 50% in renal impairment.
Adverse effects:	Headache, nausea, vomiting, elevated liver enzymes
Monitoring:	Drug interactions
Cost:	$$$$
Notes:	Diflucan is a potent P450 enzyme inhibitor. Numerous drug interactions. Consult pharmacy.

E. Asthma and COPD Agents

- Asthma education is important in overall asthma management. Patient should be educated on disease, trigger, proper inhaler technique, compliance issues, etc.
- Use stepwise approach for managing adults and children older than 5 years of age (see following chart).
- All patients should be on short-acting β_2-agonist as rescue therapy.

Step 1: Mild Intermittent	No daily medication needed
Step 2: Mild Persistent	Low-dose inhaled corticosteroids
Step 3: Moderate Persistent	Low- to medium-dose inhaled corticosteroids *and* long-acting inhaled β_2-agonists
Step 4: Severe Persistent	High-dose inhaled corticosteroids *and* long-acting inhaled β_2-agonists If needed oral corticosteroids daily

Albuterol MDI

Common trade name(s):	Proventil, Ventolin
Therapeutic class:	Bronchodilators, short-acting β_2-agonists
Indications:	Asthma—acute or rescue treatment for bronchospam COPD Bronchitis Exercise-induced bronchospasm
Dose:	2 puffs q 4–6 hr prn
Adverse effects:	Nervousness, palpitations, tachycardia, tremor
Cost:	$ (generics available)
Notes:	Monitor usage. Good asthma control means patient uses albuterol inhaler ≤2×/wk. One canister should last at least 6 months.

Albuterol + Ipratropium MDI

Common trade name(s):	Combivent
Therapeutic class:	Bronchodilator, β-agonist + anticholinergic
Indications:	COPD
Dose:	2 puffs qid
Adverse effects:	Palpitation, tremor, headache, dry mouth
Cost:	$$$$

Inhaled Corticosteroids—Fluticasone, Budesonide

Common trade name(s):	Flovent MDI (fluticasone), Pulmicort Turbuhaler (budesonide)
Therapeutic class:	Corticosteroids, anti-inflammatory
Indications:	Asthma prophylaxis/maintenance therapy
Dose:	Flovent—2 puffs bid (44 mcg is low-dose, 110 mcg is medium-dose, and 220 mcg is high-dose strength) Pulmicort—2–6 puffs per day (1–3 puffs is low-dose, 3–6 puffs is medium-dose, and >6 puffs is high-dose strength) either qd or bid regimen
Adverse effects:	Oral thrush, pharyngitis Serious and rare: adrenal suppression (high-dose strength Flovent 220 mcg or Pulmicort >6 puffs), glaucoma
Cost:	$$$$
Notes:	*Not* for acute treatment. Anti-inflammatory effect takes ≥1 week. Use spacer or rinse mouth after use to minimize oral thrush.

Salmeterol	
Common trade name(s):	Serevent Diskus
Therapeutic class:	Bronchodilator, long-acting β-agonist
Indications:	Asthma maintenance therapy, COPD
Dose:	1 puff bid
Adverse effects:	Dizziness, headache, nervousness, palpitation, tremor, throat irritation
Cost:	$$$$
Notes:	Asthma—*Not* for acute treatment of asthma; add on therapy to inhaled corticosteriods.

Fluticasone + Salmeterol	
Common trade name(s):	Advair Diskus
Therapeutic class:	Anti-inflammatory and brochodilator
Indications:	Asthma, maintenance therapy
Dose:	1 puff bid (100/50 is low-dose, 250/50 is medium-dose, and 500/50 is high-dose strength)
Adverse effects:	Headache, hoarseness, oral thrush, tachycardia, throat irritation
Monitoring:	Serious: adrenal suppression (500/50 strength), glaucoma
Cost:	$$$$
Notes:	Combination therapy with inhaled corticosteroid and long-acting β-agonist is preferred treatment in Step 3 moderate persistent asthma, more so than ICS monotherapy. Rinse mouth after use to avoid oral thrush.

Motelukast	
Common trade name(s):	Singulair
Therapeutic class:	Leukotriene inhibitors
Indications:	Asthma, maintenance therapy; allergic rhinitis
Dose:	10 mg po qd
Adverse effects:	Well-tolerated
	Serious and rare: Churg-Strauss Syndrome
Cost:	$$$$
Notes:	In asthma management, Singulair is an alternative treatment to inhaled corticosteroid therapy. Singulair is as effective as antihistamine in treatment of allergic rhinitis.

Prednisone	
Common trade name(s):	Deltasone
Therapeutic class:	Corticosteroids, systemic
Indications:	Asthma, acute exacerbation
Dose:	40–60 mg po qd × 3–10 days
Adverse effects:	CNS changes (euphoria/depression), increased appetite, GI upsets Long-term complications are avoided with short duration of use.
Cost:	$
Notes:	When given as "burst" (dose listed above), it does not cause adrenal suppression or increase asthma relapses.

F. Contraceptives and Hormone Replacement Therapy

Ethinyl Estradiol + Progestins	
Common trade name(s):	Low-dose estrogen: Alesse, Ortho Tri-cyclen Lo Medium-dose estrogen: Ortho Tri-cyclen, Lo/Ovral, Ortho Novum, Yasmin, Ortho Evra
Therapeutic class:	Combined contraceptive, systemic
Indications:	Prevention of pregnancy, acne vulgaris (Ortho Tri-cyclen)
Dose:	1 tablet po qd Ortho Evra 1 patch q wk × 3 wk then off patch × 1 wk and repeat
Dose adjustments:	Ortho Evra patch—avoid in patients weighing >98 kg (198 lb) because of decreased efficacy
Adverse effects:	Nausea, bloating, breakthrough bleeding/spotting, breast tenderness, edema, weight gain, melasma Serious: PE, DVT, stroke, gallbladder disease, HTN, MI, retinal thrombosis
Monitoring:	Annual history and physical exam with pap
Cost:	$$
Notes:	Warning signs: ACHES. A = abdominal pain, C = chest pain, H = headaches, E = eye changes, S = swelling in lower extremities. Avoid in smokers and age ≥35 yo. Low-dose estrogen products may have more breakthrough bleeding/spotting. Ortho Tri-cyclen is also indicated for acne. Yasmin has a progestin that is a spironolactone (diuretic) analog. Yasmin may have fewer bloating, weight gain, PMS issues.

Conjugated Estrogens ± Progestins	
Common trade name(s):	Premarin, Prempro
Therapeutic class:	Estrogen/hormone replacement therapy
Indications:	Vasomotor symptoms associated with menopause, vulvar and vaginal atrophy, postmenopausal osteoporosis prevention and treatment
Dose:	Premarin 0.625–1.25 mg po qd Prempro 0.3/1.5–0.625/5 mg po qd Premarin vaginal cream 0.5–2 g qhs then decrease dose and frequency (e.g., 1–3 times/wk)
Adverse effects:	Nausea, abdominal cramps, bloating, breast pain/tenderness, irregular spotting, weight gain Serious: breast cancer, gallbladder disease, pancreatitis, MI, stroke, PE, DVT
Monitoring:	Blood pressure, breast exam, pap
Cost:	$$
Notes:	Premarin therapy is reserved for patient without uterus. Prempro (estrogens + progestins) is indicated for women with intact uterus. Because of the increased risks (MI, stroke, breast cancer, PE, DVT) shown in Women's Health Initiative study, use shortest duration and lowest effective dose of Prempro 0.3/1.5 mg or 0.45/1.5 mg po qd and titrate dose if necessary. Vaginal preparations are more effective for vulvar and vaginal atrophy. HRT should not be a first-line agent for osteoporosis treatment or prevention.

G. Diabetes Agents

- All of the oral agents are indicated for monotherapy.
- Selection of agents depends on patient's characteristics and to target insulin resistance.
- Only the most commonly prescribed agents are detailed here (see chart).
- Management strategies: see figure.

Comparison of the Efficacy of Oral Agents as Monotherapy

Drug Class	⇓ in FPG (mg/dL)	⇓ in PPG (mg/dL)	⇓ in $HgbA_{1c}$ (%)
Sulfonylureas	60–70		1.0–2.0
Meglitinides	30–50	40–60	0.5–1.0
Metformin	50–70		1.5
Glitazones	20–55		0.5–1.5 (2+)*
Alpha-glucosidase inhibitor	20–40	20–75	0.5–1.0

* Variable efficacy

Type 2 DM Management Strategies[1]

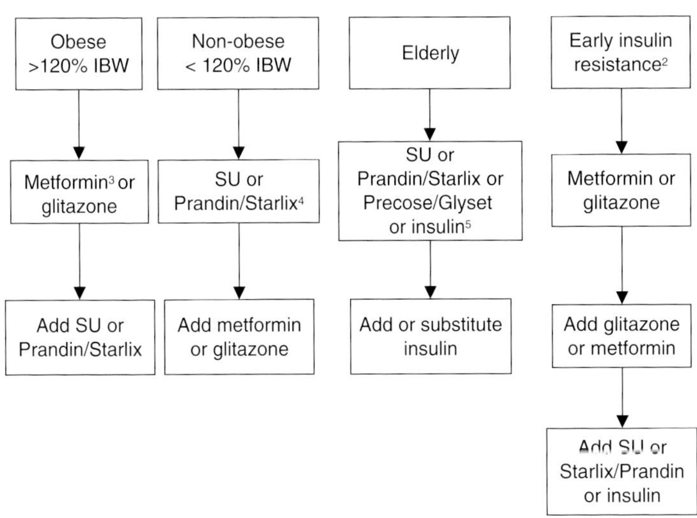

[1] At any point, in case of severe metabolic decompensation, insulin may be used.
[2] β-cell still present or IFG or IGT.
[3] Metformin is preferred if no contraindications.
[4] In nonobese patients, metformin can be considered alternative at this stage; however, because lean patients tend to have a relatively greater degree of β-cell dysfunction relative to insulin resistance, they may respond better to insulin-secreting agents.
[5] In elderly, monitor for potential hypoglycemia with these agents. If DM2 is diagnosed at old age, patient tends to be lean and have more of an insulin deficiency than resistance. Some may require insulin.

Sulfonylureas—Glipizide, Glyburide	
Common trade name(s):	Glucotrol XL (glipizide), Diabeta (glyburide)
Therapeutic class:	Sulfonylureas, hypoglycemic; insulin-secreting agent
Indications:	Type 2 DM
Dose:	Glucotrol XL 2.5–20 mg po qd Diabeta (glyburide) 1.25–20 mg po qd
Dose adjustments:	Geriatrics—conservative doses
Adverse effects:	Hypoglycemia, heartburn, nausea, rash
Cost:	$ (generics available)
Notes:	Has faster onset effects than other oral agents

Metformin	
Common trade name(s):	Glucophage
Therapeutic class:	Biguanide, insulin-sensitizing agents
Indications:	Type 2 DM, PCOS
Dose:	500 mg bid to 2500 mg per day
Dose adjustments:	Avoid in renal impairment (SCr >1.4 for women, >1.5 for men), hepatic impairment
Adverse effects:	Nausea, abdominal pain, diarrhea, weight loss Serious and rare: lactic acidosis
Monitoring:	Check serum Cr before initiation and then periodically
Cost:	$–$$
Notes:	Considered on all type 2 DM with typical insulin resistance presentation. Beneficial effects include weight loss, lipid improvement. May not be ideal in elderly population due to declining renal function. Risk factors for lactic acidosis include IV contrast dye, renal or hepatic impairment, CHF, hypoxic states, heavy alcohol consumption.

Glyburide + Metformin	
Common trade name(s):	Glucovance
Therapeutic class:	Insulin-secreting + insulin-sensitizing agent
Indications:	Type 2 DM
Dose:	1.25/250 po qd to 5/500 2 po bid
Dose adjustments:	Avoid in renal and hepatic impairment
Adverse effects:	See Sulfonylureas and Metformin.
Monitoring:	Serum SCr, liver function test
Cost:	$$
Notes:	Combination therapy provides additive effect at lower doses with reduced side effects

Glitazones—Pioglitazone, Rosiglitazone	
Common trade name(s):	Actos (pioglitazone), Avandia (rosiglitazone)
Therapeutic class:	Thiazolidinediones, insulin-sensitizing agent
Indications:	Type 2 DM
Dose:	Actos—15–45 mg po qd
	Avandia—4–8 mg po per day as qd or bid
Dose adjustments:	Avoid in hepatic impairment.
Adverse effects:	Peripheral edema, headache, myalgia, weight gain
	Serious and rare: hepatotoxicity, exacerbation of CHF
Monitoring:	Liver function test—baseline, q 2 months × 1 yr then periodically
Cost:	$$$$
Notes:	Slow onset of effect (4–12 weeks). Best used in the early stage of type 2 DM. Variable efficacy results. May decrease insulin requirement. Do not use in patient with active liver disease (ALT >2.5 × ULN) and CHF III-IV.

H. Gastrointestinal Drugs

Proton Pump Inhibitors (PPIs)— Rabeprazole, Esomeprazole, Lansoprazole, Omeprazole, Pantoprazole	
Common trade name(s):	Acidphex (rabeprazole), Nexium (esomeprazole), Prevacid (lansoprazole), Prilosec (omeprazole), Protonix (pantoprazole)
Therapeutic class:	Anti-ulcer, PPIs
Indications:	Peptic ulcer disease, GERD, erosive esophagitis, *H. pylori* eradication, hypersecretory conditions, prevention and treatment of NSAID-induced ulcer
Dose:	Aciphex—20 mg po qd
	Nexium—20–40 mg po qd
	Prevacid—15–30 mg po qd
	Prilosec—10–40 mg po qd
	Protonix—40 mg po qd
Adverse effects:	Abdominal pain, diarrhea, constipation, flatulence, headache, nausea
Cost:	$$ (Prilosec OTC)
	$$$$

Histamine H_2-Antagonists—Famotidine, Ranitidine	
Common trade name(s):	Pepcid (famotidine), Zantac (ranitidine)
Therapeutic class:	H_2-antagonists
Indications:	PUD, GERD
Dose:	Pepcid—20–40 mg po qd
	Zantac—150–300 mg po bid
Dose adjustments:	Reduce dose in renal impairment
Adverse effects:	Well-tolerated
Cost:	\$–\$\$

I. Lipid-Lowering Agents

Statins—Rosuvastatin, Atorvastatin, Pravastatin, Simvastatin	
Common trade name(s):	Crestor (rosuvastatin), Lipitor (atorvastatin), Pravachol (pravstatin), Zocor (simvastatin)
Therapeutic class:	Antihyperlipidemic, HMG-CoA reductase inhibitors
Indications:	Hypercholesterolemia, hypertriglyceridemia
Dose:	Crestor—10–40 mg po qd
	Lipitor—10–80 mg po qd
	Pravachol—40–80 mg po qd
	Zocor—20–80 mg po qd
Dose adjustments:	Avoid in severe liver disease
Adverse effects:	Nausea, headache, liver enzyme elevation, myopathy
	Serious and rare: hepatoxicity, rhabdomyolysis
Monitoring:	Lipid panel at 4–6 weeks (↓LDL 30–55%, ↓TG 7–30%, ↑HDL 5–15%). Liver function test at baseline, 3 months, then every 6 months. Consider CK enzyme in patients experiencing muscle pain or those receiving combination therapy with niacin, gemfibrozil, or fenofibrate
Cost:	\$\$\$–\$\$\$\$
Notes:	Agents of choice because of outcome data. Best drug class to target LDL. Discontinue therapy if serum transaminase levels are three times the upper limit of normal. Risk factors for myopathy include higher dose, elderly, polypharmacy, combination treatment with niacin, fibrates, and drug interactions (cyclosporine, erythromycin, azole antifungals) (switch to a different statin).

Ezetimibe

Common trade name(s):	Zetia
Therapeutic class:	Antihyperlipidemic
Indications:	Hypercholesterolemia
Dose:	10 mg po qd
Adverse effects:	Abdominal pain, diarrhea
Monitoring:	Lipid panel at 4–6 wks (↓LDL 18–20%, ↓TG 10%)
Cost:	$$$$
Notes:	Works by reducing absorption of cholesterol. Limited role in monotherapy. Useful as combination with a statin to achieve further LDL- or triglyceride-lowering effects.

Fibric Acids—Fenofibrate, Gemfibrozil

Common trade name(s):	Tricor (fenofibrate), Lopid (gemfibrozil)
Therapeutic class:	Antihyperlipidemic, fibric acid derivative
Indications:	Hypertriglyceridemia, hypercholesterolemia
Dose:	Tricor—160 mg po qd Lopid—600 mg po bid
Adverse effects:	Abdominal pain, diarrhea, muscle pain, nausea Serious and rare: hepatotoxicity
Monitoring:	Lipid panel at 4–6 wks (↓LDL 10–25%, ↓TG 40–50%, HDL ↑10–20%), liver function test (1-2x/yr)
Cost:	Tricor $$$$ Lopid $–$$ (generics available)
Notes:	Mainly used for hypertriglyceridemia and to increase HDL. LDL-lowering effect is variable, more reduction with Tricor than Lopid. Combination therapy with statin increases risk of rhabdomyolysis. Tricor may have less incidence of rhabdomyolysis.

J. Osteoporosis Drugs

Bisphosphonate—Alendronate, Risedronate	
Common trade name(s):	Fosamax (alendronate), Actonel (risedronate)
Therapeutic class:	Bisphosphonate, calcium regulator
Indications:	Osteoporosis prevention and treatment in women
	Osteoporosis treatment in men
	Glucocorticoid-induced osteoporosis
Dose:	Fosamax—35–70 mg q wk
	Actonel—35 mg q wk
Administration:	Must be taken with plain water at least 30 min before the first food, beverage, or medication of the day
	Should be swallowed upon arising for the day with 6–8 oz of water
	Should not lie down for at least 30 min
Adverse effects:	Dyspepsia, headache
	Serious: esophagitis, esophageal ulcers
Monitoring:	DEXA bone density 1–3 years after therapy
Cost:	$$$$
Notes:	Should have adequate calcium (1000–1500 mg/d) and vitamin D (400–800 IU/d) intake. Increases both vertebral and hip BMD and decreases fracture rates for both vertebral and hip. Considered first-line agent.

Raloxifene	
Common trade name(s):	Evista
Therapeutic class:	Selective estrogen receptor modulators (SERM)
Indications:	Prevention and treatment of osteoporosis
Dose:	60 mg po qd
Adverse effects:	Hot flashes, leg cramps
	Serious: DVT, PE
Cost:	$$$$
Notes:	Should have adequate calcium (1000–1500 mg/d) and vitamin D (400–800 IU/d) intake. Increases both vertebral and hip BMD but only decreases fracture rates in spine. Prevents/decreases breast cancer risks.

K. Psychiatric Agents

Selective Serotonin Re-uptake Inhibitors (SSRIs)	
Common trade name(s):	Celexa (citalopram), Lexapro (escitalopram), Paxil (paroxetine), Prozac (fluoxetine), Zoloft (sertraline)
Therapeutic class:	SSRI antidepressants
Indications:	Depression, OCD, panic disorder, PTSD, PMDD, social anxiety disorder
Dose:	Depression dose Celexa—20–60 mg po qd Lexapro—10–20 mg po qd Paxil—20–60 mg po qd Prozac—20–80 mg po qd Zoloft—50–200 mg po qd Anxiety dose—start at ½ of initial depression dose and titrate.
Dose adjustments:	Geriatrics—use lower initial dosages and titrate slowly
Adverse effects:	CNS activation (agitation, insomnia, fatigue, tremor, headache, dizziness), GI effects (nausea, vomiting, diarrhea), sexual dysfunction, serotonin withdrawal syndrome (Paxil) Serious and rare: serotonin syndrome (drug interaction with additive serotonin effects)
Monitoring:	Adverse effects, drug interactions (Prozac, Paxil)
Cost:	$$$–$$$$
Notes:	Considered first-line choice in outpatient management of depression and anxiety disorder. Relatively safe in overdose, medically ill, elderly, and heart disease patients. As a class, SSRIs may cause transient CNS activation at the beginning of treatment. Starting at ½ of depression dose and titrating upward, adding trazodone, and patient education are some of the strategies to minimize the adverse effects. Paxil and Zoloft are most studied in anxiety disorder. Full antidepressant effects usually seen at 4–6 weeks.

Venlafaxine

Common trade name(s):	Effexor XR
Therapeutic class:	Antidepressant
Indications:	Depression, generalized anxiety disorder
Dose:	37.5–75 mg po qd and titrate to response, max dose 225 mg po qd
Dose adjustments:	Reduce dose by 50% for either renal or hepatic impairment
Adverse effects:	CNS activation effects (anxiety, dizziness, insomnia, nervousness, tremor), sexual dysfunction, nausea, blood pressure elevation
Monitoring:	Blood pressure
Cost:	$$$$
Notes:	"Dual mechanism" (serotonin and norepinephrine) agent. Works like an SSRI at lower dose.

Bupropion

Common trade name(s):	Wellbutrin SR, Wellbutrin XL, Zyban
Therapeutic class:	Antidepressant
Indications:	Depression, smoking cessation
Dose:	Wellbutrin SR—150 mg qd × 3d then 150 mg bid Wellbutrin XL—150 mg qd × 3d then 300 mg qd Zyban—150 mg qd × 3d then 150 mg bid
Dose adjustments:	Reduce dose in renal or hepatic impairment.
Adverse effects:	Agitation, anxiety, confusion, constipation, dry mouth, nausea/vomiting, dizziness, headache, impaired sleep quality Serious: activation of psychosis and/or mania, HTN (in combination with nicotine patch)
Cost:	$$$$
Notes:	Contraindicated in seizure disorders, bulimia or anorexia, prior head trauma. Brand name Zyban is used for smoking cessation. Useful to treat SSRI-induced sexual dysfunction.

Mirtazapine

Common trade name(s):	Remeron
Therapeutic class:	Antidepressant
Indications:	Depression
Dose:	15–45 mg po qhs
Adverse effects:	Somnolence, increased appetite and weight gain (most common), dizziness, abnormal dreams, constipation, lipid elevations Serious and rare: agranulocytopenia
Monitoring:	If a patient develops a sore throat, fever, stomatitis or other signs of infection, along with a low WBC count, treatment should be discontinued and patient closely monitored.
Cost:	$–$$ (generics available)
Notes:	Useful in elderly patients because of its sedation and appetite-stimulant effects. Sedation effect decreases with increasing dose.

Benzodiazepines

Common trade name(s):	Xanax (alprazolam), Ativan (lorazepam), Klonopin (clonazepam)
Therapeutic class:	Antianxiety, benzodiazepines
Indications:	Anxiety, panic disorders (Xanax, Klonopin), insomnia (Ativan)
Dose:	Xanax—0.25–0.5 mg tid or prn and titrate Ativan—0.5–1 mg bid–tid or prn and titrate Klonopin—0.25–2 mg bid
Adverse effects:	Dizziness, drowsiness, impaired coordination, cognitive impairment Serious: physical dependence and addiction issues, withdrawal syndrome with abrupt discontinuance (especially Xanax)
Cost:	$–$$ (generics available)
Notes:	Recommend using these agents as PRN or for short-term basis in treatment of anxiety disorder. SSRIs should be used as maintenance treatment for anxiety disorder. Taper dose prior to discontinuation.

Hypnotic—Zolpidem, Zaleplon	
Common trade name(s):	Ambien (zolpidem), Sonata (Zalepon)
Therapeutic class:	Nonbarbiturate hypnotic
Indications:	Insomnia
Dose:	Ambien—5–10 mg po qhs prn
	Sonata—5–10 mg po qhs prn; may repeat dose × 1
Dose adjustments:	Geriatrics—use smaller dose
Adverse effects:	Drowsiness, dizziness, dry mouth, headache
Cost:	\$\$\$–\$\$\$\$
Notes:	Limit duration of use to 2 weeks if possible.

L. Thyroid Replacement Therapy

Levothyroxine	
Common trade name(s):	Levoxyl, Synthroid
Therapeutic class:	Thyroid hormone
Indications:	Hypothyroidism
Dose:	100–200 mcg po qd
Dose adjustments:	Geriatric or cardiovascular disease—start at 25–50 mcg po qd
Adverse effects:	Signs and symptoms of over-replacement (hyperthyroidism)
Monitoring:	TSH at 6–8 weeks
Cost:	\$

Index

D

G

H

I

J

K

L

M

N

Q

R

X

Z